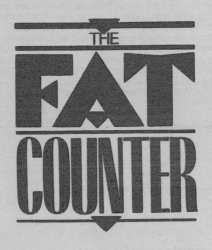

THE FAT COUNTER

ANNETTE B. NATOW, PH.D., R.D.,
—— AND ——
JO-ANN HESLIN, M.A., R.D.

POCKET BOOKS

New York   London   Toronto   Sydney   Tokyo   Singapore

An *Original* Publication of POCKET BOOKS

POCKET BOOKS, a division of Simon & Schuster Inc.
1230 Avenue of the Americas, New York, NY 10020

ISBN: 0-671-72594-7

First Pocket Books printing August 1989

10 9 8 7 6 5 4

POCKET and colophon are registered trademarks of Simon & Schuster Inc.

Printed in the U.S.A.

In his 1988 report on nutrition and health, Surgeon General C. Everett Koop said:

"Of greatest concern is our excessive intake of dietary fat and its relationship to risk for chronic diseases such as coronary heart disease, some types of cancers, diabetes, high blood pressure, strokes and obesity."

". . . the primary priority for dietary change is the recommendation to reduce intake of total fats."

The first recommendation in the Surgeon General's report is, "Reduce consumption of fat." Americans eat too much fat; 37% of all our calories are fat. Experts believe that we should be eating much less. They recommend that we reduce our fat intake by one-third.

The Food Marketing Institute in a recent survey found that the top nutritional concern of American consumers is the amount of fat in their food. Americans know that they eat more fat than is good for them. They want to do something about it.

Now it's easier to watch your fat intake—and protect your health—with the over 10,000 handy alphabetical listings in . . .

THE
FAT COUNTER

ANNETTE B. NATOW, PH.D., R.D., and JO-ANN HESLIN, M.A., R.D., are the authors of eight books on nutrition, including *The Cholesterol Counter, The Pocket Encyclopedia of Nutrition, No-Nonsense Nutrition for Kids* and *Megadoses: Vitamins as Drugs* (all available from Pocket Books). They are faculty members of Adelphi University and previously taught at Downstate Medical Center and New York University. They have held editorial positions at the *Journal of Nutrition for the Elderly, American Baby* and *Prevention* magazines, and are regular contributors to health magazines and journals.

Books by Annette B. Natow and Jo-Ann Heslin

The Cholesterol Counter
The Fat Counter
Megadoses
No-Nonsense Nutrition for Kids
The Pocket Encyclopedia of Nutrition

Published by POCKET BOOKS

To our families who support us through every project:
Harry, Allen, Irene, Sarah, Laura, Marty, George,
Emily, Steven, Joseph, Kristen, and Karen.

ACKNOWLEDGMENTS

Without the tireless cooperation of Steven, *The Fat Counter* would never have been completed. A special thanks to our editor, Claire Zion, and the Production Department of Pocket Books.

Our thanks also go to all the food manufacturers who graciously shared their data.

"Too much fat is a disadvantage . . . laying the foundation for troubles with the heart."

"Foods very high in fuel value, i.e., fats and dishes containing much fat, should be avoided."

MARY SWARTZ ROSE, PH.D.
Feeding the Family
The MacMillan Company, 1919

AUTHORS' NOTE

Sources of Data

Values in this counter have been obtained from the Composition of Foods, United States Department of Agriculture: Dairy and Egg Products, Agricultural Handbook No. 8–1; Spices and Herbs, Agricultural Handbook No. 8–2; Fats and Oils, Agricultural Handbook No. 8–4; Poultry, Agricultural Handbook No. 8–5; Soups, Sauces and Gravies, Agricultural Handbook No. 8–6; Sausages and Luncheon Meats, Agricultural Handbook No. 8–7; Fruit and Fruit Juices, Agricultural Handbook No. 8–9; Pork Products, Agricultural Handbook No. 8–10; Vegetables and Vegetable Products, Agricultural Handbook No. 8–11; Nut and Seed Products, Agricultural Handbook No. 8–12; Beef Products, Agricultural Handbook No. 8–13; Beverages, Agricultural Handbook No. 8–14; Finfish and Shellfish Products, Agricultural Handbook No. 8–15; Legumes and Legume Products, Agricultural Handbook No. 8–16.

Nutritive value of foods, United States Department of Agriculture, Home and Garden Bulletin No. 72.

Bowes & Church's Food Values of Portions Commonly Used (Philadelphia, PA: J.B. Lippincott Co., 1985).

Nutrients in Foods (Cambridge, MA: Nutrition Guild, 1983).

Information from food labels, manufacturers and processors. The values are based on research conducted prior to 1989. Manufacturers' ingredients are subject to change, so current values may vary from those listed in the book.

CONTENTS

PART II
Restaurant, Take-Out and Fast Food Chains

INTRODUCTION

FAT FACTS

Too Much Is Not Safe

High fat diets are unhealthy. Almost three-fourths of the two million Americans who died last year died from diseases linked to our high fat diet.

Eating too much fat increases the risk for:

HEART ATTACK—Americans have more than one and a quarter million heart attacks each year with more than a million deaths as a result.

STROKE—Americans have one-half million strokes each year, many of which result in death or disability.

CANCER—Studies suggest that high fat intake increases risk for breast, colon and prostate cancer.

OVERWEIGHT—Diets high in fat lead to overweight more easily than do diets high in protein or carbohydrate. High fat diets make you fatter faster.

GALLBLADDER DISEASE—People with high fat diets who are overweight have a greater risk of gallbladder trouble.

OSTEOARTHRITIS—High fat diets cause overweight, which puts more strain on the joints.

HEARING LOSS—Studies suggest that as people age, high fat and high cholesterol intakes coupled with high blood pressure can lead to hearing loss.

GOUT—A high fat diet aggravates gout.

DIABETES—High fat diets cause overweight, which increases the risk for diabetes and complicates treatment.

Most foods contain fat. Some have more, some less, few have none. Some fat can be easily seen—butter, margarine, salad oils and the fat on your steak or chop. Much of the fat you eat can't be seen. There's invisible fat in meat, milk, egg yolks, olives, walnuts, cakes, pies, cookies and candy. Whether you can see the fat or not, it adds up quickly.

FAT FACT #1—*Everyone should be eating less fat.* Americans eat too much fat. Almost forty percent of all the calories we eat are from fat! Experts agree that we should be eating much less; thirty percent of our calories should come from fat.

FAT FACT #2—*Fat makes you fatter faster.* The fat we eat gets turned into body fat much easier than the other things we eat. Fat calories make us fatter than calories from protein, sugar or starch.

FAT FACT #3—*Fat comes in three forms.* There are different kinds of fats depending on the types of fatty acids they contain: They can be saturated, polyunsaturated or monounsaturated. Most foods contain all three of these fats. Some foods have more of one type than another. For example, beef has a lot more saturated fat, margarine a lot of polyunsaturated fat and olive oil is high in monounsaturates.

Saturated Fat
How can you tell the difference between the three fats?

If you left a stick of butter on the kitchen counter all day it would soften but it wouldn't melt. Butter is high in saturated fat. Saturated fat is solid at room temperature. Research shows that eating a lot of saturated fats raises blood cholesterol levels. People with higher blood cholesterol levels are more likely to have a heart attack. Recently it has been found that not all saturated fats raise cholesterol. Even though that is true, foods we eat never contain only one type of saturated fat. All fats in foods are mixtures of fats. Foods often contain some saturated fats that raise cholesterol and other saturated fats that may not. That makes it difficult to translate these studies into food recommendations. *The safest recommendation: eat less total fat.*

FOODS HIGH IN SATURATED FATS

Whole milk	Beef	Lunch meats
Cheese	Pork	Sausage
Butter	Lamb	Chocolate
Cream	Veal	Coconut
Sour cream	Duck	Coconut oil
Whipped cream	Chicken	Palm oil
Half & Half	Fish	Palm kernel oil
Ice cream	Hot dogs	

Polyunsaturated Fat

Corn oil left out on the kitchen counter will not get solid. It doesn't even get solid in the refrigerator. Polyunsaturated fats are liquid at room temperature. These fats may help lower cholesterol levels in the blood. Research suggests that too much polyunsaturated fat may not be good. High intake may cause gallbladder disease, depress the immune system and put you at greater risk for some cancers. *The safest recommendation: eat less total fat.*

FOODS HIGH IN POLYUNSATURATED FATS

Corn oil	Salad dressing	Bluefish
Cottonseed oil	Mayonnaise	Mackerel
Sunflower oil	Walnuts	Sablefish
Safflower oil	Walnut oil	Herring
Sesame oil	Wheat germ	Whitefish
Soybean oil	Tuna	Rainbow trout
Soft margarine	Salmon	

Monounsaturated Fat

Olive oil left out on the kitchen counter never becomes solid. In the refrigerator olive oil gets cloudy as it becomes partly solid. Monounsaturated fat stays liquid at room temperature but becomes partly solid when chilled. You may have been hearing more about monounsaturated fats lately. Recent research shows these fats may help lower blood cholesterol. This sounds good, but too much of any fat is not good for you. *The safest recommendation: eat less total fat.*

FOODS HIGH IN MONOUNSATURATED FAT

Almonds	Sesame oil
Olive oil	Soybean oil
Canola oil (rapeseed oil)	Peanut oil
Cashews	Peanuts
Filberts (hazelnuts)	Peanut butter
Macadamia nuts	Chicken fat
Pignolia (pine nuts)	Olives
Pistachio nuts	Shortening made from
Soybean oil margarine	vegetable fat

FINDING FAT IN FOODS

Doesn't everybody need some fat?

Yes, you do need a small amount of fat. Fat is part of every cell in your body. It is used to make hormones. Fat cushions bones and body organs. Fat insulates the body and helps maintain normal temperature. Food fats carry fat soluble vitamins A, D, E and K. Fats stay in the stomach longer making you feel full so that you don't get hungry as soon.

Finding Food Fats

Most fruits and vegetables have little or no fat. There are a few exceptions, like avocados and olives (see page 10 and page 314).

Dried peas and beans are all pretty low in fat. Soybeans have a little more fat than other beans (see page 438). All nuts and seeds including coconut and peanuts, have a lot of fat. All these are examples of hidden fat.

Grains like oats, rice, wheat, rye and barley contain little fat. Cereals, breads and pasta made from grains are usually low in fat. Exceptions are some granola-type cereals, cookies, pies, sweet rolls and cakes. You can judge how much fat is in a cookie by how soft it is. The softer the cookie, the more fat it has. Judge your cookies by breaking them in half: A cookie that bends instead of breaking is higher in fat. Place a croissant, muffin or danish on a napkin for a few minutes. If a grease ring forms, it's high in fat.

People think of animal foods like meat, milk, cheese, eggs, poultry and fish as good protein foods. While this is true, it is also true that all animal foods contain fat. In fact an ounce of lean meat has the same amount of calories from protein as from fat. In fatty meat like spare ribs, there may be twice as many calories from fat as from protein. Meats like bacon should really be thought of as fat, not meat. The fat in one slice of bacon is equal to the fat in a pat of butter.

Choosing Low Fat Proteins

1. Choose skim or low fat milk and yogurt. Use skim milk cheese or reduced fat cheese. On occasions when you eat regular cheese, limit the portion.

2. Use low fat yogurt in place of sour cream.

3. Choose the leanest cuts of meat; remove all visible fat before cooking.

4. Choose ground beef that has as little fat as possible. Supermarkets label the ground beef with the percentage of fat; sometimes it is as low as 10%. Ground poultry is a good substitute for ground meat. It is lower in fat.

5. Roast, broil or grill meats on a rack so that fats drips off during cooking. When making soups, stews or sauces, skim fat off the top.

6. Avoid turkey and turkey breasts that are "self basted." The basting usually adds more fat.

7. Poultry skin is high in fat. Remove it before eating.

8. All fish contains less fat than most cuts of meat. Very lean fish choices are: cod, scrod, flounder, halibut, pollock, sole and haddock. Shellfish like shrimp, lobster, scallops and crab are low in fat too.

9. Choose tuna canned in water. Tuna is a low fat fish but

when it is canned in oil, this adds seven times more fat than tuna canned in water.

10. Choose poached, steamed or broiled fish instead of breaded, battered and fried.

Reading Labels

There's a lot of information on labels, but sometimes it can be confusing. Words don't always mean what you expect. "Lite" or "light" on a label can refer to color, flavor, texture, weight and not necessarily calories. It may have nothing to do with the amount of fat or calories in the food. "Lite" olive oil is lighter in color and milder in flavor than regular olive oil, but the fat and calorie content is the same in both. "Lean" is another misleading word that doesn't necessarily mean less fat unless it is applied to meat.

Many products today are labeled lowfat. The term "low-fat" has a legal meaning only when it is used to describe dairy products or meat. For milk, yogurt or cheese to be labeled lowfat it must contain between 0.4% and 2% fat by weight. For meats, descriptive terms are:

LEAN: No more than 10% fat by weight (not by calories)
EXTRA LEAN: No more than 5% fat by weight (not by calories)
LEANER: At least 25% less fat by weight than the original product

Terms used on some products can be misleading. A cheese that seems to be low fat because it is made with part skim milk may have only slightly less fat than a regular whole milk cheese.

When you want to know more about a food, look at the list of ingredients. Most of our packaged foods have ingredient listings. The first ingredient listed is the main one in the food. If it is fat, this is a high fat food. But even if fat is the second or third ingredient listed, the food is fairly high in fat.

Fats on labels can appear as any of the following:

Animal fats
(lard, suet, chicken fat)
Butter
Cocoa butter
Cream
Cheese
Whole milk
Diglycerides
Fat
Hydrogenated fat

Hydrogenated oil
Margarine
Monoglycerides
Oil
Shortening
Vegetable fat
Vegetable oil
Partially hydrogenated fat
Partially hydrogenated oil

American Heart Association
Seal of Approval

In 1989, The American Heart Association (AHA) began
a food product approval program designed to help
consumers identify heart-healthy food items. The AHA
Seal of Approval will appear on food labels of products
that are low in total fat, saturated fat, cholesterol and
sodium.

Choosing the Best Fats

Once in a while everyone feels like having some toast with
butter or margarine. In most homes you find butter, margarine and some kind of cooking oil. Even low fat recipes
occasionally call for some oil or shortening. There are some
things you should remember to help you choose the best
fats.

When selecting a margarine, choose one with a liquid oil
as the first ingredient. Avoid margarines with tropical oils,
such as palm oil and palm kernel oil. These oils are very
high in saturated fat. Our bodies make cholesterol more
easily from saturated fat. Soft tub margarines are often
highest in polyunsaturates. The nutrition label in Figure 1 is
an example of a good margarine choice. Liquid sunflower oil
is the first ingredient. This is a highly polyunsaturated oil.
The nutrition information panel lists 5 grams polyunsaturated

Figure 1   NUTRITION INFORMATION PANEL
PROMISE REGULAR MARGARINE

PROMISE
Lower in Saturated Fat
than regular margarine
No Cholesterol

72% VEGETABLE OIL SPREAD

Nutrition Information Per Serving

Serving Size	14 Grams (1 Tbsp)
Servings Per Pound	32
Calories	90
Protein	0g
Carbohydrate	0g
Fat	10g
Percent Calories From Fat	99%
Polyunsaturated**	5g
Saturated**	1g
Cholesterol** (0mg per 100g)	0mg
Sodium	90mg

Percentages of U.S. Recommended
Daily Allowances (U.S. RDA)*

Vitamin A 10%	Vitamin D 15%

*Contains less than 2 percent of the U.S. RDA of protein,
vitamin C, thiamine, riboflavin, niacin, calcium and iron.

**This information on fat and cholesterol content is provided for
individuals who on the advice of a physician are modifying their
total dietary intake of fat and cholesterol.

INGREDIENTS: LIQUID SUNFLOWER OIL, SWEET DAIRY WHEY,
PARTIALLY HYDROGENATED SOYBEAN OIL, WATER, SALT,
PARTIALLY HYDROGENATED COTTONSEED OIL, VEGETABLE
MONO AND DIGLYCERIDES, SOY LECITHIN, POTASSIUM SORBATE
AND CITRIC ACID ADDED AS PRESERVATIVES, ARTIFICIALLY
FLAVORED, COLORED WITH BETA CAROTENE, VITAMINS A
(PALMITATE) AND D_2 ADDED.

Courtesy of PROMISE® Spread

Figure 2   NUTRITION INFORMATION PANEL
PURITAN OIL

Courtesy: The Procter and Gamble Company Copyright 1989

To Open: Unscrew cap, pull white ring out, throw ring away   To Close: Replace cap

Puritan is **94% SATURATED FAT FREE**—
It has earned the acceptance of the
American College of Nutrition.

"Puritan is made from canola
oil, the vegetable oil lowest
in saturated fat. It is an
excellent choice to help meet
present dietary recommendations for reducing saturated fat and
cholesterol intake."
— American College of Nutrition

IF YOU HAVE QUESTIONS OR COMMENTS ABOUT
PURITAN, PLEASE
CALL US TOLL-
FREE IN THE CONTI-
NENTAL U.S. CALL
1-800-543-7276

PROCESSED IN
U.S.A. BY PROCTER &
GAMBLE, CINCINNATI,
OHIO 45202 FROM
CANADIAN OIL.
© 1988 P&G

NUTRITION INFORMATION PER PORTION
PORTION SIZE 1 TABLESPOON . . . . (14 g)
PORTIONS PER BOTTLE 64
CALORIES 120
PROTEIN, g 0
CARBOHYDRATE, g 0
FAT, g (100% OF CALORIES FROM FAT) 14
POLYUNSATURATED, g 4
SATURATED, g 1
CHOLESTEROL, mg (0 mg/100 g) 0

INFORMATION ON FAT AND CHOLESTEROL IS PROVIDED FOR
INDIVIDUALS WHO, ON ADVICE OF A PHYSICIAN, ARE MODIFYING
THEIR TOTAL DIETARY INTAKE OF FAT AND CHOLESTEROL
SODIUM, mg 0
PERCENTAGE OF U.S. RECOMMENDED DAILY ALLOWANCES (U.S.
RDA): LESS THAN 2% OF THE U.S. RDA OF PROTEIN, VITAMIN A,
VITAMIN C, THIAMINE, RIBOFLAVIN, NIACIN, CALCIUM AND IRON
INGREDIENT: ALL VEGETABLE CANOLA OIL.
CAUTION: ANY OIL WILL BURN IF OVERHEATED. DO NOT LEAVE UN-
ATTENDED WHILE HEATING. IF SMOKING OCCURS, REDUCE HEAT.
IF PRODUCT CATCHES FIRE, TURN OFF HEAT AND COVER POT
UNTIL COOLED. **DO NOT PUT WATER ON HOT OR FLAMING OIL.
DO NOT REFILL WITH HOT OIL OR EXPOSE PLASTIC BOTTLE TO
HEAT DAMAGE OR INJURY MAY RESULT**

oil and 1 gram saturated fat per serving, more than twice as
much polyunsaturated fat as saturated fat. This is a good
ratio. Using moderate amounts of this or a similar margarine
would be a good choice.

You may have seen one of the new butter blends. A butter
blend is a combination of some butter and some margarine.
Blends have less saturated fat than butter but more saturated
fat than margarine.

A good, all purpose cooking oil is tasteless and fries
without smoking. Corn, safflower, sunflower, soybean, cottonseed are all highly polyunsaturated oils. Peanut, olive,
and canola oil are high in polyunsaturates and monounsaturates. All are good choices. The label in Figure 2 lists as its
contents all vegetable canola oil. This oil is high in polyunsaturates and very low in saturates. Moderate amounts of
this or a similar cooking oil would be a good choice.

FINDING FAT CALORIES IN FOOD

Fat calories make you fatter faster. The food fat we eat is easily turned into body fat. You can limit fat calories by counting fat grams.

Nutrition labels can help you find out how much fat is in a food. Fat is listed in grams.

1 gram of fat = 9 calories

For example, 1 oz. of corn chips has 155 calories and 9 grams of fat.

9 grams of fat × 9 calories = 81 fat calories

More than one-half of the calories in corn chips come from fat.

Fat foods have a lot of calories. One teaspoon of fat has 45 calories. A teaspoon of protein, sugar or starch has only 20 calories.

Another example: 1 oz. of pretzels has 120 calories and 1 gram of fat.

1 gram of fat × 9 calories = 9 fat calories

Less than one-tenth of the calories in pretzels come from fat. Pretzels are a good snack choice. Less fat, less fat calories, less fattening for you.

How Much Fat Should You Eat?

Americans eat too much fat. A few years ago, the average American got over 40% of his calories from fat. We eat a little less now. But still, we get a whopping 37% of our calories from fat. Experts agree we should be eating much less.

The American Heart Association, The American Cancer Society, The American Health Foundation and the Surgeon General all recommend lowering fat intake. Americans should eat no more than 30% of their food as fat each day.

That's a good suggestion. How do you do it? The question is how many grams of fat can you eat and still limit your fat to no more than 30% of your calories? It's easy to find out.

1. *Find out how many calories you eat each day.* If your weight generally stays at around the same, you are probably eating about:

> 13 calories a pound, if you are not very active
> 15 calories a pound, if you are moderately active
> 17 calories a pound, if you are very active
> 20 calories a pound, if you are extremely active

For example, if you weigh 145 pounds and are moderately active you need 2175 calories a day (145 pounds × 15 calories = 2175 calories a day). Round that number to 2200 calories. You need 2200 calories a day to maintain your weight.

If you are overweight, estimate your desired weight and multiply that by the appropriate number of calories per pound. For example, if you would like to weigh 130 pounds and are not very active, estimate your calorie needs as follows: 130 pounds × 13 calories a pound = 1690 calories. Round answer to 1700 calories.

2. *Find out how many grams of fat you should be eating each day.* In Step 1 you found out how many calories you need each day. Find the number of calories you need each day on the list below. Next to it is the maximum grams of fat allowed for the day. For example, if you need 1800 calories a day, you should be eating no more than 60 grams of fat a day.

MAXIMUM GRAMS OF FAT ALLOWED

CALORIES	GRAMS OF FAT	CALORIES	GRAMS OF FAT
1300	43	2200	73
1400	47	2300	77
1500	50	2400	80
1600	53	2500	83
1700	57	2600	87
1800	60	2700	90
1900	63	2800	90
2000	67	2900	97
2100	70	3000	100

Now that you know how many grams of fat you should be eating each day, it's time to count up your fat.

COUNT UP YOUR FAT

We often eat on the run and pick foods high in fat. By the end of the day, we've eaten too much fat. You know you shouldn't be eating so much fat. You want to cut back. The fat counter will help you do it. For the first time it's simple to find out the amount of fat in all the foods you are eating.

Let's look at a typical day. Are the food choices familiar? Let's see how much fat this sample day has in it.

FAT COUNTING
A SAMPLE DAY OF POOR FOOD CHOICES

Breakfast	FAT (g)	CALORIES
Orange juice (½ cup)	0	55
French toast (1 slice)	7	155
Syrup (2 Tbsp)	0	122
Sausage (1 link)	5	50
Coffee w/ Half & Half (2 Tbsp)	4	40
Lunch		
Cheeseburger		
Hamburger (3 oz)	18	245
American cheese (1 slice)	9	105
Roll	2	115
Catsup (1 Tbsp)	0	15
French fries (10 strips)	8	160
Vanilla shake (10 oz)	9	315
Snack		
Doughnut	13	235
Coffee w/ Half & Half (2 Tbsp)	4	40
Dinner		
Batter dipped fried chicken (½ breast)	18	365
Baked potato &	0	145
Sour cream (2 Tbsp)	6	50
Tossed salad &	0	10
French dressing (2 Tbsp)	10	170
Apple pie (1 slice)	18	405
Tea &	0	0
Sugar (1 tsp)	0	15
TV Snack		
Rich vanilla ice cream (½ cup)	12	175
Total	**143**	**2987**

143 grams of fat × 9 calories = 1287 fat calories
Calories from fat divided by total calories = percentage of calories from fat
1287 fat calories divided by 2987 total calories = 43% fat

This is too much fat for one day—43 percent of the day's calories came from fat. Now you can see how easy it is to eat too much fat.

FAT COUNTING
A SAMPLE DAY OF WISE FOOD CHOICES

Breakfast	FAT (g)	CALORIES
Orange juice (4 oz)	0	55
All Bran &	0	70
Lowfat milk (½ cup)	1	40
Toast (1 slice) &	0	55
Jelly (1 Tbsp)	0	50
Coffee &	0	0
Lowfat milk (2 Tbsp)	0	20
Lunch		
Hamburger (3 oz)	18	245
Roll	2	115
Catsup (1 Tbsp)	0	15
French fries	8	160
Cola	0	160
Snack		
Pear	1	85
Dinner		
Roasted chicken breast, no skin		
(½ breast)	3	140
Baked potato &	0	145
Plain yogurt (2 Tbsp or 1 oz)	1	18
Tossed salad &	0	10
Oil & vinegar dressing (2 Tbsp)	16	140
Fruit cocktail (½ cup)	0	58
Tea &	0	0
Sugar (1 tsp)	0	15
TV Snack		
Vanilla ice milk (½ cup)	3	93
Total	**53**	**1689**

53 grams of fat × 9 calories = 477 fat calories
Calories from fat divided by total calories = percentage of calories from fat
477 fat calories divided by 1689 total calories = 28% fat

Wise food choices! A much healthier intake of fat for the day. When you cut down on grams of fat, you cut down on calories too. In this sample day, fat calories are only 28% of the total.

Now it's your turn to count your fat. Use the sample worksheet on the following page to note everything you eat today, then look up the fat in each food you have eaten and see how much fat you ate today. While you're at it, jot down the calories, too!

FAT COUNTING
A SAMPLE WORKSHEET FOOD AMOUNT

FOOD	PORTION	FAT (g)	CALORIES
Breakfast			
Snack			
Lunch			
Snack			
Dinner			
Snack			

TOTAL

Grams of fat × 9 calories = total fat calories
____ grams of fat × 9 calories = total fat calories
Calories from fat divided by total calories = percentage of calories from fat
____ fat calories divided by ____ total calories = ____% fat

Did you eat more than 30% fat today? If you did, you're eating too much fat. Turn back to page xxvi "Maximum Grams of Fat Allowed."

Start right now to make lower fat food choices.

TEN STEPS TO LOWER YOUR FAT INTAKE

1. Choose skim or low fat milk, evaporated milk, yogurt and cheese. Look for the words: skim, 1% fat, 2% fat, 99% fat free. *Note:* Many companies now make "imitation" cheeses with less fat. *Beware:* Cheeses labeled "made with partially skimmed milk" may contain almost as much fat as regular cheese.

2. Choose lean meats trimmed of all visible fat; poultry without skin. Choose meat and poultry labeled lean (no more than 10% fat by weight) or extra lean (no more than 5% fat by weight). *Beware:* Meat, poultry and fish contain invisible fat. Limit portion size to 4 oz., about the size of the palm of your hand.

3. Choose lean fish like cod, scrod, haddock and halibut. When using fatty fish like salmon, bluefish or mackerel, remove the skin and all visible fat.

4. Roast, broil, grill, bake or poach meat, poultry and fish, so no extra fat is added. During cooking fat drips off; discard it. *Beware:* When you add bread crumbs to ground meat for meat loaf or hamburgers, the crumbs act like a blotter, soaking up fat instead of allowing it to drip off.

5. Use jelly or jam as a spread on toast and bread instead of butter, margarine or cream cheese. Good taste and no fat.

6. Sour cream as a topping for baked potatoes is a lower fat choice than butter. Plain, lowfat yogurt is even better. Use butter flavor sprinkles.

7. Use lowfat milk in tea or coffee instead of half and half, cream or nondairy creamers (whiteners). More flavor and less fat.

8. Dress your salad with lemon juice or herb flavored vinegar instead of regular oil-based salad dressing or mayonnaise.

9. Sweet rolls, donuts and Danish pastries are high fat snacks. Try cinnamon raisin bread for a low fat sweet treat.

10. Use cooking spray to grease pans and sauté foods.

These suggestions are just a beginning. To reduce the total amount of fat you eat you have to learn how to recognize fat when you see it and even when you don't see it. It's not always easy. *The Fat Counter* will help.

PROJECT LEAN
LOW-FAT EATING FOR AMERICA NOW
Project LEAN is a national campaign sponsored by over 20 professional organizations with the purpose of helping Americans to eat a diet lower in fat. You will be seeing nutrition education messages sponsored by Project LEAN in the media and at your local supermarket, worksite cafeterias and restaurants.

WHEN IS A FAT NOT A FAT?

In spite of the fact that high fat foods make us fat and are not healthy, we love fatty foods. Fried foods, cakes, pies, cookies, butter and ice cream are favorites.

Scientists working with food manufacturers are busily developing fat substitutes that will help make our favorite high fat foods lower in calories and healthier for us.

Two new fat substitutes are currently being reviewed by the Food and Drug Administration (FDA), and are expected to be available in processed foods within the next few years.

OLESTRA (Procter and Gamble) is a calorie-free fatty substance made from soybean oil and sugar. Its technical name is sucrose polyester (SPE). Olestra looks and tastes like fat, has the same feeling in the mouth and can be used in cooking.

Olestra will not be used to replace all the fat in a food. It will be blended into cooking oils at levels of from 35% in fats for home use to 75% in commercial frying fats. These blended fats will contain only ¼ to ½ the usual calories.

Another benefit of Olestra is that it may help reduce blood cholesterol levels. Vitamin E will be added to Olestra to make up for the fact that absorption of that vitamin is reduced.

SIMPLESSE (NutraSweet Company) is a low calorie fat substitute made from egg whites or milk. One gram of Simplesse has only 1⅓ calories compared to 9 calories in a gram of fat. Simplesse becomes rubbery when it is heated so it can't be used in cooked foods.

It will be used in yogurt, ice cream, butter, margarine, cream cheese, sour cream, salad dressings, mayonnaise, dips and spreads. These foods will have the same familiar taste with only 15% of the usual fat calories. For example, 4 ounces of rich ice cream made with Simplesse has 130 calories instead of 283. One teaspoon of margarine made with Simplesse has 8 calories instead of 36.

Even though these new fat substitutes sound exciting, it may be a while before we can take advantage of them. Even then we'll still have to watch our fat intake because these new fats substitutes will replace only part of the fat in our foods.

USING YOUR FAT COUNTER

This book lists the fat and calorie content of over 10,000 foods. For the first time, information about fat values is at your fingertips. Now you will find it easy to follow a low fat diet.

Before *The Fat Counter* it was impossible to compare so many foods at one time. When you want to pick a low fat cookie, look up the cookie category, page 152. Fresh foods like meat, chicken, fish and cheese do not usually have a label. The same goes for take-out items like potato salad, coleslaw, ice cream, or foods bought at the bakery. How can you tell how much fat is in a burger or taco that you enjoy at the local fast food restaurant? *The Fat Counter* lists them all!

The Fat Counter is divided into two main sections.

Part I: Brand Name and Generic Foods lists foods alphabetically. For each group, you will find brand name foods listed first in alphabetical order, followed by an alphabetical listing of generic foods.

If you want to know how much fat is in the hamburger you are having for lunch: look under BEEF where you will find ground beef or a microwave hamburger sandwich listed. If you are making a homemade hamburger look under ROLL where you will find the hamburger roll listed alphabetically. For foods like FRENCH TOAST, SUGAR or TUNA, simply look for the specific food alphabetically in the complete listing. For example, FRENCH TOAST is found on page 217, listed alphabetically between FRENCH FRIES and FROGS' LEGS. Two slices have 14 grams of fat.

Part II: Restaurant, Take-out and Fast Food Chains contains an alphabetical listing of over 25 popular chains. Fast foods like BURGER KING, DOMINO'S PIZZA, TACO BELL and WENDY'S are listed alphabetically under the chain's name. For example MCDONALD'S is listed on page 514 under M.

If you are eating at home, simply look up the individual foods you are eating and total the fat for the meal. For example, your dinner may consist of:

	FAT (GRAMS)
Rib Lamb Chops, broiled	48
Broccoli w/ Cheese Sauce	6
(Birds Eye)	
Long Grain & Wild Rice	5
(Minute Rice)	
French Cheese Cake	13
(Sara Lee)	
Glass of White Wine	0
TOTAL FAT FOR THE MEAL =	72 g

We have tried to include all foods for which fat values are known. There will be some foods, however, that are not listed in *The Fat Counter* because the fat values are not available for that particular food.

When you can't locate your favorite brand, look at other similar foods. You will probably find a brand food, a generic product or a home recipe that is like your favorite food. For example, you may find that your favorite brand of vanilla ice cream is not listed. Look at the different ice creams listed on pages 250–259. From these entries you can quickly determine that vanilla ice cream has from 5 to 9 grams of fat in a serving. You can then assume that your favorite brand has a comparable amount.

With *The Fat Counter* as your guide, you will never again wonder how much fat is in food. You will always be able to tell if a food is high in fat, moderate in fat or low in fat. *Your goal is to pick low fat foods each time you eat.*

DEFINITIONS

as prep (as prepared): refers to food that has been prepared according to package directions

cooked: refers to food cooked without the addition of fat (oil, butter, margarine, etc.); steaming, poaching, broiling and dry roasting are examples of this type of preparation

home recipe: describes homemade dishes; those included can be used as guide to the cholesterol and calorie values of similar products you may prepare or take-out food you buy ready-to-eat

lean & fat: describes meat with some fat on its edges that is not cut away before cooking or poultry prepared with skin and fat as purchased

lean only: lean portion, trimmed of all visible fat

trace (tr): value used when a food contains less than one calorie or less than one gram (g) of fat

ABBREVIATIONS

diam	=	diameter	qt	=	quart
frzn	=	frozen	reg	=	regular
g	=	gram	sm	=	small
lb	=	pound	sq	=	square
lg	=	large	Tbsp	=	tablespoon
med	=	medium	tr	=	trace
mg	=	milligram	tsp	=	teaspoon
oz	=	ounce	w/	=	with
pkg	=	package	w/o	=	without
prep	=	prepared	"	=	inch

EQUIVALENT MEASURES

1 tablespoon	=	3 teaspoons
4 tablespoons	=	¼ cup
8 tablespoons	=	½ cup
12 tablespoons	=	¾ cup
16 tablespoons	=	1 cup
1000 milligrams	=	1 gram
28 grams	=	1 ounce

DRY MEASUREMENTS

16 ounces	=	1 pound
12 ounces	=	¾ pound
8 ounces	=	½ pound
4 ounces	=	¼ pound

LIQUID MEASUREMENTS

2 tablespoons	=	1 ounce
¼ cup	=	2 ounces
½ cup	=	4 ounces
¾ cup	=	6 ounces
1 cup	=	8 ounces
2 cups	=	1 pint
4 cups	=	1 quart

ALL FAT VALUES OF FOODS ARE GIVEN IN GRAMS (g)

PART I
Brand Name and Generic Foods

FOOD	PORTION	CALORIES	FAT

ABALONE

fried	3 oz	161	6
raw	3 oz	89	1

ACEROLA

acerola	1 fruit	2	tr
acerola juice	1 oz	6	tr

ADZUKI BEANS

CANNED
sweetened	½ cup	351	tr

DRIED
cooked	1 cup	294	tr
raw	1 cup	649	1

READY-TO-USE
yokan; sliced	¼" slice	36	tr

ALE
   (*see* BEER, ALE AND MALT LIQUOR)

ALFALFA

sprouts	1 cup	40	tr
sprouts	1 Tbsp	2	tr

ALMONDS

Almond Butter (Erewhon)	1 Tbsp	90	8
Blanched, Slivered, Whole or Sliced (Planters)	1 oz	170	15
Dry Roasted (Planters)	1 oz	170	15
Honey Roasted (Planters)	1 oz	170	13

FOOD	PORTION	CALORIES	FAT
Shelled Almonds (Dole)	1 oz	170	14
almond butter	1 Tbsp	101	10
almond butter, honey and cinnamon	1 Tbsp	96	8
almond meal, partially defatted	1 oz	116	5
almond paste	1 oz	127	8
dried, blanched	1 oz	166	15
dried, unblanched	1 oz	167	15
dried, unblanched	1 cup	837	74
dry roasted, unblanched	1 oz	167	15
oil roasted, blanched	1 oz	174	16
oil roasted, unblanched	1 oz	176	16
toasted, unblanched	1 oz	167	14
whole, dried, blanched	1 cup	850	76

AMARANTH

FOOD	PORTION	CALORIES	FAT
Amaranth Flakes (Health Valley)	1 oz	110	1
Amaranth w/ Banana (Health Valley)	1 oz	100	2
Amaranth Crunch w/ Raisins (Health Valley)	1 oz	110	3
Amaranth Pilaf (Health Valley)	7.5 oz	178	12
amaranth; cooked	½ cup	59	tr

ANCHOVY

FOOD	PORTION	CALORIES	FAT
CANNED			
in oil	3 oz	62	4
in oil	5 oz	42	2
in oil	1 can (1 ⁵ oz)	95	4

FOOD	PORTION	CALORIES	FAT
FRESH			
raw	3 oz	62	4

APPLE

FOOD	PORTION	CALORIES	FAT
CANNED			
Apple Sauce (Mott's)	4 oz	88	0
Apple Sauce (Mott's)	6 oz	132	0
Apple Sauce 100% Gravenstein Sweetened (S&W)	½ cup	90	0
Apple Sauce 100% Gravenstein Unsweetened (S&W)	½ cup	55	0
Apple Sauce Cherry Fruit Pack (Mott's)	3.75 oz	65	0
Apple Sauce, Chunky (Mott's)	4 oz	57	0
Apple Sauce, Chunky (Mott's)	6 oz	86	0
Apple Sauce, Cinnamon (Mott's)	4 oz	72	0
Apple Sauce, Cinnamon (Mott's)	6 oz	108	0
Apple Sauce, Natural (Mott's)	4 oz	44	0
Apple Sauce, Natural (Mott's)	6 oz	66	0
Apple Sauce, Natural Packed w/ Apple Juice (White House)	4 oz	50	0
Apple Sauce, Peach Fruit Pak (Mott's)	3.75 oz	70	0
Apple Sauce, Pineapple Fruit Pak (Mott's)	3.75 oz	79	0

FOOD	PORTION	CALORIES	FAT
Apple Sauce, Regular or Chunky (White House)	4 oz	80	0
Apple Sauce, Strawberry Fruit Pak (Mott's)	3.75 oz	70	0
Apple Sauce, Unsweetened (White House)	4 oz	50	0
Applesauce, Cinnamon (Seneca)	½ cup	90	0
Applesauce, Cinnamon (Tree Top)	½ cup	80	0
Applesauce, McIntosh (Seneca)	½ cup	90	0
Applesauce, Natural (Seneca)	½ cup	50	0
Applesauce, Natural (Tree Top)	½ cup	60	0
Applesauce, Original (Tree Top)	½ cup	80	0
Applesauce, Regular (Seneca)	½ cup	90	0
Baked Style Apples (White House)	3.5 oz	118	0
Fried Apples (Luck's)	8 oz	190	0
Sliced (White House)	4 oz	50	0
Spiced Apple Rings (White House)	3.5 oz	180	0
applesauce, sweetened	½ cup	97	tr
applesauce, unsweetened	½ cup	53	tr
sliced, unsweetened	½ cup	68	tr
DRIED			
Dried Apples (Mariani)	¼ cup	150	0
cooked w/ sugar	½ cup	116	tr

FOOD	PORTION	CALORIES	FAT
cooked w/o sugar	½ cup	172	tr
rings	10	155	tr
FRESH			
apple	1	81	tr
w/o skin; cooked	1	91	tr
w/o skin; microwaved	1 cup	96	tr
w/o skin; sliced	1 cup	62	tr
FROZEN			
Apple Fritters (Mrs. Paul's)	2	270	13
Apples, Glazed in Raspberry Sauce (Budget Gourmet)	5 oz	110	3
sliced	½ cup	41	tr
JUICE			
Apple (Mott's)	6 oz	88	0
Apple (Mott's)	8.5 oz	124	0
Apple (Mott's)	9.5 oz	141	0
Apple (Mott's)	10 oz	148	0
Apple (Seneca)	6 oz	90	0
Apple (Tree Top)	6 oz	90	0
Apple, frzn; as prep (Seneca)	6 oz	90	0
Apple, frzn; as prep (Tree Top)	6 oz	90	0
Apple 100% Pure (Sippin' Pak)	8.45 oz	110	0
Apple 100% Unsweetened (S&W)	6 oz	85	0

FOOD	PORTION	CALORIES	FAT
Apple Cider (Tree Top)	6 oz	90	0
Apple Cider, frzn; as prep (Tree Top)	6 oz	90	0
Apple Juice (Ocean Spray)	6 oz	90	0
Apple Juice (White House)	6 oz	87	0
Apple Juice 100% Pure (Kraft)	6 oz	80	0
Apple Natural Style (Mott's)	6 oz	88	0
Apple Unfiltered, frzn; as prep (Tree Top)	6 oz	90	0
Natural Apple, frzn; as prep (Seneca)	6 oz	90	0
apple	1 cup	116	tr
apple, frzn; as prep	1 cup	111	tr
apple, frzn; not prep	6 oz	349	1

APRICOT

FOOD	PORTION	CALORIES	FAT
CANNED Apricot Halves Unpeeled in Heavy Syrup (S&W)	½ cup	110	0
Apricots, Whole, Peeled in Heavy Syrup (S&W)	½ cup	100	0
apricots, heavy syrup w/ skin	3 halves, 1.75 Tbsp liquid	70	tr
apricots, juice pack w/ skin	3 halves, 1.75 Tbsp liquid	40	tr
apricots, light syrup w/ skin	3 halves, 1.75 Tbsp liquid	54	tr

FOOD	PORTION	CALORIES	FAT
apricots, water pack w/o skin	2 fruits, 2 Tbsp liquid	20	tr
apricots, water pack w/ skin	3 halves	22	tr
DRIED Apricots (Mariani)	¼ cup	140	0
halves	10	83	tr
halves; cooked w/o sugar	½ cup	106	tr
FRESH apricots	3	51	tr
FROZEN apricots	½ cup	119	tr
JUICE Nectar (S&W)	6 oz	100	0
nectar	1 cup	141	tr

ARROWHEAD

boiled	1 med	9	tr
raw	1 med	12	tr

ARTICHOKE

CANNED Heart Marinated (S&W)	3.5 oz	225	26
FRESH artichoke; cooked	1 med	53	tr
artichoke, raw	1 med	65	tr
hearts; cooked	½ cup	37	tr
Jerusalem, raw; sliced	½ cup	57	tr

FOOD	PORTION	CALORIES	FAT
FROZEN			
Artichoke Hearts (Birds Eye)	½ cup	32	tr
frzn; cooked	9 oz pkg	108	1.2
frzn; not prep	9 oz pkg	96	1

ASPARAGUS

FOOD	PORTION	CALORIES	FAT
CANNED			
Cut Spears (Owatonna)	½ cup	20	0
Spears, Colossal Fancy (S&W)	½ cup	20	0
Spears, Fancy (S&W)	½ cup	18	0
spears	½ cup	24	1
FRESH			
asparagus, raw	½ cup	15	tr
asparagus; cooked	½ cup	22	tr
asparagus; cooked	4 spears	15	tr
FROZEN			
Cut (Birds Eye)	½ cup	23	tr
Spears (Birds Eye)	½ cup	24	tr
frzn; cooked	4 spears	17	tr
frzn; not prep	10 oz	69	1

AVOCADO

FOOD	PORTION	CALORIES	FAT
Avocado (California Avocados)	½	153	14
Avocado; mashed (California Avocados)	1 cup	407	36
avocado	1	324	31

FOOD	PORTION	CALORIES	FAT

BABY FOOD

CEREAL

FOOD	PORTION	CALORIES	FAT
Baby Cereal (Health Valley)	1 oz	60	1
Baby Cereal, Brown Rice (Health Valley)	1 oz	60	1
Barley (Beech-Nut)	½ oz	50	0
Mixed Cereal (Beech-Nut)	½ oz	50	1
Mixed Cereal w/ Applesauce & Bananas (Beech-Nut)	4.5 oz	80	0
Oatmeal (Beech-Nut)	½ oz	50	1
Oatmeal Cereal w/ Applesauce & Bananas (Beech-Nut)	4.5 oz	90	1
Oatmeal Cereal w/ Bananas (Beech-Nut)	½ oz	50	1
Rice (Beech-Nut)	½ oz	60	1
Rice Cereal w/ Apples (Beech-Nut)	½ oz	60	0
Rice Cereal w/ Applesauce & Bananas (Beech-Nut)	4.5 oz	100	0
Rice Cereal w/ Bananas (Beech-Nut)	½ oz	60	0

BAKED GOODS

FOOD	PORTION	CALORIES	FAT
Animal Shaped Cookies (Gerber)	2	60	2
Arrowroot Cookies (Gerber)	2	50	2
Pretzels (Gerber)	2	50	0

FOOD	PORTION	CALORIES	FAT
Toddler Biter Biscuits (Gerber)	1	50	1
Zwieback Toast (Gerber)	2	60	2
CHUNKY FOODS			
Beef Stew (Beech-Nut)	6 oz	140	4
Heart Chicken w/ Stars Soup (Beech-Nut)	6 oz	180	9
Homestyle Noodles & Beef (Gerber)	6 oz	150	6
Macaroni Alphabets w/ Beef & Tomato Sauce (Gerber)	6.25 oz	130	3
Noodles & Chicken w/ Carrots & Peas (Gerber)	6 oz	100	2
Rice w/Beef & Tomato Sauce (Gerber)	6.25 oz	150	5
Saucy Rice w/ Chicken (Gerber)	6 oz	150	5
Spaghetti Tomato Sauce & Beef (Gerber)	6.25 oz	160	5
Spaghetti Rings In Meat Sauce (Beech-Nut)	6 oz	160	4
Vegetable Stew w/ Chicken (Beech-Nut)	6 oz	190	8
Vegetables & Beef (Gerber)	6.25 oz	140	5
Vegetables & Chicken (Gerber)	6.25 oz	140	5
Vegetables & Ham (Gerber)	6.25 oz	120	4
Vegetables & Turkey (Gerber)	6.25 oz	110	3

FOOD	PORTION	CALORIES	FAT
JUICE			
Apple (Beech-Nut)	4.2 oz	60	0
Juice Plus (Beech-Nut)	4 oz	80	0
Pear (Beech-Nut)	4.2 oz	60	0
White Grape (Beech-Nut)	4.2 oz	80	0
JUNIOR AND TODDLER MEATS			
Beef (Gerber)	3.5 oz	110	5
Chicken (Gerber)	3.5 oz	140	9
Chicken Sticks (Gerber)	2.5 oz	120	8
Ham (Gerber)	3.5 oz	120	7
Lamb (Gerber)	3.5 oz	100	5
Meat Sticks (Gerber)	2.5 oz	110	7
Turkey (Gerber)	3.5 oz	130	8
Turkey Sticks (Gerber)	2.5 oz	120	9
Veal (Gerber)	3.5 oz	100	5
JUNIOR DESSERTS			
Cottage Cheese w/ Pineapple (Beech-Nut)	7.5 oz	190	2
Dutch Apple (Gerber)	6 oz	128	2
Fruit Dessert (Gerber)	6 oz	128	tr

FOOD	PORTION	CALORIES	FAT
Hawaiian Delight (Gerber)	6 oz	105	tr
Mixed Fruit & Yogurt (Beech-Nut)	7.5 oz	170	1
Peach Cobbler (Gerber)	6 oz	128	tr
Vanilla Custard Pudding (Beech-Nut)	7.5 oz	210	5
Vanilla Custard Pudding (Gerber)	6 oz	128	2
JUNIOR DINNERS Beef Egg Noodle Dinner (Gerber)	7.5 oz	140	4
Beef With Vegetables (Gerber)	4.5 oz	130	7
Chicken Noodle Dinner (Gerber)	7.5 oz	120	3
Chicken With Vegetables (Gerber)	4.5 oz	130	7
Ham With Vegetables (Gerber)	4.5 oz	110	4
Macaroni Tomato Beef Dinner (Gerber)	7.5 oz	130	3
Spaghetti Tomato Sauce Beef Dinner (Gerber)	7.5 oz	140	2
Split Peas With Ham Dinner (Gerber)	7.5 oz	150	3
Turkey Rice Dinner (Gerber)	7.5 oz	120	4
Turkey With Vegetables (Gerber)	4.5 oz	140	8
Vegetable Bacon Dinner (Gerber)	7.5 oz	180	8
Vegetable Beef Dinner (Gerber)	7.5 oz	140	4

FOOD	PORTION	CALORIES	FAT
Vegetable Chicken Dinner (Gerber)	7.5 oz	120	3
Vegetable Ham Dinner (Gerber)	7.5 oz	140	4
Vegetable Lamb Dinner (Gerber)	7.5 oz	140	5
Vegetable Turkey Dinner (Gerber)	7.5 oz	120	3
STRAINED DESSERTS			
Banana Pineapple Dessert (Beech-Nut)	4.5 oz	100	0
Banana Apple (Gerber)	4.5 oz	90	1
Banana Custard Pudding (Beech-Nut)	4.5 oz	120	1
Cherry Vanilla Pudding (Gerber)	4.5 oz	90	1
Chocolate Custard Pudding (Gerber)	4.5 oz	110	2
Cottage Cheese w/ Pineapple (Beech-Nut)	4.5 oz	110	1
Dutch Apple (Gerber)	4.5 oz	100	2
Dutch Apple Dessert (Beech-Nut)	4.5 oz	80	0
Fruit Dessert (Beech-Nut)	4.5 oz	80	0
Fruit Dessert (Gerber)	4.5 oz	100	1
Guava Tropical Fruit Dessert (Beech-Nut)	4.5 oz	100	0
Hawaiian Dessert (Gerber)	4.5 oz	120	1
Mango Tropical Fruit Dessert (Beech-Nut)	4.5 oz	90	0

FOOD	PORTION	CALORIES	FAT
Mixed Fruit & Yogurt (Beech-Nut)	4.5 oz	110	1
Orange Pudding (Gerber)	4.5 oz	110	1
Papaya Tropical Fruit Dessert (Beech-Nut)	4.5 oz	80	0
Peach Cobbler (Gerber)	4.5 oz	100	1
Peaches & Yogurt (Beech-Nut)	4.5 oz	110	1
Vanilla Custard Pudding (Beech-Nut)	4.5 oz	130	3
Vanilla Custard Pudding (Gerber)	4.5 oz	100	1
STRAINED DINNERS Beef Egg Noodle Dinner (Gerber)	4.5 oz	90	3
Beef & Egg Noodles w/ Vegetables (Beech-Nut)	4.5 oz	90	4
Beef Supreme (Beech-Nut)	4.5 oz	120	7
Beef With Vegetables (Gerber)	4.5 oz	120	6
Chicken & Rice w/ Vegetables (Beech-Nut)	4.5 oz	80	3
Chicken Noodle Dinner (Gerber)	4.5 oz	80	2
Chicken Noodle w/ Vegetables (Beech-Nut)	4.5 oz	90	3
Chicken With Vegetables (Gerber)	4.5 oz	140	8
Ham With Vegetables (Gerber)	4.5 oz	100	4
Macaroni Cheese Dinner (Gerber)	4.5 oz	90	3

FOOD	PORTION	CALORIES	FAT
Macaroni Tomato Beef Dinner (Gerber)	4.5 oz	90	3
Macaroni, Tomato & Beef (Beech-Nut)	4.5 oz	90	3
Turkey Rice Dinner (Gerber)	4.5 oz	80	3
Turkey Rice w/ Vegetables (Beech-Nut)	4.5 oz	70	2
Turkey Supreme (Beech-Nut)	4.5 oz	110	5
Turkey With Vegetables (Gerber)	4.5 oz	130	7
Vegetable Bacon Dinner (Gerber)	4.5 oz	100	5
Vegetable Beef Dinner (Gerber)	4.5 oz	80	3
Vegetable Chicken (Beech-Nut)	4.5 oz	90	3
Vegetable Chicken Dinner (Gerber)	4.5 oz	80	2
Vegetable Ham Dinner (Gerber)	4.5 oz	80	3
Vegetable Lamb Dinner (Gerber)	4.5 oz	90	4
Vegetable Liver Dinner (Gerber)	4.5 oz	60	1
Vegetable Turkey Dinner (Gerber)	4.5 oz	7	2
Vegetable Beef (Beech-Nut)	4.5 oz	90	3
Vegetable Ham (Beech-Nut)	4.5 oz	90	3
Vegetable Lamb (Beech-Nut)	4.5 oz	90	3
STRAINED FRUITS AND VEGETABLES Apples & Strawberries (Beech-Nut)	½ oz	90	0

FOOD	PORTION	CALORIES	FAT
Apples, Mandarin Oranges & Bananas (Beech-Nut)	4.5 oz	90	0
Apples, Peaches & Strawberries (Beech-Nut)	4.5 oz	100	0
Apples, Pears & Bananas (Beech-Nut)	4.5 oz	90	0
Applesauce, Golden Delicious (Beech-Nut)	2.8 oz	45	0
Applesauce, Golden Delicious (Beech-Nut)	4.5 oz	60	0
Applesauce & Apricots (Beech-Nut)	4.5 oz	60	0
Applesauce & Bananas (Beech-Nut)	4.5 oz	60	0
Applesauce & Cherries (Beech-Nut)	4.5 oz	70	0
Apricots w/ Pears & Applesauce (Beech-Nut)	4.5 oz	70	0
Bananas, Chiquita (Beech-Nut)	2.8 oz	60	0
Bananas, Chiquita (Beech-Nut)	4.5 oz	100	0
Bananas w/ Pears & Applesauce (Beech-Nut)	4.5 oz	90	0
Bartlett Pears (Beech-Nut)	2.8 oz	50	0
Bartlett Pears & Pineapple (Beech-Nut)	4.5 oz	80	0
Butternut Squash (Beech-Nut)	2.8 oz	20	0
Butternut Squash (Beech-Nut)	4.5 oz	40	0
Carrots (Beech-Nut)	4.5 oz	40	0
Creamed Corn (Beech-Nut)	4.5 oz	90	0

FOOD	PORTION	CALORIES	FAT
Garden Vegetables (Beech-Nut)	4.5 oz	60	0
Green Beans (Beech-Nut)	4.5 oz	40	0
Mixed Vegetables (Beech-Nut)	4.5 oz	50	0
Peaches, Yellow Cling (Beech-Nut)	2.8 oz	40	0
Peaches, Yellow Cling (Beech-Nut)	4.5 oz	60	0
Pears & Applesauce (Beech-Nut)	4.5 oz	70	0
Pears, Bartlett (Beech-Nut)	4.5 oz	60	0
Peas (Beech-Nut)	4.5 oz	70	0
Peas & Carrots (Beech-Nut)	4.5 oz	60	0
Plums w/ Rice (Beech-Nut)	4.5 oz	110	0
Prunes (Beech-Nut)	4.5 oz	130	0
Prunes w/ Pears (Beech-Nut)	4.5 oz	120	0
Regal Imperial Carrots (Beech-Nut)	2.8 oz	20	0
Sweet Potatoes (Beech-Nut)	4.5 oz	70	0
Yellow Wax Beans (Beech-Nut)	4.5 oz	30	0

STRAINED MEATS AND EGG YOLKS

FOOD	PORTION	CALORIES	FAT
Beef (Beech-Nut)	2.8 oz	100	7
Beef (Gerber)	3.5 oz	100	5

FOOD	PORTION	CALORIES	FAT
Chicken (Beech-Nut)	2.8 oz	90	6
Chicken (Gerber)	3.5 oz	100	4
Egg Yolks (Gerber)	2.25 oz	128	13
Ham (Gerber)	3.5 oz	110	6
Lamb (Beech-Nut)	2.8 oz	90	6
Lamb (Gerber)	3.5 oz	100	5
Pork (Gerber)	3.5 oz	110	6
Turkey (Beech-Nut)	2.8 oz	100	6
Turkey (Gerber)	3.5 oz	130	8
Veal (Beech-Nut)	2.8 oz	100	7
Veal (Gerber)	3.5 oz	100	5

BACON
(*see also* BACON SUBSTITUTE)

FOOD	PORTION	CALORIES	FAT
Armour Lower Salt; cooked	1 strip	38	3
Armour Star; cooked	1 strip	38	3
Oscar Mayer; cooked	1 strip (6 g)	35	3
Oscar Mayer Center Cut; cooked	1 strip (4.6 g)	24	2
Oscar Mayer Lower Salt; cooked	1 strip (6.1 g)	33	3
bacon; cooked	3 strips (9 g)	109	9
breakfast strips, beef; cooked	3 strips (34 g)	153	12
breakfast strips, pork, raw	3 slices (3 oz)	264	25
breakfast strips; cooked	3 strips (34 g)	156	12

FOOD	PORTION	CALORIES	FAT
canadian bacon; grilled	2 slices (1.7 oz)	86	4
canadian bacon; unheated	1 pkg (6 oz)	268	12
pork	3 slices (2 oz)	378	39

BACON SUBSTITUTE

Bacon Bits (Oscar Mayer)	¼ oz	21	1
Breakfast Strips Lean 'N Tasty Beef; cooked (Oscar Mayer)	1 strip (12 g)	46	4
Breakfast Strips Lean 'N Tasty Pork; cooked (Oscar Mayer)	1 strip (12 g)	54	5
Strips; frozen (Morningstar Farms)	3.5 oz	333	25
bacon substitute	1 strip	25	2
breakfast strips, beef, raw	3 strips	276	26

BAGEL

Big 'N Crusty (Lenders)	1	230	1
Blueberry (Lenders)	1	190	2
Cinnamon & Raisin (Sara Lee)	1	240	2
Egg (Sara Lee)	1	250	2
Onion (Sara Lee)	1	230	1
Plain (Lenders)	1	150	1
Plain (Sara Lee)	1	230	1
Poppy Seed (Sara Lee)	1	230	1

FOOD	PORTION	CALORIES	FAT
Sesame Seed (Sara Lee)	1	260	3

BAKING POWDER

Calumet	1 tsp	3	tr
Davis	1 tsp	8	0

BAKING SODA

Arm & Hammer (Church Dwight)	1 tsp	0	0

BAMBOO SHOOTS

CANNED			
Bamboo Shoots (La Choy)	¼ cup	6	tr
bamboo shoots; sliced	1 cup	25	1
FRESH			
cooked	½ cup	15	tr
raw	½ cup	21	tr

BANANA

DRIED			
dehydrated powder	1 Tbsp	21	tr
FRESH			
Chiquita	1 (3.5 oz)	110	0
banana	1	105	tr

BASS

freshwater	1 fillet (2.7 oz)	903	3
freshwater	3 oz	97	3
sea; cooked	3 oz	105	2
sea; cooked	1 fillet (3.5 oz)	125	3

FOOD	PORTION	CALORIES	FAT
sea, raw	1 fillet (4.5 oz)	125	3
sea, raw	3 oz	82	2
striped, raw	3 oz	82	2
striped, raw	1 fillet (5.6 oz)	154	4

BEANS
(*see also* INDIVIDUAL NAMES)

FOOD	PORTION	CALORIES	FAT
CANNED			
Baked Beans, Brick Oven (S&W)	½ cup	160	2
Barbecue Beans (Campbell)	7⅞ oz	250	4
Barbecue Beans, Texas Style (S&W)	½ cup	135	1
Barbeque Baked Beans (B&M)	⅞ cup	310	6
Boston Baked Beans (Health Valley)	4 oz	110	1
Cut Green & Shelled Beans Seasoned w/ Pork (Luck's)	7.25 oz	200	6
Cut Green & Shelled Beans Seasoned w/ Pork (Luck's)	7.25 oz	200	8
Cut Green Beans (Hanover)	½ cup	20	0
Four Bean Salad (Hanover)	½ cup	80	0
Home Style Beans (Campbell)	8 oz	270	4
Honey Baked Beans (B&M)	⅞ cup	280	2
Maple Sugar Beans (S&W)	½ cup	150	1
Mixed Bean Salad, Marinated (S&W)	½ cup	90	1

FOOD	PORTION	CALORIES	FAT
Mixed Beans Seasoned w/Pork (Luck's)	7.25 oz	200	5
Old Fashioned Beans in Molasses & Brown Sugar (Campbell)	8 oz	270	3
Pork & Beans in Tomato Sauce (Campbell)	8 oz	240	3
Pork & Molasses (Libby)	½ cup	140	2
Pork & Tomato Sauce (Libby)	½ cup	140	2
Pork & Tomato Sauce (Seneca)	½ cup	140	2
Pork 'N Beans (S&W)	½ cup	130	2
Ranch Style (Ranch Style)	7.5 oz	200	4
Ranchero Beans (Campbell)	7⅞ oz	220	5
Refried Beans & Green Chili (Little Pancho)	½ cup	80	0
Smokey Ranch Beans (S&W)	½ cup	130	2
Tomato Baked Beans (B&M)	⅞ cup	270	3
Vegetarian (Libby)	½ cup	130	1
Vegetarian (Seneca)	½ cup	130	1
Vegetarian Baked Beans (B&M)	⅞ cup	250	2
Vegetarian w/ Miso (Health Valley)	4 oz	90	1
baked beans, plain	½ cup	118	1
baked beans, vegetarian	½ cup	118	1
baked beans, w/ beef	½ cup	161	5

FOOD	PORTION	CALORIES	FAT
baked beans, w/ franks	½ cup	182	8
baked beans, w/ pork	½ cup	133	2
baked beans, w/ pork & sweet sauce	½ cup	140	2
baked beans, w/ pork & tomato sauce	½ cup	123	1
FROZEN Romano Bean Medley (Hanover)	½ cup	25	0
HOME RECIPE baked beans	½ cup	190	6
refried beans	½ cup	43	2
three bean salad	¾ cup	230	11
SPROUTS canned	½ cup	8	tr

BEECHNUTS

dried	1 oz	164	14

BEEF

(*see also* BEEF DISHES, VEAL)

Beef is graded according to its marbling, the little flecks of fat in the muscle. Beef graded "Prime" has the highest percentage of fat, followed by "Choice" with less fat and "Select" with the least fat.

CANNED			
corned beef	1 oz	71	4
corned beef	1 slice (21 g)	53	3

FRESH
Note that the values for cooked beef may differ slightly from values for raw beef. When meat is cooked some moisture and fat is lost, changing the nutrition value slightly. As a rule of thumb it can be assumed that a 4 oz raw portion will equal a 3 oz cooked portion of meat.

New York Strip Steak, raw (Dakota Lean Meats)	3 oz	101	1

FOOD	PORTION	CALORIES	FAT
bottom round, lean & fat, Choice, raw	4 oz	256	7
bottom round, lean & fat, Choice; braised	3 oz	224	13
bottom round, lean & fat, Prime; braised	3 oz	253	16
bottom round, lean & fat, Prime, raw	4 oz	256	17
bottom round, lean & fat, Select, raw	4 oz	244	16
bottom round, lean & fat, Select; braised	3 oz	215	25
bottom round, lean only, Choice, raw	4 oz	172	7
bottom round, lean only, Choice; braised	3 oz	191	8
bottom round, lean only, Prime, raw	4 oz	180	8
bottom round, lean only, Prime; braised	3 oz	212	11
bottom round, lean only, Select, raw	4 oz	164	7
bottom round, lean only, Select; braised	3 oz	182	7
brisket, flat half, lean & fat; braised	3 oz	347	30
brisket, flat half, lean only; braised	3 oz	223	14
brisket, point half, lean & fat, raw	4 oz	336	28
brisket, point half, lean only, raw	4 oz	152	6
brisket, point half, lean only; braised	3 oz	181	7
brisket, point half; braised	3 oz	311	25
brisket, whole, lean & fat; braised	3 oz	332	28
brisket, whole, lean only, braised	3 oz	205	11
chuck arm pot roast, lean & fat, Choice; braised	3 oz	301	23
chuck arm pot roast, lean & fat, Choice, raw	4 oz	296	23

FOOD	PORTION	CALORIES	FAT
chuck arm pot roast, lean & fat, Prime, raw	4 oz	332	27
chuck arm pot roast, lean & fat, Prime; braised	3 oz	332	26
chuck arm pot roast, lean & fat, Select, raw	4 oz	268	20
chuck arm pot roast, lean & fat, Select; braised	3 oz	287	21
chuck arm pot roast, lean only, Choice; braised	3 oz	199	9
chuck arm pot roast, lean only, Choice, raw	4 oz	156	6
chuck arm pot roast roast, lean only, Prime; braised	3 oz	222	11
chuck arm pot roast, lean only, Prime, raw	4 oz	176	8
chuck arm pot roast, lean only, Select; braised	3 oz	189	8
chuck arm pot roast, lean only, Select, raw	4 oz	148	5
chuck blade roast, Select	4 oz	296	24
chuck blade roast, lean only, Choice; braised	3 oz	234	13
chuck blade roast, lean only, Prime; braised	3 oz	270	17
chuck blade roast, lean only, Select; braised	3 oz	218	12
chuck blade roast, lean & fat, Choice, raw	4 oz	328	28
chuck blade roast, lean & fat, Choice; braised	3 oz	330	26
chuck blade roast, lean & fat, Prime, raw	4 oz	372	32
chuck blade roast, lean & fat, Prime; braised	3 oz	354	29

FOOD	PORTION	CALORIES	FAT
chuck blade roast, lean & fat, Select; braised	3 oz	311	24
chuck blade roast, lean only, Choice, raw	4 oz	192	11
chuck blade roast, lean only, Prime, raw	4 oz	232	15
chuck blade roast, lean only, Select, raw	4 oz	172	9
corned beef brisket, raw	4 oz	224	17
corned beef brisket; cooked	3 oz	213	16
eye of round, lean & fat, Choice, raw	4 oz	228	15
eye of round, lean & fat, Choice; roasted	3 oz	207	12
eye of round, lean & fat, Prime, raw	4 oz	252	17
eye of round, lean & fat, Select, raw	4 oz	212	12
eye of round, lean & fat, Select; roasted	3 oz	201	12
eye of round, lean & fat, Prime; roasted	3 oz	213	13
eye of round, lean only, Choice, raw	4 oz	152	5
eye of round, lean only, Choice; roasted	3 oz	156	6
eye of round, lean only, Prime; roasted	3 oz	168	7
eye of round, lean only, Select, raw	4 oz	144	4
eye of round, lean only, Select; roasted	3 oz	151	5
eye of round, lean only, Prime, raw	4 oz	168	7
flank, lean & fat, Choice, raw	4 oz	220	14
flank, lean & fat, Choice; braised	3 oz	218	13
flank, lean & fat, Choice; broiled	3 oz	216	14
flank, lean only, Choice; boiled	3 oz	207	13
flank, lean only, Choice, raw	3 oz	192	11

FOOD	PORTION	CALORIES	FAT
flank, lean only, Choice; braised	3 oz	208	12
ground, extra lean, raw	4 oz	265	19
ground, extra lean; cooked medium	3 oz	213	14
ground, extra lean; cooked well-done	3 oz	232	14
ground, lean, raw	4 oz	298	23
ground, lean; cooked medium	3 oz	227	16
ground, lean; cooked well-done	3 oz	248	16
ground, regular, raw	4 oz	351	30
ground, regular; cooked medium	3 oz	244	18
ground, regular; cooked well-done	3 oz	269	18
lungs, raw	4 oz	104	3
lungs; braised	3 oz	102	3
pancreas, raw	4 oz	265	21
pancreas; braised	3 oz	230	15
porterhouse steak, lean & fat, Choice, raw	4 oz	324	26
porterhouse steak, lean & fat, Choice; broiled	3 oz	254	21
porterhouse steak, lean only, Choice, raw	4 oz	180	9
porterhouse steak, lean only, Choice; broiled	3 oz	185	9
rib eye small end, lean & fat, Choice, raw	4 oz	284	22
rib eye small end, lean & fat, Choice; broiled	3 oz	250	18
rib eye small end, lean only, Choice, raw	4 oz	184	10
rib large end, lean & fat Choice, raw	4 oz	404	36
rib large end, lean & fat, Choice; broiled	3 oz	327	28

FOOD	PORTION	CALORIES	FAT
rib large end, lean & fat, Choice; roasted	3 oz	316	26
rib large end, lean & fat, Prime; broiled	3 oz	361	32
rib large end, lean & fat, Prime, raw	4 oz	436	40
rib large end, lean & fat, Prime; roasted	3 oz	346	29
rib large end, lean & fat, Select, raw	4 oz	372	33
rib large end, lean & fat, Select; broiled	3 oz	301	25
rib large end, lean & fat, Select; roasted	3 oz	304	19
rib large end, lean only, Choice, raw	4 oz	196	11
rib large end, lean only, Choice; broiled	3 oz	203	13
rib large end, lean only, Choice; roasted	3 oz	210	12
rib large end, lean only, Prime; broiled	3 oz	250	18
rib large end, lean only, Prime; roasted	3 oz	241	16
rib large end, lean only, Select, raw	4 oz	180	9
rib large end, lean only, Select; broiled	3 oz	183	10
rib large end, lean only, Select; roasted	3 oz	197	11
rib large end, lean only, Prime, raw	4 oz	240	16
rib small end, lean & fat, Choice, raw	4 oz	356	30
rib small end, lean & fat, Choice; broiled	3 oz	282	22
rib small end, lean & fat, Choice; roasted	3 oz	312	26
rib small end, lean & fat, Prime, raw	4 oz	396	35

FOOD	PORTION	CALORIES	FAT
rib small end, lean & fat, Prime; broiled	3 oz	309	25
rib small end, lean & fat, Prime; roasted	3 oz	357	31
rib small end, lean & fat, Select, raw	4 oz	324	27
rib small end, lean & fat, Select; broiled	3 oz	263	19
rib small end, lean & fat, Select; roasted	3 oz	283	22
rib small end, lean only, Choice, raw	4 oz	184	10
rib small end, lean only, Choice; broiled	3 oz	191	10
rib small end, lean only, Choice; broiled	3 oz	191	10
rib small end, lean only, Choice; roasted	3 oz	206	12
rib small end, lean only, Prime; broiled	3 oz	221	13
rib small end, lean only, Prime; roasted	3 oz	259	18
rib small end, lean only, Select, raw	4 oz	168	8
rib small end, lean only, Select; broiled	3 oz	178	8
rib small end, lean only, Select; roasted	3 oz	183	10
rib small end, lean only, Prime, raw	4 oz	228	14
rib whole, lean & fat, Choice, raw	4 oz	384	34
rib whole, lean & fat, Choice; broiled	3 oz	313	26
rib whole, lean & fat, Choice; roasted	3 oz	328	28
rib whole, lean & fat, Prime, raw	4 oz	420	38
rib whole, lean & fat, Prime; broiled	3 oz	347	30
rib whole, lean & fat, Prime; roasted	3 oz	361	31
rib whole, lean & fat, Select, raw	4 oz	352	30

FOOD	PORTION	CALORIES	FAT
rib whole, lean & fat, Select; broiled	3 oz	289	23
rib whole, lean & fat, Select; roasted	3 oz	306	25
rib whole, lean only, Choice, raw	4 oz	192	11
rib whole, lean only, Choice; broiled	3 oz	198	12
rib whole, lean only, Choice; roasted	3 oz	209	12
rib whole, lean only, Prime, raw	4 oz	232	15
rib whole, lean only, Prime; broiled	3 oz	238	16
rib whole, lean only, Prime; roasted	3 oz	248	17
rib whole, lean only, Select, raw	4 oz	172	9
rib whole, lean only, Select; broiled	3 oz	181	10
rib whole, lean only, Select; roasted	3 oz	191	10
round, lean & fat, Choice, raw	4 oz	272	20
round, lean & fat, Choice; broiled	3 oz	233	16
round, lean & fat, Select, raw	4 oz	260	19
round, lean & fat, Select; broiled	3 oz	222	14
round, lean only, Choice, raw	4 oz	156	6
round, lean only, Choice; broiled	3 oz	165	7
round, lean only, Select, raw	4 oz	152	5
round, lean only, Select; broiled	3 oz	157	6
shank, crosscut, lean & fat, Choice, raw	4 oz	180	9
shank, crosscut, lean & fat, Choice; simmered	3 oz	208	10
shank, crosscut, lean only, Choice; raw	4 oz	144	4
shank, crosscut, lean only, Choice; simmered	3 oz	171	5
short loin tenderloin, lean & fat, Choice, raw	1 steak (6.6 oz)	391	29
short loin tenderloin, lean & fat, Prime, raw	1 steak (5.5 oz)	450	37
short loin tenderloin, lean & fat, Prime; broiled	1 steak (4 oz)	362	27

FOOD	PORTION	CALORIES	FAT
short loin tenderloin, lean & fat, Select, raw	1 steak (5.5 oz)	364	26
short loin tenderloin, lean & fat, Select; broiled	1 steak (4 oz)	286	18
short loin tenderloin, lean only, Choice, raw	4 oz	168	8
short loin tenderloin, lean only, Prime, raw	4 oz	192	10
short loin tenderloin, lean only, Select, raw	4 oz	160	7
short loin top loin, lean & fat, Choice, raw	1 steak (10.7 oz)	886	72
short loin top loin, lean & fat, Choice; broiled	1 steak (8.2 oz)	672	46
short loin top loin, lean & fat, Prime, raw	1 steak (10.7 oz)	980	83
short loin top loin, lean & fat, Prime; broiled	1 steak (8 oz)	774	59
short loin top loin, lean & fat, Select, raw	1 steak (10.7 oz)	804	63
short loin top loin, lean & fat, Select; broiled	1 steak (8.1 oz)	603	39
short loin top loin, lean only, Choice, raw	4 oz	176	8
short loin top loin, lean only, Prime, raw	4 oz	212	12
short loin top loin, lean only, Select, raw	4 oz	156	6
short loin, tenderloin, lean & fat, Choice; broiled	3 oz	230	15
short loin, tenderloin, lean & fat, Choice; roasted	3 oz	262	19
short loin, tenderloin, lean & fat, Choice; broiled	1 steak (4.1 oz)	314	21
short loin, tenderloin, lean & fat, Prime; broiled	3 oz	270	20

FOOD	PORTION	CALORIES	FAT
short loin, tenderloin, lean & fat, Prime; roasted	3 oz	305	24
short loin, tenderloin, lean & fat, Select; broiled	3 oz	216	13
short loin, tenderloin, lean & fat, Select; roasted	3 oz	245	17
short loin, tenderloin, lean only, Choice; broiled	3 oz	176	8
short loin, tenderloin, lean only, Choice; roasted	3 oz	189	10
short loin, tenderloin, lean only, Prime; broiled	3 oz	197	11
short loin, tenderloin, lean only, Prime; roasted	3 oz	217	13
short loin, tenderloin, lean only, Select; broiled	3 oz	167	7
short loin, tenderloin, lean only, Select; roasted	3 oz	177	9
short loin, top loin, lean & fat, Choice; roasted	3 oz	243	17
short loin, top loin, lean & fat, Prime; broiled	3 oz	288	22
short loin, top loin, lean & fat, Select; broiled	3 oz	223	14
short loin, top loin, lean only, Choice; broiled	3 oz	176	8
short loin, top loin, lean only, Prime; broiled	3 oz	208	12
short loin, top loin, lean only, Select; broiled	3 oz	162	6
shortribs, lean & fat, Choice, raw	4 oz	440	41
shortribs, lean & fat, Choice; braised	3 oz	400	36
shortribs, lean only, Choice, raw	4 oz	196	12
shortribs, lean only, Choice; braised	3 oz	251	15

FOOD	PORTION	CALORIES	FAT
sirloin, wedge-bone, lean & fat, Choice; broiled	3 oz	240	16
sirloin, wedge-bone, lean & fat, Choice; pan-fried	3 oz	288	21
sirloin, wedge-bone, lean & fat, Prime; broiled	3 oz	271	19
sirloin, wedge-bone, lean & fat, Select; broiled	3 oz	232	15
sirloin, wedge-bone, lean only, Choice; broiled	3 oz	180	26
sirloin, wedge-bone, lean only, Choice; pan-fried	3 oz	202	28
sirloin, wedge-bone, lean only, Prime; broiled	3 oz	201	26
sirloin, wedge-bone, lean only, Select; broiled	3 oz	170	7
sirloin, wedge-bone, lean only, Choice, raw	4 oz	156	6
sirloin, wedge-bone, lean only, Prime, raw	4 oz	176	8
sirloin, wedge-bone, lean only, Select, raw	4 oz	148	5
sirloin, wedge bone, lean & fat, Choice, raw	4 oz	300	32
sirloin, wedge bone, lean & fat, Prime, raw	4 oz	328	27
sirloin, wedge bone, lean & fat, Select, raw	4 oz	280	21
spleen, raw	4 oz	119	3
spleen; braised	3 oz	123	4
T-bone steak, lean & fat, Choice, raw	4 oz	348	30
T-bone steak, lean only, Choice, raw	4 oz	180	9
T-bone steak, lean & fat, Choice, broiled	3 oz	276	21

FOOD	PORTION	CALORIES	FAT
T-bone steak, lean only, Choice, broiled	3 oz	182	9
thymus, raw	4 oz	266	23
thymus; braised	3 oz	271	21
tip round, lean & fat, Choice, raw	4 oz	240	24
tip round, lean & fat, Choice; roasted	3 oz	216	13
tip round, lean & fat, Prime, raw	4 oz	256	18
tip round, lean & fat, Prime; roasted	3 oz	242	16
tip round, lean & fat, Select, raw	4 oz	220	14
tip round, lean & fat, Select; roasted	3 oz	205	12
tip round, lean only, Choice, raw	4 oz	152	5
tip round, lean only, Choice; roasted	3 oz	164	7
tip round, lean only, Prime, raw	4 oz	164	7
tip round, lean only, Prime; roasted	3 oz	181	9
tip round, lean only, Select, raw	4 oz	144	4
tip round, lean only, Select; roasted	3 oz	156	6
top round, lean & fat, Choice, raw	4 oz	196	10
top round, lean & fat, Choice; pan fried	3 oz	246	15
top round, lean & fat, Choice; roasted	3 oz	181	8
top round, lean & fat, Prime, raw	4 oz	212	12
top round, lean & fat, Prime; broiled	3 oz	201	10
top round, lean & fat, Select, raw	4 oz	188	9
top round, lean & fat, Select; broiled	3 oz	176	7
top round, lean only, Choice, raw	4 oz	152	5
top round, lean only, Choice; broiled	3 oz	165	5
top round, lean only, Choice; pan-fried	3 oz	193	7
top round, lean only, Prime, raw	4 oz	176	7
top round, lean only, Prime; broiled	3 oz	183	27

FOOD	PORTION	CALORIES	FAT
top round, lean only, Select; raw	4 oz	144	4
top round, lean only, Select; broiled	3 oz	156	5
tripe, raw	4 oz	111	4
FROZEN Cheeseburger (Micro Magic)	1 (4.75 oz)	450	25
Hamburger (Micro Magic)	1 (4.75 oz)	350	18
ground patties, frzn, raw	4 oz	319	26
patties; cooked medium	3 oz	240	17

BEEF DISHES

FOOD	PORTION	CALORIES	FAT
CANNED Beef Stew (Chef Boy.ar.dee)	7 oz	220	13
Beef Stew (Estee)	7.5 oz	210	9
Meat Ball Stew (Chef Boy.ar.dee)	8 oz	330	21
stew w/ vegetables	1 cup	186	7
FROZEN Beef w/ Barbecue Sauce (Chefwich)	1	400	10
HOME RECIPE stew w/ vegetables	1 cup	209	10
stroganoff	¾ cup	260	19
swiss steak	4.6 oz	214	9
MIX Hamburger Helper Beef Noodle; as prep (General Mills)	6 oz	326	15
Hamburger Helper Cheeseburger Macaroni; as prep (General Mills)	6 oz	366	18

FOOD	PORTION	CALORIES	FAT
Hamburger Helper Chili Tomato; as prep (General Mills)	6 oz	336	18
Hamburger Helper Lasagne; as prep (General Mills)	6 oz	336	15

BEER, ALE AND MALT LIQUOR

Amstel Light	12 oz	95	0
Anheuser Busch Natural Light	12 oz	110	0
Bud Light	12 oz	108	0
Coors Light	12 oz	105	0
Guiness Kaliber (nonalcoholic)	12 oz	43	0
Michelob Light	12 oz	134	0
Miller Lite	12 oz	96	0
Molson Light	12 oz	109	0
Piels Light	12 oz	136	0
Schaefer Light	12 oz	112	0
Schlitz Light	12 oz	96	0
Schmidts Light	12 oz	96	0
ale	12 oz	155	0
beer, light	12 oz	100	0
beer, regular	12 oz	146	0
malt beverage	12 oz	32	0

BEETS

CANNED			
Cuts (Libby)	½ cup	35	0
Cuts (Seneca)	½ cup	35	0
Diced (Libby)	½ cup	35	0

FOOD	PORTION	CALORIES	FAT
Diced (Seneca)	½ cup	35	0
Diced Tender (S&W)	½ cup	40	0
Harvard (Libby)	½ cup	80	0
Harvard (Seneca)	½ cup	80	0
Julienne French Style (S&W)	½ cup	40	0
Pickled (Libby)	½ cup	35	0
Pickled (Seneca)	½ cup	35	0
Sliced (Libby)	½ cup	35	0
Sliced (Seneca)	½ cup	35	0
Sliced Pickled w/ Red Wine Vinegar (S&W)	½ cup	70	0
Sliced Small Premium (S&W)	½ cup	40	0
Whole (Libby)	½ cup	35	0
Whole (Seneca)	½ cup	35	0
Whole Extra Small Pickled (S&W)	½ cup	70	0
Whole Small (S&W)	½ cup	40	0
beets, harvard	½ cup	89	tr
beets, pickled	½ cup	75	tr
beets, sliced	½ cup	27	tr
FRESH beet greens, chopped, raw	½ cup	4	tr

FOOD	PORTION	CALORIES	FAT
beet greens; cooked	½ cup	20	tr
cooked	½ cup	26	tr
raw	2 (5.7 oz)	30	tr

BEVERAGES

(*see* BEER, ALE AND MALT LIQUOR, COFFEE, DRINK MIXER, FRUIT DRINKS, LIQUOR/LIQUEUR, MINERAL/BOTTLED WATER, SODA, TEA/HERBAL TEA, WINE, WINE COOLERS)

BISCUIT

MIX

FOOD	PORTION	CALORIES	FAT
Buttermilk Biscuit Mix; not prep (Health Valley)	1 oz	100	1

HOME RECIPE

FOOD	PORTION	CALORIES	FAT
biscuit	1.5 oz	155	10

REFRIGERATED

FOOD	PORTION	CALORIES	FAT
1896 Brand Baking Powder	2	210	10
1896 Brand Butter Tastin'	2	210	25
1896 Brand Buttermilk	2	210	10
Ballard Ovenready	2	100	1
Ballard Ovenready Buttermilk	2	100	1
Big Country Southern Style	2	200	8
Hungry Jack Butter Tastin' Flaky	2	180	9
Hungry Jack Buttermilk Flaky	2	170	7
Hungry Jack Buttermilk Fluffy	2	180	8
Hungry Jack Extra Rich Buttermilk	2	110	3
Hungry Jack Flaky	2	170	7
Pillsbury Big Country Buttermilk	2	200	8
Pillsbury Big Country Buttertastin'	2	190	8
Pillsbury Big Tenderflake Baking Powder Dinner	2	110	5
Pillsbury Big Tenderflake Buttermilk	2	110	5

FOOD	PORTION	CALORIES	FAT
Pillsbury Butter	2	100	1
Pillsbury Buttermilk	2	100	1
Pillsbury Country	2	100	1
Pillsbury Deluxe Heat 'n Eat Buttermilk	2	280	15
Pillsbury Extra Lights Flaky Buttermilk	2	110	4
Pillsbury Good 'N Buttery Fluffy	2	180	10
Pillsbury Heat 'N Eat Buttermilk	2	170	5

BLACK BEANS

FOOD	PORTION	CALORIES	FAT
cooked	1 cup	227	1
raw	1 cup	661	3

BLACKBERRIES

FOOD	PORTION	CALORIES	FAT
CANNED in heavy syrup	½ cup	118	tr
FRESH blackberries	½ cup	37	tr
FROZEN blackberries	1 cup	97	1

BLACKEYE PEAS

FOOD	PORTION	CALORIES	FAT
CANNED Blackeye Peas (Ranch Style)	7.5 oz	170	2
Blackeye Peas & Beans Seasoned w/ Pork (Luck's)	7.25 oz	200	6
Blackeyes w/ Jalapeno (Ranch Style)	7.5 oz	180	2
DRIED Blackeye (Hurst Brand)	1 cup	233	1

FOOD	PORTION	CALORIES	FAT

BLINTZE

FOOD	PORTION	CALORIES	FAT
cheese (home recipe)	2	186	6

BLUEBERRIES

FOOD	PORTION	CALORIES	FAT
CANNED Blueberries in Heavy Syrup (S&W)	½ cup	111	0
in heavy syrup	½ cup	112	tr
FRESH blueberries	1 cup	82	1
FROZEN unsweetened	1 cup	78	1
sweetened	1 cup	187	tr

BLUEFISH

FOOD	PORTION	CALORIES	FAT
raw	3 oz	105	4
raw	1 fillet (5.3 oz)	186	6

BORAGE

FOOD	PORTION	CALORIES	FAT
cooked; chopped	3.5 oz	25	1
raw; chopped	½ cup	9	tr

BOYSENBERRIES

FOOD	PORTION	CALORIES	FAT
CANNED in heavy sirup	½ cup	113	tr
FROZEN unsweetened	1 cup	66	tr
JUICE Boysenberry (Smucker's)	8 oz	120	0

FOOD	PORTION	CALORIES	FAT
BRAINS			
beef; pan-fried	3 oz	167	11
beef, raw	4 oz	142	10
beef; simmered	3 oz	136	11
pork; braised	3 oz	117	8
pork, raw	3 oz	108	8

BRAN
(*see* CEREAL)

BRAZILNUTS

FOOD	PORTION	CALORIES	FAT
dried, unblanched	1 oz	186	19

BREAD
(*see also* BAGEL, BISCUIT, BREADSTICK, CROISSANT, ENGLISH MUFFIN, MUFFIN, ROLL, SCONE)

FOOD	PORTION	CALORIES	FAT
CANNED			
Brown Bread (B&M)	½ slice	80	tr
Brown Bread New England Recipe (S&W)	2 slices	76	0
Brown Bread w/ Raisins (B&M)	½ slice	80	tr
FROZEN			
OH Boy! Garlic Bread	2 oz	202	11
HOME RECIPE			
banana	½″ slice	116	6
cornbread	2″x2″ piece (1.4 oz)	107	2
cornstick	1 (1.3 oz)	101	4
date-nut	½″ slice	92	3
hush puppies	1 (2 oz)	147	7

FOOD	PORTION	CALORIES	FAT
nut	1 slice (1.5 oz)	127	4
pita, whole wheat	1, 6" diam	247	1
pumpkin	1 slice (1.5 oz)	127	5
raisin	1 slice (1.5 oz)	140	2
whole wheat	1 slice	71	tr
MIX			
Corn Bread, as prep (Dromedary)	1 piece (2" × 2")	130	3
Cornbread Blue Cornmeal; as prep (Zia Foods)	1 piece (1.2 oz)	110	6
READY-TO-EAT			
Bran'nola Country Oat (Arnold)	1 slice	90	2
Bran'nola Dark Wheat (Arnold)	1 slice	80	1
Bran'nola Hearty Wheat (Arnold)	1 slice	90	2
Bran'nola Nutty Grains (Arnold)	1 slice	90	1
Bran'nola Original (Arnold)	1 slice	70	1
Butter Crust (Freihofer's)	1 slice	70	1
Canadian Oat (Freihofer's)	1 slice	80	1
Cinnamon (Pepperidge Farm)	2 slices	170	5
Cinnamon Oatmeal (Oatmeal Goodness)	1 slice	90	2
Club Pullman (Freihofer's)	1 slice	70	1
Cracked Wheat (Pepperidge Farm)	2 slices	140	2
Cracked Wheat (Roman Meal)	1 slice	66	tr

FOOD	PORTION	CALORIES	FAT
Dijon Rye (Pepperidge Farm)	2 slices	160	2
Family Pumpernickel (Pepperidge Farm)	2 slices	160	2
Garlic Bread (Arnold)	1 slice	80	3
Harvest Recipe 100% Whole Wheat (Roman Meal)	1 slice	66	tr
Hi-Fibre (Monks' Bread)	1 slice	50	1
Honey Bran (Pepperidge Farm)	2 slices	190	2
Honey Wheat Berry (Pepperidge Farm)	2 slices	140	2
Honey Wheat Berry (Roman Meal)	1 slice	66	1
Honey Wheatberry Light (Roman Meal)	1 slice	40	tr
Honeybran Light (Roman Meal)	1 slice	40	tr
Italian, Francisco (Arnold)	1 slice	70	1
Italian, Francisco Thick Sliced (Arnold)	1 slice	70	1
Italian, Light (Arnold)	1 slice	40	tr
Italian, No Seeds (Freihofer's)	1 slice	70	1
Italian, Seeded (Freihofer's)	1 slice	70	1
Italian, Stick, Unsliced (Arnold)	1 oz	90	1
Lite Diet (Freihofer's)	1 slice	40	0
Multi-Grain Very Thin (Pepperidge Farm)	2 slices	80	1

FOOD	PORTION	CALORIES	FAT
Oat (Roman Meal)	1 slice	71	1
Oat, Milk & Honey (Arnold)	1 slice	60	1
Oatmeal (Pepperidge Farm)	2 slices	140	3
Oatmeal & Bran (Oatmeal Goodness)	1 slice	90	2
Oatmeal & Sunflower Seeds (Oatmeal Goodness)	1 slice	90	2
Oatmeal, Light (Arnold)	1 slice	40	tr
Old Fashioned (Freihofer's)	1 slice	70	1
Party Pumpernickel (Pepperidge Farm)	4 slices	70	1
Party Dijon Slices (Pepperidge Farm)	4 slices	70	1
Party Rye (Pepperidge Farm)	4 slices	60	1
Pita, White Large Size (Sahara Bread)	1 pocket (3 oz)	240	2
Pita, White Mini Loaf (Sahara Bread)	1 pocket (1 oz)	80	1
Pita, White Regular Size (Sahara Bread)	1 pocket (2 oz)	160	1
Pita, Whole Wheat Mini Loaf (Sahara Bread)	1 pocket (1 oz)	80	1
Pita, Whole Wheat Regular Size (Sahara Bread)	1 pocket (2 oz)	150	2
Pumpernickel (Arnold)	1 slice	80	1
Pumpernickel, Levy's (Arnold)	1 slice	80	1
Raisin (Monks' Bread)	1 slice	70	2

FOOD	PORTION	CALORIES	FAT
Raisin (Monks' Bread)	1 slice	70	2
Raisin Orange (Arnold)	1 slice	70	1
Raisin Sun Maid (Arnold)	1 slice	70	1
Raisin Tea Loaf (Arnold)	1 slice	70	1
Raisin w/ Cinnamon (Pepperidge Farm)	2 slices	150	3
Rite Diet (Freihofer's)	2 slices	90	1
Rite Diet Wheat (Freihofer's)	2 slices	90	1
Round Top (Roman Meal)	1 slice	67	tr
Rye, Dill, Seeded (Arnold)	1 slice	80	1
Rye, Jewish, Seeded (Arnold)	1 slice	80	1
Rye, Jewish, Unseeded (Arnold)	1 slice	80	1
Rye, Levy's Real Jewish, Seeded (Arnold)	1 slice	80	1
Rye, Levy's Real Jewish, Unseeded (Arnold)	1 slice	80	1
Rye, Melba Thin (Arnold)	1 slice	40	tr
Rye, Stub Pullman (Freihofer's)	1 slice	70	1
Sandwich Bread (Roman Meal)	1 slice	55	tr
Sandwich White (Pepperidge Farm)	2 slices	130	2
Seeded Family Rye (Pepperidge Farm)	2 slices	80	1

FOOD	PORTION	CALORIES	FAT
Seedless Rye (Pepperidge Farm)	2 slices	160	2
Seven Grain (Roman Meal)	1 slice	68	tr
Seven Grain Light (Roman Meal)	1 slice	40	tr
Soft Rye Dill & Onion (Freihofer's)	1 slice	70	1
Soft Rye Pumpernickel (Freihofer's)	1 slice	70	1
Soft Rye No Seeds (Freihofer's)	1 slice	70	1
Soft Rye Seeded (Freihofer's)	1 slice	70	1
Split Top Wheat (Freihofer's)	1 slice	70	1
Split Top White (Freihofer's)	1 slice	70	1
Sun Grain (Roman Meal)	1 slice	68	1
Sunbeam King (Freihofer's)	1 slice	70	1
Sunflower & Bran (Monks, Bread)	1 slice	70	1
The Original (Freihofer's)	1 slice	70	1
Toasting White (Pepperidge Farm)	2 slices	170	2
Wheat (Freihofer's)	1½ slices	70	1
Wheat (Fresh Horizons)	1 slice	49	tr
Wheat (Pepperidge Farm)	2 slices	190	3
Wheat Berry, Honey (Arnold)	1 slice	80	2

FOOD	PORTION	CALORIES	FAT
Wheat Germ (Pepperidge Farm)	2 slices	130	1
Wheat Light (Roman Meal)	1 slice	40	tr
Wheat Oatmeal (Oatmeal Goodness)	1 slice	90	2
Wheat, Brick Oven (Arnold)	1 slice of 8 oz loaf	60	2
Wheat, Brick Oven (Arnold)	1 slice of 16 oz loaf	60	2
Wheat, Brick Oven (Arnold)	1 slice of 32 oz loaf	90	2
Wheat, Cottage (America's Own)	1 slice	70	1
Wheat, Golden Light (Arnold)	1 slice	40	tr
Wheat, Less (Arnold)	1 slice	40	tr
Wheat, Small (Freihofer's)	1½ slices	70	1
Wheat, Stone Ground 100% Whole (Arnold)	1 slice	50	1
Wheat, Stub Pullman (Freihofer's)	1 slice	70	1
Wheat, Very Thin (Arnold)	1 slice	40	1
White (Freihofer's)	1 slice	70	1
White (Fresh Horizons)	1 slice	50	tr
White (Monks' Bread)	1 slice	60	1
White (Pepperidge Farm)	2 slices	145	3

FOOD	PORTION	CALORIES	FAT
White (Roman Meal)	1 slice	71	tr
White ½" Stub Pullman (Freihofer's)	1 slice	70	1
White Light (Roman Meal)	1 slice	40	tr
White, 7/16" Stub Pullman (Freihofer's)	1½ slices	70	1
White, Brick Oven (Arnold)	1 slice of 8 oz loaf	60	1
White, Brick Oven (Arnold)	1 slice of 16 oz loaf	60	1
White, Brick Oven (Arnold)	1 slice of 32 oz loaf	90	1
White, Cottage (America's Own)	1 slice	70	1
White, Country (Arnold)	1 slice	100	2
White, Less (Arnold)	1 slice	40	tr
White, Milk & Honey (Arnold)	1 slice	60	1
White, Very Thin (Arnold)	1 slice	40	1
Whole Wheat (Pepperidge Farm)	2 slices	130	2
Whole Wheat 100% (Freihofer's)	1 slice	75	1
Whole Wheat 100% Stone Ground (Monks' Bread)	1 slice	70	1
Whole Wheat Very Thin (Pepperidge Farm)	2 slices	80	2
whole wheat	1 slice	56	tr

FOOD	PORTION	CALORIES	FAT
REFRIGERATED			
Crusty French (Pillsbury)	1" slice	60	1
Pipin'Hot Wheat Loaf (Pillsbury)	1" slice	80	24
Pipin'Hot White Loaf (Pillsbury)	1" slice	80	24

BREAD COATING

FOOD	PORTION	CALORIES	FAT
Oven Fry Extra Crispy Recipe for Chicken (General Foods)	4 pkg (1 oz)	111	2
Oven Fry Extra Crispy Recipe for Pork (General Foods)	¼ pkg (1 oz)	115	2
Oven Fry Light Crispy Homestyle Recipe (General Foods)	¼ pkg (1 oz)	107	3
Shake 'N Bake Country Mild Recipe	¼ pkg (½ oz)	65	3
Shake 'N Bake Italian Herb	¼ pkg (½ oz)	75	1
Shake 'N Bake Original Barbecue Recipe for Chicken	¼ pkg (½ oz)	90	2
Shake 'N Bake Original Barbecue Recipe for Pork	¼ pkg (½ oz)	75	2
Shake 'N Bake Original Recipe for Chicken	¼ pkg (½ oz)	75	2
Shake 'N Bake Original Recipe for Fish	¼ pkg (½ oz)	74	1
Shake 'N Bake Original Recipe for Pork	¼ pkg (½ oz)	80	1

BREAD CRUMBS

FOOD	PORTION	CALORIES	FAT
Contadina Seasoned	1 rounded Tbsp	35	tr
Contadina Seasoned	1 cup	426	4
Friday's Seasoned	1 oz	56	tr

FOOD	PORTION	CALORIES	FAT
BREADFRUIT			
breadfruit	¼ sm	99	tr
breadfruit	3.5 oz	109	tr
seeds; roasted	1 oz	59	tr
BREADSTICK			
Cheese Breadsticks (Lance)	2	20	1
Dunking Sticks (Lance)	1⅜ oz	190	10
Garlic Breadsticks (Lance)	2	30	1
Onion (Stella D'Oro)	1	38	1
Plain (Stella D'Oro)	1	41	1
Plain (Lance)	2	30	1
Plain Dietetic (Stella D'Oro)	1	43	1
Sesame (Stella D'Oro)	1	50	2
Sesame (Lance)	2	30	1
Soft Bread Sticks (Pillsbury)	1	100	2
breadstick, onion poppyseed (home recipe)	1 med	19	tr
BREAKFAST BAR			
(*see also* BREAKFAST DRINK, NUTRITIONAL SUPPLEMENTS)			
Chocolate Chip (Carnation)	1 bar (1.44 oz)	200	11
Chocolate Crunch (Carnation)	1 bar (1.34 oz)	190	10

FOOD	PORTION	CALORIES	FAT
Oat Bran Fruit Bar (Health Valley)	1.5 oz	140	4
Peanut Butter Crunch (Carnation)	1 bar (1.35 oz)	190	11
Peanut Butter w/ Chocolate Chips (Carnation)	1 bar (1.39 oz)	200	11

BREAKFAST DRINK
 (*see also* BREAKFAST BAR, NUTRITIONAL SUPPLEMENTS)

FOOD	PORTION	CALORIES	FAT
Chocolate Instant Breakfast (Carnation)	1 pkg (1.25)	130	tr
Chocolate Instant Breakfast; as prep w/ whole milk (Carnation)	1 pkg + 8 oz milk	280	8
Chocolate Instant Breakfast; as prep w/ skim milk (Carnation)	1 pkg + 8 oz milk	220	1
Chocolate Instant Breakfast; as prep w/ whole milk (Pillsbury)	1 pkg + 8 oz milk	290	9
Chocolate Instant Breakfast No Sugar Added (Carnation)	1 pkg (.69 oz)	70	1
Chocolate Instant Breakfast No Sugar Added; as prep w/ skim milk (Carnation)	1 pkg + 8 oz milk	160	2
Chocolate Malt Instant Breakfast (Carnation)	1 pkg (1.24 oz)	130	1
Chocolate Malt Instant Breakfast; as prep w/ whole milk (Carnation)	1 pkg + 8 oz milk	280	9
Chocolate Malt Instant Breakfast; as prep w/ skim milk (Carnation)	1 pkg + 8 oz milk	220	2
Chocolate Malt Instant Breakfast; as prep w/ whole milk (Pillsbury)	1 pkg + 8 oz milk	290	9

FOOD	PORTION	CALORIES	FAT
Chocolate Malt Instant Breakfast No Sugar Added (Carnation)	1 pkg (.71 oz)	70	1
Chocolate Malt Instant Breakfast No Sugar Added; as prep w/ skim milk (Carnation)	1 pkg + 8 oz milk	160	2
Coffee Instant Breakfast (Carnation)	1 pkg (1.26 oz)	130	tr
Coffee Instant Breakfast; as prep w/ skim milk (Carnation)	1 pkg + 8 oz milk	220	1
Coffee Instant Breakfast; as prep w/ whole milk (Carnation)	1 pkg + 8 oz milk	280	8
Eggnog Instant Breakfast (Carnation)	1 pkg (1.2 oz)	130	tr
Eggnog Instant Breakfast; as prep w/ skim milk (Carnation)	1 pkg + 8 oz milk	220	1
Eggnog Instant Breakfast; as prep w/ whole milk (Carnation)	1 pkg + 8 oz milk	280	8
Strawberry Instant Breakfast (Carnation)	1 pkg (1.25 oz)	130	tr
Strawberry Instant Breakfast No Sugar Added (Carnation)	1 pkg (.68 oz)	70	0
Strawberry Instant Breakfast; as prep w/ skim milk (Carnation)	1 pkg + 8 oz milk	220	1
Strawberry Instant Breakfast; as prep w/ whole milk (Pillsbury)	1 pkg + 8 oz milk	290	9
Strawberry Instant Breakfast; as prep w/ whole milk (Carnation)	1 pkg + 8 oz milk	280	8
Strawberry Instant Breakfast No Sugar Added; as prep w/ skim milk (Carnation)	1 pkg + 8 oz milk	160	1

FOOD	PORTION	CALORIES	FAT
Vanilla Instant Breakfast; as prep w/ whole milk (Pillsbury)	1 pkg + 8 oz milk	300	9
Vanilla Instant Breakfast No Sugar Added (Carnation)	1 pkg (.67 oz)	70	0
Vanilla Instant Breakfast No Sugar Added; as prep w/ skim milk (Carnation)	1 pkg + 8 oz milk	160	1
Vanilla Instant Breakfast (Carnation)	1 pkg (1.23 oz)	130	tr
Vanilla Instant Breakfast; as prep w/ skim milk (Carnation)	1 pkg + 8 oz milk	220	1
Vanilla Instant Breakfast; as prep w/ whole milk (Carnation)	1 pkg + 8 oz milk	280	8
orange drink powder; as prep w/ water	6 oz	86	0
orange drink, powder	3 rounded tsp	93	0

BROAD BEANS

CANNED			
broadbeans	1 cup	183	1
DRIED			
cooked	1 cup	86	1
raw	1 cup	511	2
FRESH			
cooked	3½ oz	56	tr
raw	1 cup	79	1

BROCCOLI

FRESH			
raw; chopped	½ cup	12	tr
whole; cooked	½ cup	23	tr

FOOD	PORTION	CALORIES	FAT
FROZEN			
Baby Spears (Birds Eye)	⅔ cup	29	tr
Broccoli (Health Valley)	3 oz	24	tr
Broccoli Vegetable Crisp (Ore Ida)	3 oz	190	11
Broccoli With Cheese (Pepperidge Farm)	1 cup	250	17
Broccoli w/ Cheese Sauce (Birds Eye)	½ cup	115	6
Broccoli w/ Creamy Italian Cheese Sauce (Birds Eye)	½ cup	90	6
Chopped (Birds Eye)	⅔ cup	26	tr
Cut (Hanover)	½ cup	25	0
Cuts (Birds Eye)	⅔ cup	25	tr
Florets (Birds Eye)	⅔ cup	26	tr
Florets (Hanover)	½ cup	30	0
Spears (Birds Eye)	⅔ cup	26	tr
frzn; cooked	½ cup	25	tr
frzn; not prep	10 oz pkg	75	1
spears; cooked	½ cup	69	tr
spears; not prep	10 oz pkg	84	1

BROWNIE

FOOD	PORTION	CALORIES	FAT
FROZEN			
Chocolate Brownie (Weight Watchers)	1	100	4

FOOD	PORTION	CALORIES	FAT
HOME RECIPE			
brownie w/ nuts	1 (.8 oz)	97	5
MIX			
Black Forest Brownie; as prep (Pillsbury)	2" sq	160	6
Chewy Recipe Fudge Brownie Mix; as prep (Duncan Hines)	1	130	5
Double Fudge Brownie; as prep (Pillsbury)	2" sq	160	6
Estee Brownie Mix; as prep	2" sq	45	2
Family-Size Fudge Brownie; as prep (Pillsbury)	2" sq	150	7
Family-Size Walnut Brownie; as prep (Pillsbury)	2" sq	150	8
Fudge Brownie; as prep (Pillsbury)	2" sq	150	6
Gourmet Truffle Brownie Mix; as prep (Duncan Hines)	1	280	13
Gourmet Turtle Brownie Mix; as prep (Duncan Hines)	1	240	10
Gourmet Vienna White Brownie Mix; as prep (Duncan Hines)	1	240	12
Milk Chocolate Brownie Mix; as prep (Duncan Hines)	1	160	7
Original Fudge Brownie Mix; as prep (Duncan Hines)	1	160	7
Peanut Butter Chocolate Brownie Mix; as prep (Duncan Hines)	1	150	8
Rocky Road Fudge Brownie; as prep (Pillsbury)	2" sq	170	7

FOOD	PORTION	CALORIES	FAT
READY-TO-EAT			
Fudge Walnut (Tastykake)	1	373	10
Lance Brownie	1 pkg (1.7 oz)	200	6
Little Debbie Fudge Brownies	1 pkg (2 oz)	240	8
Little Debbie Fudge Brownies	1 pkg (2.9 oz)	350	12

BRUSSELS SPROUTS

FOOD	PORTION	CALORIES	FAT
FRESH			
cooked	½ cup	30	tr
raw	½ cup	19	tr
FROZEN			
Baby Brussels Sprouts w/ Cheese Sauce (Birds Eye)	½ cup	113	6
Brussels Sprouts (Birds Eye)	½ cup	37	tr
Brussels Sprouts (Hanover)	½ cup	40	0
frzn; cooked	½ cup	33	tr
frzn; not prep	10 oz	116	1

BULGUR

FOOD	PORTION	CALORIES	FAT
bulgur; not prep	1 cup	605	3

BURBOT (FISH)

FOOD	PORTION	CALORIES	FAT
raw	1 fillet (4.1 oz)	104	1
raw	3 oz	76	1

BURDOCK ROOT

FOOD	PORTION	CALORIES	FAT
cooked	1 cup	110	tr
raw	1 cup	85	tr

FOOD	PORTION	CALORIES	FAT

BUTTER
(*see also* BUTTER BLENDS, BUTTER SUBSTITUTE, MARGARINE)

REGULAR
Hotel Bar	1 tsp	35	4
Land O'Lakes, Lightly Salted	1 Tbsp	100	11
Land O'Lakes, Unsalted	1 Tbsp	100	11
butter	1 tsp, 1 pat	36	4
butter	4 oz	813	92
butter	1 pat	36	4
butter	1 stick	813	92
butter oil	1 cup	1795	204
butter oil	1 Tbsp	112	13
clarified butter	3.5 oz	876	99

WHIPPED
Land O'Lakes, Lightly Salted	1 Tbsp	60	7
Land O'Lakes, Unsalted	1 Tbsp	60	7
butter	1 tsp	27	3
butter	4 oz	542	61

BUTTER BEANS

CANNED
Butter Beans (Hanover)	½ cup	80	0
Butter Beans In Sauce (Hanover)	½ cup	100	0
Butter Beans Tender Cooked (S&W)	½ cup	100	0
Speckled Butter Beans, Seasoned w/ Pork (Luck's)	7.5 oz	230	8

FOOD	PORTION	CALORIES	FAT

BUTTER BLENDS
(*see also* BUTTER, BUTTER SUBSTITUTE, MARGARINE)

FOOD	PORTION	CALORIES	FAT
REGULAR			
Blue Bonnet	1 Tbsp	90	11
Blue Bonnet, Unsalted	1 Tbsp	90	11
Country Morning Blend, Lightly Salted	1 Tbsp	100	11
Country Morning Blend, Unsalted	1 Tbsp	100	11
SOFT			
Blue Bonnet	1 Tbsp	90	11
Country Morning Blend, Lightly Salted Soft	1 Tbsp	90	10
Country Morning Blend, Unsalted, Soft	1 Tbsp	90	10
Downey's Cinnamon Honey-Butter	1 Tbsp	34	5
Downey's Original Honey-Butter	1 Tbsp	34	5

BUTTER SUBSTITUTE
(*see also* BUTTER BLENDS, MARGARINE)

FOOD	PORTION	CALORIES	FAT
Butter Buds	⅛ oz	12	0
Butter Buds Sprinkles	½ tsp	4	0
Molly McButter All Natural Butter Flavor Sprinkles	½ tsp	4	0
Molly McButter Natural Sour Cream & Butter Flavor Sprinkles	½ tsp	4	0

BUTTERFISH

FOOD	PORTION	CALORIES	FAT
raw	3 oz	124	7
raw	1 fillet (1.1 oz)	47	3

BUTTERNUTS

FOOD	PORTION	CALORIES	FAT
dried	1 oz	174	16

FOOD	PORTION	CALORIES	FAT

CABBAGE

FRESH
chinese cabbage, (pak-choi), shredded, raw	1 cup	9	tr
chinese cabbage, (pak-choi), shredded; cooked	½ cup	10	tr
chinese cabbage, (pe-tsai), shredded, raw	1 cup	12	tr
chinese cabbage, (pe-tsai), shredded; cooked	1 cup	16	tr
coleslaw	½ cup	42	tr
green, shredded, raw	½ cup	8	tr
green, shredded; cooked	½ cup	16	tr
red, shredded, raw	½ cup	10	tr
red, shredded; cooked	½ cup	16	tr
savoy, shredded, raw	½ cup	10	tr
savoy, shredded; cooked	½ cup	18	tr

HOME RECIPE
stuffed cabbage	1 (6 oz)	373	22

CAKE
(see also BROWNIE, COOKIE, DANISH PASTRY, DOUGHNUT, PIE)

FROSTING/ICING
Cake & Cookie Decorator, Chocolate (Pillsbury)	1 Tbsp	60	2
Cake & Cookie Decorator, all flavors but chocolate (Pillsbury)	1 Tbsp	70	2
Caramel Pecan Frosting Supreme (Pillsbury)	for 1/12 cake	160	8
Chocolate Chip Frosting Supreme (Pillsbury)	for 1/12 cake	150	5
Chocolate Creamy Frosting (Duncan Hines)	1/12 pkg	160	7

FOOD	PORTION	CALORIES	FAT
Chocolate Fudge Frosting Supreme (Pillsbury)	for 1/12 cake	150	6
Chocolate Mint Frosting Supreme (Pillsbury)	for 1/12 cake	150	7
Coconut Almond Frosting Mix; as prep (Pillsbury)	for 1/12 cake	160	10
Coconut Almond Frosting Supreme (Pillsbury)	for 1/12 cake	150	9
Coconut Pecan Frosting Mix; as prep (Pillsbury)	for 1/12 cake	150	7
Coconut Pecan Frosting Supreme (Pillsbury)	for 1/12 cake	160	10
Cream Cheese Frosting Supreme (Pillsbury)	for 1/12 cake	160	6
Dark Dutch Fudge Creamy Frosting (Duncan Hines)	1/12 pkg	160	7
Double Dutch Frosting Supreme (Pillsbury)	for 1/12 cake	140	6
Fluffy White Frosting Mix; as prep (Pillsbury)	for 1/12 cake	60	0
Frosting Mix; as prep (Estee)	1.5 Tbsp	50–60	1–2
Lemon Frosting Supreme (Pillsbury)	for 1/12 cake	160	6
Milk Chocolate Creamy Frosting (Duncan Hines)	1/12 pkg	160	7
Milk Chocolate Frosting Supreme (Pillsbury)	for 1/12 cake	150	6
Mocha Frosting Supreme (Pillsbury)	for 1/12 cake	150	6
Sour Cream Vanilla Frosting Supreme (Pillsbury)	for 1/12 cake	160	6
Strawberry Frosting Supreme (Pillsbury)	for 1/12 cake	160	6

FOOD	PORTION	CALORIES	FAT
Vanilla Creamy Frosting (Duncan Hines)	1/12 pkg	160	7
Vanilla Frosting Supreme (Pillsbury)	for 1/12 cake	160	6
caramel (home recipe)	1 cup	895	26
chocolate (home recipe)	1 cup	1123	37
coconut fluff (home recipe)	1 cup	533	36
white boiled (home recipe)	1 cup	247	0
white uncooked (home recipe)	1 cup	813	21
FROZEN			
All Butter Coffee Cake, Butter Streusel (Sara Lee)	1 slice (40.8 g)	160	7
All Butter Coffee Cake, Cheese (Sara Lee)	1 slice (56.7 g)	210	12
All Butter Coffee Cake, Pecan (Sara Lee)	1 slice (40.8 g)	160	8
All Butter Pound Cake, Family Size (Sara Lee)	1 slice (30.5 g)	130	7
All Butter Pound Cake, Original (Sara Lee)	1 slice (30.5 g)	130	7
Apple Criss-Cross Pastry (Pepperidge Farm)	2 oz	170	8
Apple Strudel (Pepperidge Farm)	3 oz	240	10
Apple Turnover (Pepperidge Farm)	1	300	17
Better Than Cheesecake, Blueberry (Tofutti)	2 oz	160	10
Better Than Cheesecake, Chocolate Brownie (Tofutti)	2 oz	160	10
Better Than Cheesecake, Classic (Tofutti)	2 oz	160	10
Black Forest Cake (Weight Watchers)	1	180	5

FOOD	PORTION	CALORIES	FAT
Blueberry Turnovers (Pepperidge Farm)	1	310	19
Boston Cream (Pepperidge Farm)	2⅞ oz	290	14
Butter Pound (Pepperidge Farm)	1 oz	120	6
Butterscotch Pecan (Pepperidge Farm)	1⅝ oz	160	7
Carrot Cake (Weight Watchers)	1	170	6
Carrot w/ Cream Cheese Icing (Pepperidge Farm)	1⅜ oz	130	7
Cheesecake (Weight Watchers)	1	220	7
Cherry Turnover (Pepperidge Farm)	1	310	19
Chocolate (Pepperidge Farm)	2⅞ oz	300	16
Chocolate Cake (Weight Watchers)	1	180	5
Chocolate Fudge (Pepperidge Farm)	1⅝ oz	180	9
Chocolate Mint (Pepperidge Farm)	1⅝ oz	170	9
Coconut (Pepperidge Farm)	1⅝ oz	180	8
Devil's Food (Pepperidge Farm)	1⅝ oz	170	8
Dutch Chocolate (Pepperidge Farm)	1.75 oz	190	10
Fruit Squares, Apple (Pepperidge Farm)	1	220	12
Fruit Squares, Blueberry (Pepperidge Farm)	1	220	11
Fruit Squares, Cherry (Pepperidge Farm)	1	230	12

FOOD	PORTION	CALORIES	FAT
German Chocolate (Pepperidge Farm)	1⅝ oz	180	10
German Chocolate Cake (Weight Watchers)	1	190	7
Golden (Pepperidge Farm)	1⅝ oz	180	9
Grand Marnier (Pepperidge Farm)	1.5 oz	160	18
Individual Danish, Apple (Sara Lee)	1	120	6
Individual Danish, Cheese (Sara Lee)	1	130	8
Individual Danish, Cinnamon Raisin (Sara Lee)	1	150	8
Individual Danish, Raspberry (Sara Lee)	1	130	6
Lemon Coconut (Pepperidge Farm)	3 oz	280	13
Light Classics, Frehch Cheese (Sara Lee)	1 slice (66.6 g)	200	13
Light Classics, Strawberry French Cheese (Sara Lee)	1 slice (73.7 g)	200	11
Peach Melba (Pepperidge Farm)	3⅛ oz	270	7
Peach Turnover (Pepperidge Farm)	1	310	19
Pineapple Cream (Pepperidge Farm)	2 oz	190	7
Pound Cake, Cholesterol Free (Pepperidge Farm)	1 slice (1 oz)	110	6
Pound Cake w/ Blueberry Topping (Weight Watchers)	1	180	6
Raspberry Turnovers (Pepperidge Farm)	1	310	17
Raspberry Mocha (Pepperidge Farm)	3⅛ oz	310	14

FOOD	PORTION	CALORIES	FAT
Single Layer Iced Cakes, Banana (Sara Lee)	1 slice (48.6 g)	170	6
Single Layer Iced Cakes, Carrot (Sara Lee)	1 slice (67.3 g)	260	13
Strawberry Cheesecake (Weight Watchers)	1	180	5
Strawberry Cream (Pepperidge Farm)	2 oz	190	7
Strawberry Shortcake (Weight Watchers)	1	160	4
Turnover, Apple; frzn (Lamb-Weston)	3 oz	230	10
Turnover, Blueberry; frzn (Lamb-Weston)	3 oz	260	11
Turnover, Cherry; frzn (Lamb-Weston)	3 oz	260	11
Two Layer Cake, Black Forest (Sara Lee)	1 slice (71 g)	190	8
Two Layer Cake, Strawberry Shortcake (Sara Lee)	1 slice (71 g)	190	8
Vanilla (Pepperidge Farm)	1⅝ oz	170	8
eclair w/ chocolate icing & custard filling; frzn	1	205	10
HOME RECIPE			
apple cake	1.5 oz piece	145	7
baklava	1 oz	126	9
boston creme	⅛ of 9" cake	433	17
carrot w/ cream cheese icing	1 cake 10" diam tube	6175	328
carrot w/ cream cheese icing	1/16 of cake	385	21
chocolate cupcake	1 (1.1 oz)	103	5
chocolate cupcake w/ chocolate icing	1 (1.6 oz)	175	8

FOOD	PORTION	CALORIES	FAT
cobbler, peach	½ cup	201	6
cream puff, shell only	1 (2.3 oz)	156	12
hot cross bun	1 (1.8 oz)	172	7
kuchen	2¼" × 2¼" (3.3 oz)	315	13
peanut butter	1 piece (1.8 oz)	211	11
spice w/ caramel icing	1/10 of 9" cake	411	16
sponge	1/12 of 8½" cake	135	36
strudel	1 piece (4.1 oz)	272	8
torte, chocolate	1/16 of 8½" diam (3.2 oz)	317	22
white cupcake	1 (1.1 oz)	114	5
white cupcake w/ white icing	1 (1.6 oz)	164	6
yellow cupcake	1 (1.1 oz)	127	5
yellow cupcake w/ chocolate icing	1 (1.6 oz)	186	7
MIX			
Angel Food, Chocolate (General Mills)	1/12 cake	150	0
Angel Food, Confetti (General Mills)	1/12 cake	160	0
Angel Food, Lemon Custard (General Mills)	1/12 cake	150	0
Angel Food, Strawberry (General Mills)	1/12 cake	150	0
Angel Food, Traditional (General Mills)	1/12 cake	130	0
Angel Food, White (General Mills)	1/12 cake	150	0
Apple Cinnamon Coffee Cake; as prep (Pillsbury)	1/8 cake	240	7
Applesauce; as prep (Pillsbury Plus)	1/12 cake	250	11

FOOD	PORTION	CALORIES	FAT
Applesauce Spice; as prep (Pillsbury Plus)	1/12 cake	250	11
Applesauce Spice Quick Bread; as prep (Pillsbury)	1/12 loaf	150	3
Apricot Nut Quick Bread; as prep (Pillsbury)	1/12 loaf	160	4
Banana; as prep (Pillsbury Plus)	1/12 cake	250	11
Banana Quick Bread; as prep (Pillsbury)	1/12 loaf	160	5
Bisquick (General Mills)	2 oz	230	7
Black Forest Cherry Bundt; as prep (Pillsbury)	1/16 cake	240	9
Blueberry Nut Quick Bread; as prep (Pillsbury)	1/12 loaf	150	4
Boston Cream Bundt; as prep (Pillsbury)	1/16 cake	270	10
Butter Recipe; as prep (Pillsbury Plus)	1/12 cake	260	13
Butter Recipe Fudge; as prep (Duncan Hines)	1/12 cake	270	13
Butter Recipe Golden; as prep (Duncan Hines)	1/12 cake	270	13
Carrot 'N Spice; as prep (Pillsbury Plus)	1/12 cake	260	11
Carrot Nut Quick Bread; as prep (Pillsbury)	1/12 loaf	150	4
Cheesecake No Bake Dessert; as prep (Jell-O)	1/8 cake	281	13
Cherry Nut Quick Bread; as prep (Pillsbury)	1/12 loaf	180	5
Chocolate; as prep (Estee)	1/10 cake	100	2

FOOD	PORTION	CALORIES	FAT
Chocolate Chip; as prep (Pillsbury Plus)	1/12 cake	270	14
Chocolate Chip Oatmeal Fudge Jumbles; as prep (Pillsbury)	1 bar	100	4
Chocolate Lite Cake & Frosting Mix (Batter Lite)	1/9 of cake	110	2
Chocolate Macaroon Bundt; as prep (Pillsbury)	1/16 cake	270	9
Chocolate Mint; as prep (Pillsbury Plus)	1/12 cake	250	12
Chocolate Mousse Bundt; as prep (Pillsbury)	1/16 cake	230	9
Cinnamon Streusel Swirl; as prep (Pillsbury)	1/16 cake	260	11
Cranberry Quick Bread; as prep (Pillsbury)	1/12 loaf	160	3
Dark Chocolate; as prep (Pillsbury Plus)	1/12 cake	250	12
Dark Dutch Fudge; as prep (Duncan Hines)	1/12 cake	280	15
Date Nut Roll; as prep (Dromedary)	1/2" slice	80	2
Date Quick Bread; as prep (Pillsbury)	1/12 loaf	160	3
Devil's Food; as prep (Duncan Hines)	1/12 cake	280	15
Devil's Food; as prep (Pillsbury Plus)	1/12 cake	270	14
Dutch Apple Streusel Swirl; as prep (Pillsbury)	1/16 cake	260	11
French Vanilla; as prep (Duncan Hines)	1/12 cake	260	11
Fudge Marble; as prep (Pillsbury Plus)	1/12 cake	270	12

FOOD	PORTION	CALORIES	FAT
Fudge Marble; as prep (Duncan Hines)	1/12 cake	260	11
German Chocolate; as prep (Pillsbury Plus)	1/12 cake	250	11
Gingerbread; as prep (Dromedary)	1 piece (2" × 2")	100	2
Gingerbread; as prep (Pillsbury)	3" sq	190	4
Honey Granola Quick Bread; as prep (Pillsbury)	1/12 loaf	170	4
Lemon Streusel Swirl; as prep (Pillsbury)	1/16 cake	270	11
Lemon Supreme; as prep (Duncan Hines)	1/12 cake	260	11
Lemon Blueberry Bundt; as prep (Pillsbury)	1/16 cake	200	8
Lemon; as prep (Pillsbury Plus)	1/12 cake	220	9
Mocha; as prep (Pillsbury Plus)	1/12 cake	250	12
Nut Quick Bread; as prep (Pillsbury)	1/12 loaf	170	6
Peanut Butter Oatmeal Fudge Jumbles; as prep (Pillsbury)	1 bar	100	4
Pecan Brown Sugar Streusel Swirl; as prep (Pillsbury)	1/16 cake	260	11
Pineapple Cream Bundt; as prep (Pillsbury)	1/16 cake	260	10
Pineapple Supreme; as prep (Duncan Hines)	1/12 cake	260	11
Pound Bundt; as prep (Pillsbury)	1/16 cake	230	9
Pound Cake; as prep (Dromedary)	1/2" slice	150	6

FOOD	PORTION	CALORIES	FAT
Spice; as prep (Duncan Hines)	1/12 cake	260	11
Strawberry; as prep (Pillsbury Plus)	1/12 cake	260	11
Strawberry Supreme; as prep (Duncan Hines)	1/12 cake	260	11
Swiss Chocolate; as prep (Duncan Hines)	1/12 cake	280	15
Tunnel of Fudge Bundt; as prep (Pillsbury)	1/16 cake	270	12
Tunnel of Lemon Bundt; as prep (Pillsbury)	1/16 cake	270	9
White; as prep (Duncan Hines)	1/12 cake	250	10
White; as prep (Pillsbury Plus)	1/12 cake	240	10
White Lite Cake & Frosting (Batter Lite)	1/9 of cake	110	2
Yellow; as prep (Duncan Hines)	1/12 cake	260	11
yellow w/ chocolate frosting; as prep	1 cake 9" diam	3735	125
yellow w/ chocolate frosting; as prep	1/16 of cake	235	8
READY-TO-USE			
Cheesecake La Creame, Amaretto Almond (Formagg)	2 oz	115	6
Cheesecake La Creame, Pineapple (Formagg)	2 oz	115	6
Cheesecake La Creame, Plain (Formagg)	2 oz	115	6
Cheesecake La Creame, Strawberry (Formagg)	2 oz	115	6
angelfood	1 cake 9¾" diam	1510	2
angelfood	1/12 of cake	125	tr

FOOD	PORTION	CALORIES	FAT
cheesecake	1 cake 9" diam	3350	213
cheesecake	1/12 of cake	280	18
cream puff w/ custard filling	1 (4.6 oz)	303	18
crumb coffeecake	1 cake 7¾" × 5⅝"	1385	41
crumb coffeecake	⅙ of cake	230	7
devil's cupcake w/ chocolate frosting	1	120	4
devil's food w/ chocolate frosting	1 cake, 2 layers	3755	136
devil's food w/ chocolate frosting	1/16 of cake	235	8
fruitcake, dark	1 cake 7½" × 2¼" tube	5185	228
fruitcake, dark	⅔" slice	165	7
gingerbread	1 cake 8" sq	1575	39
gingerbread	⅑ cake	175	4
pound	1 loaf 8½" × 3½"	1935	94
sheet cake w/ white frosting	⅑ of cake	445	14
sheet cake w/ white frosting	1 cake 9" sq	4020	129
sheet cake w/o frosting	1 cake 9" sq	2830	108
sheet cake w/o frosting	⅑ of cake	315	12
REFRIGERATED Apple Danish w/ Icing (Pillsbury Best)	1	240	11
Apple Turnovers (Pillsbury)	1	170	8
Blueberry Turnovers (Pillsbury)	1	170	8
Caramel Danish w/ nuts (Pillsbury)	2	310	16
Cherry Turnovers (Pillsbury)	1	170	8

FOOD	PORTION	CALORIES	FAT
Cinnamon Raisin Danish w/ Icing (Pillsbury)	2	290	14
Orange Danish w/ Icing (Pillsbury)	2	290	14
SNACK			
All Butter Pound Cake (Sara Lee)	1	200	11
Apple Delights (Little Debbie)	1 pkg (1.25 oz)	140	4
Apple Toastettes (Nabisco)	1	200	5
Banana Slices (Little Debbie)	1 pkg (3 oz)	340	12
Banana Twins (Little Debbie)	1 pkg (2.2 oz)	250	9
Be My Valentine (Little Debbie)	1 pkg (2.5 oz)	330	17
Big Wheels (Hostess)	2	345	20
Blueberry Frosted Toastettes (Nabisco)	1	200	5
Blueberry Toastettes (Nabisco)	1	200	5
Brown Sugar Cinnamon Frosted Toastettes (Nabisco)	1	200	5
Caravella (Little Debbie)	1 pkg (1.2 oz)	170	9
Cherry Frosted Toastettes (Nabisco)	1	200	5
Cherry Cordials (Little Debbie)	1 pkg (1.2 oz)	160	8
Cherry Toastettes (Nabisco)	1	200	5
Choc-O-Jel (Little Debbie)	1 pkg (1.16 oz)	150	7

FOOD	PORTION	CALORIES	FAT
Chocolate Cakes (Little Debbie)	1 pkg (2.4 oz)	320	16
Chocolate Cupcake (Tastykake)	1	113	3
Chocolate Fudge Cake (Sara Lee)	1	190	10
Chocolate Twins (Little Debbie)	1 pkg (2.2 oz)	240	7
Christmas Tree Cakes (Little Debbie)	1 pkg (1.6 oz)	220	11
Classic Cheesecake (Sara Lee)	1	200	14
Coconut Crunch (Little Debbie)	1 pkg (2 oz)	320	19
Coconut Rounds (Little Debbie)	1 pkg (1.13 oz)	150	7
Coffee Cake, Apple Cinnamon (Sara Lee)	1	290	13
Coffee Cake, Butter Streusel (Sara Lee)	1	230	12
Coffee Cake, Pecan (Sara Lee)	1	280	16
Cream Filled Butter Cream Cupcake (Tastykake)	1	125	3
Cream Filled Chocolate Cupcake (Tastykake)	1	130	4
Creamies, Banana Treat (Tastykake)	1	138	3
Creamies, Chocolate (Tastykake)	1	174	7
Creamies, Vanilla (Tastykake)	1	182	8
Crumb Cake (Hostess)	2 cakes	259	8
Cupcake, Chocolate (Hostess)	2 cupcakes	314	9

FOOD	PORTION	CALORIES	FAT
Cupcake, Orange (Hostess)	2 cupcakes	294	8
Debbie Doodle Dandies (Little Debbie)	1 pkg (2.5 oz)	320	16
Deluxe Carrot Cake (Sara Lee)	1	180	7
Dessert Cups (Little Debbie)	1 pkg (.79 oz)	80	1
Devil Cremes (Little Debbie)	1 pkg (1.3 oz)	160	7
Devil Slices (Little Debbie)	1 pkg (3 oz)	320	9
Devil Squares (Little Debbie)	1 pkg (2.2 oz)	270	11
Devil's Food Cupcakes (Hostess)	1 (1.5 oz)	136	4
Ding Dongs (Hostess)	2	345	20
Dutch Apple (Little Debbie)	1 pkg (2.17 oz)	230	8
Dutch Apple (Little Debbie)	1 pkg (2.5 oz)	270	8
Easter Bunny Cakes (Little Debbie)	1 pkg (2.5 oz)	320	15
Fancy Cakes (Little Debbie)	1 pkg (2.6 oz)	340	16
Fig Cake (Lance)	2⅛ oz	210	3
Figaroos (Little Debbie)	1 pkg (1.5 oz)	160	4
Fudge Frosted Toastettes (Nabisco)	1	200	6
Fudge Crispy (Little Debbie)	1 pkg (2.08 oz)	260	7
Fudge Rounds (Little Debbie)	1 pkg (1.19 oz)	150	6

FOOD	PORTION	CALORIES	FAT
Fudge Rounds (Little Debbie)	1 pkg (2.75 oz)	330	12
Golden Cremes (Little Debbie)	1 pkg (1.4 oz)	150	6
Golden Cremes (Little Debbie)	1 pkg (2.5 oz)	270	11
Hoho (Hostess)	1 (1 oz)	119	6
Holiday Cakes, Chocolate (Little Debbie)	1 pkg (2.5 oz)	320	15
Holiday Cakes, Vanilla (Little Debbie)	1 pkg (2.5 oz)	320	16
Honeybuns, Glazed (Tastykake)	1	330	13
Honeybuns, Iced (Tastykake)	1	342	12
Ice Cream Cups (Little Debbie)	1 pkg (.15 oz)	15	tr
Jelly Rolls (Little Debbie)	1 pkg (2.2 oz)	250	9
Juniors, Chocolate (Tastykake)	1	364	8
Juniors, Coconut (Tastykake)	1	317	4
Juniors, Koffee Kake (Tastykake)	1	317	12
Kandy Kakes, Chocolate (Tastykake)	1	99	4
Kandy Kakes, Peanut Butter (Tastykake)	1	103	5
Koffe Kakes, Cream Filled (Tastykake)	1	143	6
Krimpets, Butterscotch (Tastykake)	1	118	2
Krimpets, Cream Filled Chocolate (Tastykake)	1	142	4

FOOD	PORTION	CALORIES	FAT
Krimpets, Cream Filled Vanilla (Tastykake)	1	139	4
Krimpets, Jelly (Tastykake)	1	96	tr
Lemon Stix (Little Debbie)	1 pkg (1.5 oz)	220	10
Marshmallow Supremes (Little Debbie)	1 pkg (1.1 oz)	130	5
Mint Sprints (Little Debbie)	1 pkg (1.33 oz)	200	10
Nutty Bar (Little Debbie)	1 pkg (2 oz)	310	20
Nutty Bar (Little Debbie)	1 pkg (2.5 oz)	390	23
Nutty Wafers (Little Debbie)	1 pkg (2 oz)	310	19
PB Krunch (Tastykake)	1	292	13
Peanut Butter Bars (Little Debbie)	1 pkg (1.83 oz)	260	13
Peanut Butter Bars (Little Debbie)	1 pkg (2.5 oz)	370	18
Peanut Clusters (Little Debbie)	1 pkg (1.5 oz)	220	11
Pecan Twins (Little Debbie)	1 pkg (2 oz)	220	10
Pumpkin Delights (Little Debbie)	1 pkg (1.1 oz)	140	6
Snack Cakes, Chocolate (Little Debbie)	1 pkg (2.5 oz)	320	14
Snack Cakes, Chocolate (Little Debbie)	1 pkg (3 oz)	390	19
Snack Cakes, Vanilla (Little Debbie)	1 pkg (2.6 oz)	330	16
Snack Cakes, Vanilla (Little Debbie)	1 pkg (3 oz)	390	19

FOOD	PORTION	CALORIES	FAT
Snoball (Hostess)	1 (1.5 oz)	136	4
Spice Cakes (Little Debbie)	1 pkg (2.2 oz)	270	11
Star Crunch (Little Debbie)	1 pkg (1.08 oz)	150	6
Strawberry Frosted Toastettes (Nabisco)	1	200	5
Strawberry Toastettes (Nabisco)	1	200	5
Swiss Cake Roll (Little Debbie)	1 pkg (2.17 oz)	270	12
Swiss Rolls (Little Debbie)	1 pkg (2.25 oz)	280	12
Swiss Rolls (Tastykake)	1	130	6
Tasty Twists (Tastykake)	1 pkg	211	8
Tempty (Tastykake)	1	94	2
Twinkie (Hostess)	1 (1.5 oz)	144	4
Vanilla Cups (Tastykake)	1	116	3
Yodel's (Drake's)	1 (.9 oz)	115	5
toaster pastries	1 (1.9 oz)	210	6

CANADIAN BACON

Oscar Mayer	1 slice (28 g)	35	1
canadian bacon; unheated	2 slices (1.9 oz)	89	4

CANDY

3 Musketeers Bar	2.1	260	8
Baby Ruth (Nabisco)	1 oz	130	6

FOOD	PORTION	CALORIES	FAT
Baby Ruth (Pearson's)	½ bar	130	6
Bar None Candy Bar (Hershey)	1.5 oz	240	14
Barat Bar	1 (2 oz)	340	24
Beech-Nut Cough Drops	1	10	0
Bonkers! All Flavors	1	20	0
Breath Savers Sugar Free All Flavors	1	8	0
Bridge Mix (Nabisco)	1 oz	126	5
Butter Mints (Kraft)	1	8	0
Butterfinger (Pearson's)	½ bar	130	6
Caramels (Kraft)	1	35	1
Charleston Chew!, Chocolate (Pearson's)	½ bar	120	3
Charleston Chew!, Strawberry (Pearson's)	½ bar	120	3
Charleston Chew!, Vanilla (Pearson's)	½ bar	120	3
Chocolate Bar (Estee)	2 squares	60	4–6
Chocolate Coated Raisins (Estee)	6 pieces	30	2
Chocolate Covered Cherries (Cella's)	1 oz	126	4
Chocolate Covered Peanuts (Life Saver)	14 pieces	160	9
Chocolate Covered Raisins (Life Saver)	29 pieces	130	5
Chocolate Fudgies (Kraft)	1	35	1

FOOD	PORTION	CALORIES	FAT
Chocolate Parfait (Pearson's)	4 pieces	120	3
Chocolaty Peanut Bar (Lance)	2 oz	320	18
Coffioca Parfait (Pearson's)	4 pieces	120	3
Crunch Chocolate Bar (Estee)	2 squares	45	3
Crunch 'N Munch Candied (Franklin)	1.25 oz	170	7
Crunch 'N Munch Caramel (Franklin)	1.25 oz	160	5
Crunch 'N Munch Maple Walnut (Franklin)	1.25 oz	160	6
Crunch 'N Munch Toffee (Franklin's)	1.25 oz	160	5
Estee-ets (Estee)	5 pieces	35	2
Fruit & Nut Bar (Cadbury)	1 oz	150	8
Fruit and Nut Mix (Estee)	4 pieces	35	2
Gum Drops (Estee)	4 pieces	25	0
Gummy Bears (Estee)	4 pieces	20	0
Hard Candy (Estee)	2	25	0
Hard Candy Sugar Free (Louis Sherry)	2 pieces	25	0
Hershey's Kisses	9 pieces	220	13
Holidays, Plain, red & green or pastels	1 oz	140	6
Honey Roasted Peanut Bar (Planters)	1.6 oz	230	13
Junior Mints	12 pieces	120	3

FOOD	PORTION	CALORIES	FAT
Kit Kat Wafer (Hershey)	1.65 oz	250	13
Krackel Chocolate Bar (Hershey)	1.65 oz	250	14
Life Saver	1 piece	8	tr
Life Saver Lollipops All Flavors	1	45	0
Life Saver Sugar Free	1	8	0
Lollipops (Estee)	2	12	0
Lollipops Sugar Free (Louis Sherry)	1	18	0
M&M's, Peanut	1.7 oz	250	13
M&M's, Plain	1.7 oz	240	10
Mars Bar	1.8 oz	240	12
Milk Chocolate Bar (Hershey)	1.65 oz	250	14
Milk Chocolate Bar With Almonds (Hershey)	1.55 oz	250	15
Milk Chocolate Stars (Life Saver)	13 pieces	160	8
Milky Way Bar	2.2 oz	290	11
Mint Parfait (Pearson's)	4 pieces	120	3
Mints (Estee)	1	4	1
Mr. GoodBar Chocolate Bar (Hershey)	1.85 oz	300	20
Munch Bar	1.4 oz	220	14
NECCO Mint Lozenges	1 piece	12	tr
Nip, Carmel (Pearson's)	4 pieces	120	3
Nip, Coffee (Pearson's)	4 pieces	120	3

FOOD	PORTION	CALORIES	FAT
Nip, Licorice (Pearson's)	4 pieces	120	3
Old Fashioned Peanut Candy (Planters)	1 oz	140	9
Party Mints (Kraft)	1	8	0
Peanut Bar (Lance)	1.75	260	14
Peanut Bar (Planters)	1.6 oz	230	11
Peanut Brittle (Estee)	¼ oz	35	1
Peanut Brittle (Kraft)	1 oz	140	5
Peanut Butter Cups (Estee)	1	45	3
Peanut Butter Parfait (Pearson's)	4 pieces	120	3
Peppermint Pattie, Chocolate Covered (Nabisco)	1 (½ oz)	64	1
Reese's Peanut Butter Cups (Hershey)	2 cups	280	7
Reese's Pieces Candy (Hershey)	1.95 oz	270	11
Rolo Carmels in Milk Chocolate (Hershey)	9 pieces	270	12
Skittles	2 oz	320	5
Skor Toffee Bar (Hershey)	1.4 oz	220	14
Snickers Bar	2.2 oz	290	14
Special Dark Sweet Chocolate Bar (Hershey)	1.45	220	12
Starburst Fruit Chews	2 oz	240	5

FOOD	PORTION	CALORIES	FAT
Starburst Fruit Chews, Strawberry	2.07 oz	240	5
Sugar Babies Tidbits	1 pkg	180	2
Sugar Daddy	1 pop	150	1
Sweet 'n Crunchy Peanut Bar (Planters)	1.6 oz	250	15
Thin Mint (Nabisco)	1 (10 g)	42	1
Toffee (Kraft)	1	30	1
Tootsie Roll Miniature	1 (6 g)	24	tr
Twix Cookie Bar, Caramel	2 oz (2 bars)	140	7
Twix Cookie Bar, Peanut Butter	1.8 oz (2 bars)	130	7
Velamints	1 mint	9	0
Velamints, Cocoamint	1 mint	8	0
Whatchamacallit Candy Bar (Hershey)	1.8 oz	270	15
Y&S Bites Cherry Candy (Hershey)	1 oz	100	tr
Y&S Twizzlers Strawberry Candy (Hershey)	1 oz	100	tr
candy corn	¼ cup	182	1
chocolate covered raisins	1 oz	121	5
gum drop	1	7	tr
hard candy ball	1	19	tr
jelly beans	¼ cup	202	tr
licorice	1 stick (10 g)	35	tr
lollipop	1 (1 oz)	110	tr
malted milk balls, chocolate coated	1	25	2
mint fondant pattie	1 (9 g)	32	tr
peanut brittle	1 oz	120	3

FOOD	PORTION	CALORIES	FAT
CANTALOUPE			
Chiquita	1 cup	70	0
cantaloupe	½	94	1
cubed	1 cup	57	tr
CARAMBOLA			
carambola	1	42	tr
CARDOON			
cooked	3.5 oz	22	tr
raw; shredded	1 cup	36	tr
CAROB			
carob flavor mix; as prep w/ whole milk	8 oz	195	8
carob mix	3 tsp	45	0
flour	1 cup	185	1
flour	1 Tbsp	14	tr
CARP			
cooked	3 oz	138	6
cooked	1 fillet (6 oz)	276	12
raw	1 fillet (7.6 oz)	276	12
raw	3 oz	108	5
roe, raw	3.5 oz	130	2
CARROT			
CANNED Diced (Libby)	½ cup	20	0
Diced (Seneca)	½ cup	20	0

FOOD	PORTION	CALORIES	FAT
Diced Fancy (S&W)	½ cup	30	0
Julienne French Style Fancy (S&W)	½ cup	30	0
Sliced (Libby)	½ cup	20	0
Sliced (Seneca)	½ cup	20	0
Whole Tiny Fancy (S&W)	½ cup	30	0
carrots	½ cup	17	tr
FRESH cooked	½ cup	35	tr
raw	1	31	tr
FROZEN Crinkle Sliced (Hanover)	½ cup	35	0
Whole Baby (Birds Eye)	½ cup	40	tr
cooked	½ cup	26	tr
frzn sliced; not prep	½ cup	25	tr
JUICE carrot juice	6 fl oz	73	tr

CASABA

cubed	1 cup	45	tr

CASHEWS

Cashews (Beer Nuts)	1 oz	170	13
Cashews (Lance)	1⅛ oz	190	15
Cashews-Long Tube (Lance)	1.25 oz	200	16

FOOD	PORTION	CALORIES	FAT
Dry Roasted (Planters)	1 oz	160	13
Dry Roasted, Unsalted (Planters)	1 oz	160	13
Fancy, Oil Roasted (Planters)	1 oz	170	14
Halves, Oil Roasted, Unsalted (Planters)	1 oz	170	14
Halves, Oil Roasted (Planters)	1 oz	170	14
Honey Roasted (Planters)	1 oz	170	12
Honey Toasted (Lance)	1⅛ oz	200	14
Honey Toasted Tube (Lance)	1¹⁄₁₆ oz	200	13
Whole Salted (Guy's)	1 oz	170	14
cashew butter	1 oz	167	14
cashew butter	1 Tbsp	94	8
dry roasted	1 oz	163	13
oil roasted	1 oz	163	14

CASSAVA

raw	3.5 oz	120	tr

CATFISH

FRESH			
channel, raw	1 fillet (2.8 oz)	92	3
channel, raw	3 oz	99	4
FROZEN Catfish Fillets (Mrs. Paul's)	1 fillet	220	10

FOOD	PORTION	CALORIES	FAT
Catfish Strips (Mrs. Paul's)	4 oz	240	13
HOME RECIPE channel; breaded & fried	3 oz	194	11
channel; breaded & fried	1 fillet (3.1 oz)	199	12

CATSUP

Estee	1 Tbsp	6	0
Health Valley	1 Tbsp	16	tr
Health Valley, No Salt Added	1 Tbsp	16	tr
Smucker's	1 tsp	8	0
Tillie Lewis, Low Sodium, Low Calorie	1 Tbsp	8	tr

CAULIFLOWER

FRESH cooked	½ cup	15	tr
raw	½ cup	12	tr
FROZEN Cauliflower (Birds Eye)	⅔ cup	23	tr
Cauliflower (Hanover)	½ cup	20	0
Cauliflower Vegetable Crisp (Ore Ida)	3 oz	150	9
Cauliflower In Cheddar Cheese Sauce (Budget Gourmet)	5 oz	110	5
Cauliflower w/ Cheese Sauce (Pepperidge Farm)	1	210	13
Cauliflower w/ Cheese Sauce (Birds Eye)	½ cup	113	6
Florets (Hanover)	½ cup	20	0

FOOD	PORTION	CALORIES	FAT
frzn; cooked	½ cup	17	tr
frzn; not prep	½ cup	16	tr

CAVIAR

red granular	1 Tbsp	40	3
red granular	1 oz	71	5
sturgeon, granular	1 Tbsp	42	2

CELERIC

cooked	3.5 oz	25	tr
raw	½ cup	31	tr

CELERY

diced; cooked	½ cup	11	tr
raw	1 stalk	6	tr

CELTUCE

raw	3.5 oz	22	tr

CEREAL
(*see also* GRANOLA)

Cup measurements represent approximately a 1 oz serving

COOKED			
Barley Plus (Erewhon)	1 oz	110	1
Brown Rice Cream (Erewhon)	1 oz	110	1
Cream of Rice (Nabisco)	1 oz	100	0
Cream of Wheat, Instant (Nabisco)	¾ cup	110	tr
Cream of Wheat, Instant (Nabisco)	1 oz	100	0

FOOD	PORTION	CALORIES	FAT
Cream of Wheat Mix 'n Eat, Apple & Cinnamon (Nabisco)	1.25 oz	130	0
Cream of Wheat Mix 'n Eat, Brown Sugar Cinnamon (Nabisco)	1.25 oz	130	0
Cream of Wheat Mix 'n Eat, Maple Brown Sugar (Nabisco)	1 pkg (1.25 oz)	130	0
Cream of Wheat Mix 'n Eat, Our Original (Nabisco)	1 pkg (1.25 oz)	100	0
Cream of Wheat Mix 'n Eat, Peach (Nabisco)	1 pkg (1.25 oz)	140	2
Cream of Wheat Mix 'n Eat, Strawberry (Nabisco)	1 pkg (1.25 oz)	140	2
Cream of Wheat Quick (Nabisco)	¾ cup	110	tr
Cream of Wheat Quick, Apples, Raisin and Spice (Nabisco)	1 oz	110	1
Cream of Wheat Quick, Maple Brown Sugar (Nabisco)	1 oz	110	1
Cream of Wheat Quick, Regular (Nabisco)	1 oz	100	0
Cream of Wheat Regular (Nabisco)	¾ cup	114	tr
Farina; as prep (Pillsbury)	⅔ cup	80	tr
Farina Hot 'n Creamy; not prep (Quaker)	1 oz	101	tr
Hominy Quick Grits; uncooked (Albers)	¼ cup	150	0
Maltex (Standard Milling)	½ cup	86	tr

FOOD	PORTION	CALORIES	FAT
Maypo, 30 Second (Standard Milling)	½ cup	110	1
Maypo, Vermont Style (Standard Milling)	½ cup	90	tr
Oat Bran; not prep (Quaker)	⅓ cup	90	2
Oat Bran Hot Cereal (Health Valley)	1 oz	100	1
Oat Bran With Toasted Wheat Germ (Erewhon)	1 oz	115	2
Oatmeal, Instant; not prep (Quaker)	1 pkg (½ oz)	105	2
Oatmeal, Instant; not prep (Ralston)	1 pkg (1 oz)	110	2
Oatmeal, Instant Apple Cinnamon (Erewhon)	1 oz	145	3
Oatmeal, Instant Apple Raisin (Erewhon)	1 oz	150	3
Oatmeal, Instant Maple Spice (Erewhon)	1 oz	140	3
Oatmeal, Instant w/ Apples & Cinnamon; not prep (Quaker)	1 pkg (1.25 oz)	133	2
Oatmeal, Instant w/Cinnamon & Spices; not prep (Quaker)	1 pkg (1⅝ oz)	176	2
Oatmeal, Instant w/Cinnamon Spice; not prep (Ralston)	1 pkg (1⅝ oz)	176	2
Oatmeal, Instant w/ Maple & Brown Sugar; not prep (Quaker)	1 pkg (1.5 oz)	161	2
Oatmeal, Instant w/ Maple & Brown Sugar; not prep (Ralston)	1 pkg (1⅝ oz)	175	1
Oatmeal, Quick or Old Fashoned; not prep (Quaker)	1 cup	307	5

FOOD	PORTION	CALORIES	FAT
Oatmeal, Quick or Regular; not prep (Quaker)	1 cup	442	7
Oats, Old Fashioned; not prep (Roman Meal)	⅓ cup (1 oz)	100	4
Oats, Quick; not prep (Roman Meal)	⅓ cup (1 oz)	100	2
Oats, Quick & Regular (Ralston)	⅔ cup	110	1
Oats, Wheat, Dates, Raisins, Almonds Cereal; not prep (Roman Meal)	⅓ cup (1.3 oz)	140	3
Oats, Wheat, Honey, Coconut, Almonds Cereal; not prep (Roman Meal)	⅓ cup (1.3 oz)	150	6
Oats, Wheat, Rye, Flax Cereal; not prep (Roman Meal)	⅓ cup (1 oz)	90	1
Original Cereal w/ Wheat, Rye, Bran, Flax; not prep (Roman Meal)	⅓ cup (1 oz)	80	tr
Pettijohns (Quaker)	½ cup	93	tr
Ralston, Instant & Regular (Ralston)	¾ cup	110	1
Total Oatmeal, Apple Cinnamon Almond Instant (General Mills)	1.5 oz pkg	150	4
Total Oatmeal, Apple Cinnamon Instant (General Mills)	1.25 oz pkg	130	2
Total Oatmeal, Mixed Nut Instant (General Mills)	1.3 oz pkg	140	4
Total Oatmeal, Quick (General Mills)	1 oz pkg	90	2
Total Oatmeal, Regular Flavor Instant (General Mills)	1 oz pkg	90	2
Wheat Hearts; as prep (General Mills)	¾ cup	110	1

FOOD	PORTION	CALORIES	FAT
Wheatena (Standard Milling)	½ cup	79	tr
barley, pearled light; not prep	2 tsp (1 oz)	99	tr
bulgur	¼ cup	63	tr
corn grits	½ cup	54	tr
corn grits, instant; as prep	1 pkg (.8 oz)	82	tr
corn grits, instant; not prep	1 pkg (.8 oz)	82	tr
corn grits, regular & quick; cooked	1 cup	146	tr
corn grits, regular & quick; not prep	1 Tbsp	36	tr
corn grits, regular & quick; not prep	1 cup	579	2
cornmeal, white or yellow	½ cup	60	tr
READY-TO-EAT 100% Bran (Nabisco)	1 oz	110	2
7-Grain Crunchy (Loma Linda)	½ cup	110	1
7-Grain No Sugar Added (Loma Linda)	1 cup	110	1
All-Bran (Kellogg's)	⅓ cup	70	1
All-Bran Fruit & Almonds (Kellogg's)	⅔ cup	100	2
All-Bran with Extra Fiber (Kellogg's)	½ cup	60	I
Alpha-Bits (Post)	1 cup	112	tr
Apple Cinnamon Squares (Kellogg's)	½ cup	90	0
Apple Jacks (Kellogg's)	1 cup	110	0
Apple Raisin Crisp (Kellogg's)	⅔ cup	130	0
Aztec Corn and Amaranth (Erewhon)	1 oz	100	0

FOOD	PORTION	CALORIES	FAT
BooBerry (General Mills)	1 cup	110	1
Bran (Loma Linda)	⅓ cup	90	tr
Bran Buds (Kellogg's)	⅓ cup	70	1
Bran Cereal w/ Raisins (Health Valley)	1 oz	70	1
Bran Flakes (Kellogg's)	⅔ cup	90	0
Brown Sugar & Honey Body Buddies (General Mills)	1 cup	110	tr
Cap'n Crunch (Quaker)	¾ cup	120	3
Cap'n Crunch's Crunchberries (Quaker)	¾ cup	127	2
Cheerios (General Mills)	1.25 cup	110	2
Chex (Ralston)	⅔ cup	90	tr
Cinnamon Toast Crunch (General Mills)	1 cup	120	3
Circus Fun (General Mills)	1 cup	110	1
Clusters (General Mills)	½ cup	100	3
Cocoa Krispies (Kellogg's)	¾ cup	110	0
Cocoa Pebbles (Post)	⅞ cup	112	1
Cocoa Puffs (General Mills)	1 cup	110	1
Corn Flakes (Kellogg's)	1 cup	100	0
Corn Flakes Blue (Health Valley)	1 oz	90	1

FOOD	PORTION	CALORIES	FAT
Corn Pops (Kellogg's)	1 cup	110	0
Country Corn Flakes (General Mills)	1 cup	110	tr
Cracklin' Oat Bran (Kellogg's)	½ cup	110	4
Crispix (Kellogg's)	1 cup	110	0
Crispy Brown Rice Cereal (Erewhon)	1 oz	110	1
Crispy Brown Rice Cereal, Low Sodium (Erewhon)	1 oz	110	1
Crispy Critters (Post)	1 cup	112	tr
Crispy Wheats 'n Raisins (General Mills)	¾ cup	110	1
Fiber 7 Flakes (Health Valley)	1 oz	100	1
Fortified Oat Flakes (Post)	⅔ cup	105	tr
Frankenberry (General Mills)	1 cup	110	1
Froot Loops (Kellogg's)	1 cup	110	1
Frosted Flakes (Kellogg's)	¾ cup	110	0
Frosted Krispies (Kellogg's)	¾ cup	110	0
Frosted Mini-Wheats (Kellogg's)	4 biscuits	100	0
Fruit & Fiber, Dates, Raisins & Walnuts (Post)	½ cup	89	tr
Fruit & Fiber, Harvest Medley (Post)	½ cup	88	tr

FOOD	PORTION	CALORIES	FAT
Fruit & Fiber, Mountain Trail (Post)	½ cup	87	1
Fruit & Fiber, Peach Raisin Almond (Post)	½ cup	85	tr
Fruit & Fiber, Tropical Fruit (Post)	½ cup	90	1
Fruit 'n Wheat (Erewhon)	1 oz	100	1
Fruit Wheats, Apple (Nabisco)	1 oz	100	0
Fruit Wheats, Raisin (Nabisco)	1 oz	100	0
Fruit Wheats, Strawberry (Nabisco)	1 oz	100	0
Fruitful Bran (Kellogg's)	⅔ cup	110	0
Fruity Marshmallow Krispies (Kellogg's)	1.25 cups	140	0
Fruity Pebbles (Post)	⅞ cup	112	1
Golden Grahams (General Mills)	¾ cup	110	1
Grape-Nuts (Post)	¼ cup	104	tr
Grape-Nuts Flakes (Post)	⅞ cup	104	tr
Healthy Crunch w/ Almonds & Dates (Health Valley)	1 oz	110	3
Healthy Crunch w/ Apples & Cinnamon (Health Valley)	1 oz	110	3
Heartland, Natural (Pet)	¼ cup	112	tr
Honey Buc Wheat Crisp (General Mills)	¾ cup	110	tr
Honey Nut Cheerios (General Mills)	1 cup	110	1

FOOD	PORTION	CALORIES	FAT
Honey Smacks (Kellogg's)	¾ cup	110	1
Honeycomb Post (Post)	1⅓ cups	110	tr
Ice Cream Cones Chocolate Chip (General Mills)	¾ cup	110	2
Ice Cream Cones, Vanilla (General Mills)	¾ cup	110	2
Just Right Nugget & Flake (Kellogg's)	⅔ cup	100	1
Just Right Fruit Nut & Flake (Kellogg's)	¾ cup	140	1
Kaboom (General Mills)	1 cup	110	1
Lucky Charms (General Mills)	1 cup	110	1
Muesli (Ralston)	½ cup	160	3
Muesli, Sweetened (Kentaur)	1.2 oz	120	3
Muesli, Unsweetened (Kentaur)	1.2 oz	120	4
Mueslix Bran (Kellogg's)	½ cup	130	2
Mueslix Five Grain (Kellogg's)	½ cup	150	2
Natural Bran Flakes (Post)	⅔ cup	87	tr
Natural Raisin Bran (Post)	½ cup	83	tr
Natural Sugar & Honey Body Buddies (General Mills)	1 cup	110	1
Nut & Honey Crunch (Kellogg's)	⅔ cup	110	1
Nutri-Grain Almond Raisin (Kellogg's)	⅔ cup	140	2

FOOD	PORTION	CALORIES	FAT
Nutri-Grain Corn (Kellogg's)	½ cup	100	1
Nutri-Grain Nuggets (Kellogg's)	¼ cup	90	0
Nutri-Grain Wheat (Kellogg's)	⅔ cup	100	0
Nutri-Grain Wheat & Raisin (Kellogg's)	⅔ cup	130	0
Nutrific (Kellogg's)	1 cup	120	2
Oat Bran Flakes (Health Valley)	1 oz	110	tr
Oat Bran Flakes w/ Almonds & Dates (Health Valley)	1 oz	100	tr
Oat Bran Flakes w/ Raisins (Health Valley)	1 oz	100	tr
Oat Bran O's (Health Valley)	1 oz	90	2
Oat Bran O's Fruit & Nuts (Health Valley)	1 oz	90	2
Pac-Man (General Mills)	1 cup	110	tr
Post Toasties (Post)	1.25 cup	108	tr
Pro Grain (Kellogg's)	¾ cup	100	0
Product 19 (Kellogg's)	1 cup	100	0
Puffed Corn (Health Valley)	½ oz	50	0
Puffed Rice (Health Valley)	½ oz	50	0
Puffed Rice (Quaker)	1 cup	40	tr
Puffed Wheat (Health Valley)	½ oz	50	0

FOOD	PORTION	CALORIES	FAT
Puffed Wheat (Quaker)	1 cup	35	tr
Quisp (Quaker)	1⅛ cup	121	2
Raisin Bran (Erewhon)	1 oz	100	0
Raisin Bran (Kellogg's)	¾ cup	120	1
Raisin Bran (Quaker)	½ cup	90	2
Raisin Bran (Skinner's)	1 oz	100	1
Raisin Bran Flakes (Health Valley)	1 oz	100	0
Raisin Bran, No Salt Added (Skinner's)	1 oz	100	1
Raisin Grape-Nuts (Post)	¼ cup	101	tr
Raisin Squares (Kellogg's)	½ cup	90	0
Rice Crispy (Ralston)	1 cup	110	tr
Rice Krispies (Kellogg's)	1 cup	110	0
Rice Toasties (Post)	¾ oz	81	tr
Ruskets Biscuits (Loma Linda)	2 biscuits	110	tr
Shredded Wheat (Nabisco)	1 biscuit	84	tr
Shredded Wheat (Sunshine)	1 biscuit	90	1
Shredded Wheat Bite Size (Sunshine)	⅔ cup	110	1
Shredded Wheat 'n Bran (Nabisco)	1 oz	110	1

FOOD	PORTION	CALORIES	FAT
Shredded Wheat Spoon Size (Nabisco)	1 oz	110	1
Special K (Kellogg's)	1 cup	110	0
Sporting (Kentaur)	1.47 oz	140	1
Sprouts 7 w/ Raisins (Health Valley)	1 oz	90	1
Stoned Wheat Flakes (Health Valley)	1 oz	100	0
Strawberry Squares (Kellogg's)	½ cup	90	0
Sugar Frosted Flakes (Ralston)	¾ cup	110	tr
Sugar Sparkled Flakes (Post)	¾ cup	108	tr
Super Golden Crisp (Post)	⅞ cup	104	tr
Swiss Breakfast Raisin Nut (Health Valley)	1 oz	100	3
Swiss Breakfast Tropical Fruit (Health Valley)	1 oz	100	3
Team (Nabisco)	1 oz	110	1
Toasted Wheat and Raisins (Nabisco)	1.4 oz	140	2
Total (General Mills)	1 cup	110	1
Total Corn Flakes (General Mills)	1 cup	110	1
Trix (General Mills)	1 cup	110	1
Uncle Sam Cereal (US Mills)	1 oz	110	1
Wheat Bran Millers Flakes (Health Valley)	1 oz	70	2

FOOD	PORTION	CALORIES	FAT
Wheat Flakes (Erewhon)	1 oz	100	0
Wheaties (General Mills)	1 cup	110	1
WITH 1% MILK			
Cheerios (General Mills)	1 cup + ½ cup milk	160	3
Crispy Wheats 'n Raisins (General Mills)	¾ cup + ½ cup milk	160	3
Honey Buc Wheat Crisp (General Mills)	¾ cup + ½ cup milk	160	2
Honey Nut Cheerios (General Mills)	1 cup + ½ cup milk	160	3
Total (General Mills)	1 cup + ½ cup milk	160	3
Total Corn Flakes (General Mills)	1 cup + ½ cup milk	160	3
Trix (General Mills)	1½ cup + ½ cup milk	160	2
Wheaties (General Mills)	1 cup + ½ cup milk	160	3
WITH 2% MILK			
Alpha-Bits (Post)	1 cup + ½ cup milk	172	3
BooBerry (General Mills)	1 cup + ½ cup milk	170	4
Cinnamon Toast Crunch (General Mills)	1 cup + ½ cup milk	180	6
Cocoa Puffs (General Mills)	1 cup + ½ cup milk	170	4
Frankenberry (General Mills)	1 cup + ½ cup milk	170	4
Fruity Pebbles (Post)	⅞ cup + ½ cup milk	173	3
Honeycomb (Post)	1⅓ cups + ½ cup milk	171	3

FOOD	PORTION	CALORIES	FAT
Oats, Old Fashioned; as prep (Roman Meal)	⅓ cup + ½ cup milk	160	4
Oats, Quick; as prep (Roman Meal)	⅓ cup + ½ cup milk	160	4
Oats, Wheat, Dates, Raisins, Almonds Cereal; as prep (Roman Meal)	⅓ cup + ½ cup milk	170	4
Oats, Wheat, Honey, Coconut, Almonds Cereal; as prep (Roman Meal)	⅓ cup + ½ cup milk	190	7
Oats, Wheat, Rye, Flax Cereal; as prep (Roman Meal)	⅓ cup + ½ cup milk	120	3
Original Cereal w/ Wheat, Rye, Flax; a prep (Roman Meal)	⅓ cup + ½ cup milk	120	2
Pac-Man (General Mills)	1 cup + ½ cup milk	170	3
Shredded Wheat (Sunshine)	1 + ½ cup milk	150	4
Shredded Wheat Bite Size (Sunshine)	⅔ cup + ½ cup milk	170	4
Total Oatmeal, Apple Cinnamon Almond Instant (General Mills)	1.5 oz pkg + ½ cup milk	210	7
Total Oatmeal, Apple Cinnamon Instant (General Mills)	1.25 oz pkg + ½ cup milk	190	5
Total Oatmeal, Quick (General Mills)	1 oz pkg + ½ cup milk	150	5
Total Oatmeal, Regular Flavor Instant (General Mills)	1 oz pkg + ½ cup milk	150	5
WITH SKIM MILK 100% Bran (Nabisco)	1 oz + ½ cup milk	110	2

FOOD	PORTION	CALORIES	FAT
BooBerry (General Mills)	1 cup + ½ cup milk	150	1
Brown Sugar & Honey Body Buddies (General Mills)	1 cup + ½ cup milk	150	1
Cheerios (General Mills)	1 cup + ½ cup milk	150	2
Circus Fun (General Mills)	1 cup + ½ cup milk	150	1
Clusters (General Mills)	½ cup + ½ cup milk	140	3
Cocoa Puffs (General Mills)	1 cup + ½ cup milk	150	1
Count Chocula (General Mills)	1 cup + ½ cup milk	150	1
Country Corn Flakes (General Mills)	1 cup + ½ cup milk	150	1
Crispy Wheats 'n Raisins (General Mills)	¾ cup + ½ cup milk	150	1
Frankenberry (General Mills)	1 cup + ½ cup milk	150	1
Fruit & Fiber, Harvest Medley (Post)	½ cup + ½ cup milk	131	1
Fruit & Fiber, Peach Raisin Almond (Post)	½ cup + ½ cup milk	129	1
Fruit Wheats, Apple (Nabisco)	1 oz + ½ cup milk	140	tr
Fruit Wheats, Raisins (Nabisco)	1 oz + ½ cup milk	140	tr
Fruit Wheats, Strawberry (Nabisco)	1 oz + ½ cup milk	140	tr
Golden Grahams (General Mills)	¾ cup + ½ cup milk	150	1
Grape-Nuts (Post)	¼ cup + ½ cup milk	148	tr
Honey Buc Wheat Crisp (General Mills)	¾ cup + ½ cup milk	150	1

FOOD	PORTION	CALORIES	FAT
Honey Nut Cheerios (General Mills)	1 cup + ½ cup milk	150	1
Ice Cream Cones, Chocolate Chip (General Mills)	¾ cup + ½ cup milk	150	2
Ice Cream Cones, Vanilla (General Mills)	¾ cup + ½ cup milk	150	2
Kaboom (General Mills)	1 cup + ½ cup milk	150	1
Lucky Charms (General Mills)	1 cup + ½ cup milk	150	1
Muesli (Ralston)	½ cup + ½ cup milk	200	3
Natural Raisin Bran (Post)	½ cup + ½ cup milk	127	tr
Natural Sugar & Honey Body Buddies (General Mills)	1 cup + ½ cup milk	150	1
Oat Bran; as prep (Quaker)	⅓ cup + ½ cup milk	140	3
Oatmeal Raisin Crisp (General Mills)	½ cup + ½ cup milk	150	2
Pac-Man (General Mills)	1 cup + ½ cup milk	150	1
Raisin Grape Nuts (Post)	¼ cup + ½ cup milk	144	tr
Shredded Wheat 'n Bran (Nabisco)	1 oz + ½ cup milk	150	1
Shredded Wheat (Nabisco)	1 oz + ½ cup milk	130	1
Shredded Wheat (Sunshine)	1 + ½ cup milk	135	1
Shredded Wheat, Bite Size (Sunshine)	⅔ cup + ½ cup milk	200	1
Shredded Wheat, Spoon Size (Nabisco)	1 oz + ½ cup milk	150	1
Team (Nabisco)	1 oz + ½ cup milk	150	1

FOOD	PORTION	CALORIES	FAT
Toasted Wheat and Raisins (Nabisco)	1 oz + ½ cup milk	180	1
Total (General Mills)	1 cup + ½ cup milk	150	1
Total Corn Flakes (General Mills)	1 cup + ½ cup milk	150	1
Total Oatmeal, Apple, Cinnamon, Almond Instant (General Mills)	1.5 oz pkg + ½ cup milk	190	4
Total Oatmeal, Apple, Cinnamon Instant (General Mills)	1.25 oz pkg + ½ cup milk	170	2
Total Oatmeal, Mixed Nut Instant (General Mills)	1.3 oz pkg + ½ cup milk	180	4
Total Oatmeal, Quick (General Mills)	1 oz pkg + ½ cup milk	130	2
Total Oatmeal, Regular Flavor Instant (General Mills)	1 oz pkg + ½ cup milk	130	2
Trix (General Mills)	1 cup + ½ cup milk	150	1
Wheaties (General Mills)	1 cup + ½ cup milk	150	1
WITH WHOLE MILK			
Brown Sugar & Honey Body Buddies (General Mills)	1 cup + ½ cup milk	185	4
Circus Fun (General Mills)	1 cup + ½ cup milk	185	5
Clusters (General Mills)	½ cup + ½ cup milk	175	7
Country Corn Flakes (General Mills)	1 cup + ½ cup milk	185	4
Cream of Rice (Nabisco)	1 oz + ¼ cup milk	140	2
Cream of Wheat, Instant (Nabisco)	1 oz + ¼ cup milk	140	2

FOOD	PORTION	CALORIES	FAT
Cream of Wheat Mix 'n Eat, Apple & Cinnamon (Nabisco)	1¼ oz + ¼ cup milk	170	2
Cream of Wheat Mix 'n Eat, Brown Sugar Cinnamon (Nabisco)	1¼ oz + ¼ cup milk	170	2
Cream of Wheat Mix 'n Eat, Maple Brown Sugar (Nabisco)	1¼ oz + ¼ cup milk	170	2
Cream of Wheat Mix 'n Eat, Our Original (Nabisco)	1¼ oz + ¼ cup milk	140	2
Cream of Wheat Mix 'n Eat, Peach (Nabisco)	1¼ oz + ¼ cup milk	180	4
Cream of Wheat Mix 'n Eat, Strawberry (Nabisco)	1¼ oz + ¼ cup milk	180	4
Cream of Wheat Quick, Maple Brown Sugar (Nabisco)	1 oz + ¼ cup milk	150	3
Cream of Wheat Quick, Raisin, Apples & Spice (Nabisco)	1 oz + ¼ cup milk	150	3
Cream of Wheat Quick, Regular (Nabisco)	1 oz + ¼ cup milk	140	2
Cream of Wheat, Regular (Nabisco)	1 oz + ¼ cup milk	140	2
Fortified Oat Flakes (Post)	⅔ cup + ½ cup milk	181	5
Fruit Wheats, Apple (Nabisco)	1 oz + ½ cup milk	180	4
Fruit Wheats, Raisin (Nabisco)	1 oz + ½ cup milk	180	4
Fruit Wheats, Strawberry (Nabisco)	1 oz + ½ cup milk	180	4
Golden Grahams (General Mills)	¾ cup + ½ cup milk	185	5

FOOD	PORTION	CALORIES	FAT
Ice Cream Cones, Chocolate Chip (General Mills)	¾ cup + ½ cup milk	185	6
Ice Cream Cones, Vanilla (General Mills)	¾ cup + ½ cup milk	185	6
Kaboom (General Mills)	1 cup + ½ cup milk	185	5
Lucky Charms (General Mills)	1 cup + ½ cup milk	185	5
Oatmeal Raisin Crisp (General Mills)	½ cup + ½ cup milk	185	6
Shredded Wheat (Sunshine)	1 biscuit + ½ cup milk	165	5
Sugar Sparkled Flakes (Post)	¾ cup + ½ cup milk	184	4
Total Oatmeal, Mixed Nut Instant (General Mills)	1.3 oz pkg + ½ cup milk	215	8
Trix (General Mills)	1 cup + ½ cup milk	185	5

CHAYOTE

cooked, cut up	1 cup	38	1
raw, cut up	1 cup	32	tr

CHEESE
(*see also* CHEESE DISHES, CHEESE SUBSTITUTE, COTTAGE CHEESE, CREAM CHEESE)

NATURAL

Babybel (Fromageries Bel)	8 oz	726	57
Babybel (Fromageries Bel)	1 oz	91	7
Babybel, Mini (Fromageries Bel)	¾ oz	74	6
Blue (Kraft)	1 oz	100	9

FOOD	PORTION	CALORIES	FAT
Blue (Sargento)	1 oz	100	8
Blue Spread (Roka Brand)	1 oz	70	6
Bonbel (Fromageries Bel)	1 oz	100	8
Bonbel (Fromageries Bel)	8 oz	790	65
Bonbel, Mini (Fromageries Bel)	¾ oz	74	6
Bonbino (Fromageries Bel)	8 oz	822	68
Bonbino (Fromageries Bell)	1 oz	103	9
Brick (Kraft)	1 oz	110	9
Brick (Land O'Lakes)	1 oz	110	8
Brick (Sargento)	1 oz	105	8
Brie (Sargento)	1 oz	95	8
Burger Cheese (Sargento)	1 oz	106	9
Cajun (Sargento)	1 oz	110	9
Camembert (Sargento)	1 oz	85	7
Caraway (Kraft)	1 oz	100	8
Cheddar (Alpine Lace)	1 oz	97	8
Cheddar (Armour)	1 oz	110	9
Cheddar (Fromageries Bel)	1 oz	110	9

FOOD	PORTION	CALORIES	FAT
Cheddar (Fromageries Bel)	8 oz	883	73
Cheddar (Kraft)	1 oz	110	9
Cheddar (Sargento)	1 oz	114	9
Cheddar, Lower Salt (Armour)	1 oz	110	9
Cheddar, New York (Sargento)	1 oz	114	9
Cheddar, Port Wine w/ Almonds Cheese Log (Cracker Barrel)	1 oz	90	6
Cheddar, Sharp Nut Log (Sargento)	1 oz	97	7
Cheddar, Sharp w/ Almonds Cheese Ball (Cracker Barrel)	1 oz	90	6
Cheddar, Sharp w/ Almonds Cheese Log (Cracker Barrel)	1 oz	90	6
Cheddar, Shredded (Polly-O)	1 oz	110	9
Cheddar, Shredded (Weight Watchers)	1 oz	80	5
Cheddar, Smokey w/ Almonds Cheese Log (Cracker Barrel)	1 oz	90	6
Cheddar-Jack, Light Natural (Dorman's)	1 oz	90	7
Colby (Alpine Lace)	1 oz	85	5
Colby (Kraft)	1 oz	110	9
Colby (Land O'Lakes)	1 oz	110	9

FOOD	PORTION	CALORIES	FAT
Colby (Sargento)	1 oz	112	9
Colby, Lower Salt (Armour)	1 oz	110	9
Colby-Jack (Sargento)	1 oz	109	9
Edam (Fromageries Bel)	1 oz	97	8
Edam (Fromageries Bel)	1 oz	100	8
Edam (Holland Farm)	1 oz	97	8
Edam (Kraft)	1 oz	90	7
Edam (Land O'Lakes)	1 oz	110	8
Edam (May-Bud)	1 oz	100	8
Edam (Sargento)	1 oz	101	8
Farmer (Friendship)	4 oz	160	12
Farmer (Holland Farm)	1 oz	102	8
Farmer No Salt Added (Friendship)	4 oz	160	12
Farmers Cheese (May-Bud)	1 oz	90	7
Farmers Cheese (White Clover)	1 oz	90	7
Farmers Cheese (White Clover)	1 oz	81	5
Farmer's Cheese (Sargento)	1 oz	102	8
Feta (Sargento)	1 oz	75	6

FOOD	PORTION	CALORIES	FAT
Feta (White Clover)	1 oz	90	7
Finland Swiss (Sargento)	1 oz	107	8
Fior di Latte (Polly-O)	1 oz	80	6
Fontina (Sargento)	1 oz	110	9
Gjetost (Sargento)	1 oz	132	8
Gorgonzola (Sargento)	1 oz	100	8
Gouda (Fromageries Bel)	1 oz	110	9
Gouda (Fromageries Bel)	8 oz	880	73
Gouda (Holland Farm)	1 oz	103	8
Gouda (Kraft)	1 oz	110	9
Gouda (Land O'Lakes)	1 oz	110	8
Gouda (May-Bud)	1 oz	100	8
Gouda (Sargento)	1 oz	101	8
Gouda, Mini (Fromageries Bel)	¾ oz	80	6
Gouda, Mini Reduced Calorie (Fromageries Bel)	¾ oz	45	3
Grated (Polly-O)	1 oz	130	10
Gruyere (Sargento)	1 oz	117	9
Havarti (Casino)	1 oz	120	11

FOOD	PORTION	CALORIES	FAT
Havarti (Sargento)	1 oz	118	11
Hoop (Friendship)	4 oz	84	tr
Italian Style Grated Cheese (Sargento)	1 oz	108	8
Jack Slim Light Natural (Dorman's)	1 oz	90	7
Jarlsberg	1 oz	100	7
Jarlsberg (Sargento)	1 oz	100	7
Limburger (Sargento)	1 oz	93	8
Limburger Natural Little Gem Size (Mohawk Valley)	1 oz	90	8
Lorraine (Universal Food)	1 oz	100	8
Monterey Jack (Alpine Lace)	1 oz	80	4
Monterey Jack (Armour)	1 oz	110	9
Monterey Jack (Holland Farm)	1 oz	102	9
Monterey Jack (Kraft)	1 oz	110	9
Monterey Jack (Land O'Lakes)	1 oz	110	9
Monterey Jack (May-Bud)	1 oz	100	9
Monterey Jack (Sargento)	1 oz	106	9
Monterey Jack, Lower Salt (Armour)	1 oz	110	9
Monterey Jack w/ Jalapeno Peppers (Kraft)	1 oz	110	9

FOOD	PORTION	CALORIES	FAT
Monterey Jack w/ Peppers, Mild (Kraft)	1 oz	110	9
Mozzarella (Alpine Lace)	1 oz	72	4
Mozzarella (M.H. Greenbaum, Inc.)	3.5 oz	334	25
Mozzarella, Lite Sandwich Slices (Polly-O)	1 oz	70	4
Mozzarella, Low Moisture (Casino)	1 oz	90	7
Mozzarella, Low Moisture, Part-Skim (Sargento)	1 oz	79	5
Mozzarella, Low Moisture, Whole Milk (Sargento)	1 oz	90	7
Mozzarella, Low-Sodium Light (Dorman's)	1 oz	80	5
Mozzarella, Part Skim (Polly-O)	1 oz	80	5
Mozzarella, Part skim (Land O'Lakes)	1 oz	80	5
Mozzarella, Park Skim, Low Moisture (Kraft)	1 oz	80	5
Mozzarella, Part Skim, Shredded (Polly-O)	1 oz	80	6
Mozzarella, Part-Skim, Low Moisture String Cheesew/ Jalapeno Peppers (Kraft)	1 oz	80	5
Mozzarella, Smoked (Polly-O)	1 oz	85	7
Mozzarella, Whole Milk (Polly-O)	1 oz	90	6
Mozzarella, Whole Milk Sandwich Slices (Polly-O)	1 oz	90	6

FOOD	PORTION	CALORIES	FAT
Mozzarella, Whole Milk, Shredded (Polly-O)	1 oz	90	6
Mozzarella w/ Pizza Spices (Sargento)	1 oz	79	5
Muenster (Alpine Lace)	1 oz	104	8
Muenster (Holland Farm)	1 oz	102	9
Muenster (Kraft)	1 oz	110	9
Muenster (Land O'Lakes)	1 oz	100	9
Muenster, Red Rind (Sargento)	1 oz	104	9
Nacho (Sargento)	1 oz	106	9
Naturally Slender (Northfield)	1 oz	90	7
Parmesan & Romano, Grated (Sargento)	1 oz	111	7
Parmesan, Grated (Kraft)	1 oz	130	9
Parmesan, Grated (Polly-O)	1 oz	130	9
Parmesan, Natural (Kraft)	1 oz	110	7
Parmesan-Fresh (Sargento)	1 oz	111	7
Parmesan-Grated (Sargento)	1 oz	129	9
Port Wine Nut Log (Sargento)	1 oz	97	7
Provolone (Alpine Lace)	1 oz	85	7
Provolone (Kraft)	1 oz	100	7

FOOD	PORTION	CALORIES	FAT
Provolone (Land O'Lakes)	1 oz	100	8
Provolone (Sargento)	1 oz	100	8
Provolone, Low Sodium Light Natural (Dorman's)	1 oz	90	7
Queso Blanco (Sargento)	1 oz	104	9
Queso de Papa (Sargento)	1 oz	114	9
Ricotta Lite (Polly-O)	2 oz	80	4
Ricotta Lite (Sargento)	1 oz	25	tr
Ricotta, Part Skim (Polly-O)	2 oz	90	6
Ricotta, Part Skim (Sargento)	1 oz	32	2
Ricotta, Part Skim, No Salt (Polly-O)	2 oz	90	6
Ricotta, Whole Milk (Polly-O)	2 oz	100	7
Ricotta, Whole Milk (Sargento)	1 oz	53	4
Ricotta, Whole Milk & Whey (Sargento)	1 oz	40	3
Ricotta, Whole Milk, No Salt (Polly-O)	2 oz	100	7
Romano (Sargento)	1 oz	110	8
Romano, Grated (Casino)	1 oz	130	9
Romano, Grated (Polly-O)	1 oz	130	10
Romano Natural (Casino)	1 oz	100	7

FOOD	PORTION	CALORIES	FAT
Scamorze, Part Skim, Low Moisture (Kraft)	1 oz	80	5
Smokestick (Sargento)	1 oz	103	7
String Cheese (Polly-O)	1 oz	90	6
String Cheese (Sargento)	1 oz	79	5
String Cheese, Smoked (Sargento)	1 oz	79	5
Swiss (Alpine Lace)	1 oz	100	8
Swiss (Kraft)	1 oz	110	8
Swiss (Land O'Lakes)	1 oz	110	8
Swiss (M.H.Greenbaum, Inc.)	1 oz	106	8
Swiss (Sargento)	1 oz	107	8
Swiss Almond Nut Log (Sargento)	1 oz	94	7
Swiss, Aged (Kraft)	1 oz	110	8
Taco (Sargento)	1 oz	109	9
Taco, Shredded (Kraft)	1 oz	110	9
Tilsiter (Sargento)	1 oz	96	7
Tybo, Red Wax (Sargento)	1 oz	98	7
blue	1 oz	100	8
blue, crumbled	1 cup	477	39
brick	1 oz	105	8

FOOD	PORTION	CALORIES	FAT
brie	1 oz	95	8
camembert	1 oz	85	7
caraway	1 oz	107	8
cheddar	1 oz	114	9
cheshire	1 oz	110	9
colby	1 oz	112	9
edam	1 oz	101	8
feta	1 oz	75	6
fontina	1 oz	110	9
gjetost	1 oz	132	8
gouda	1 oz	101	8
gruyere	1 oz	117	9
limburger	1 oz	93	8
monterey	1 oz	106	9
mozzarella	1 oz	80	6
mozzarella	1 lb	1276	98
mozzarella, low moisture	1 oz	90	7
mozzarella, low moisture, part skim	1 oz	79	5
mozzarella, part skim	1 oz	72	5
muenster	1 oz	104	9
parmesan, grated	1 Tbsp	23	2
parmesan, grated	1 oz	129	9
parmesan, hard	1 oz	111	7
port du salut	1 oz	100	8
provolone	1 oz	100	8
ricotta, part skim	½ cup	171	10
ricotta, part skim	1 cup	340	19
ricotta, whole milk	½ cup	216	16
ricotta, whole milk	1 cup	428	32
romano	1 oz	110	8

FOOD	PORTION	CALORIES	FAT
roquefort	1 oz	105	9
swiss	1 oz	107	8
tilsit	1 oz	96	7
yogurt cheese (home recipe)	1 oz	20	0
PROCESSED American (Alpine Lace)	1 oz	80	7
American Cheese, Colored (Hoffman's)	1 oz	100	7
American Cheese, White (Hoffman's)	1 oz	110	9
Borden American Singles	1 oz	90	7
Borden American Slices	1 oz	110	9
Borden Lite Line American	1 oz	50	2
Borden Lite Line American, Sodium Lite	1 oz	70	4
Borden Lite Line Cheddar Sharp Natural, Shredded, Reduced Fat	1 oz	80	5
Borden Lite Line Mozzarella	1 oz	50	2
Borden Lite Line Sharp Cheddar	1 oz	50	2
Borden Lite Line Swiss	1 oz	50	2
Borden Swiss Slices	1 oz	100	8
Cheddar Cheese Wedges (Fromageries Bel)	1 oz	72	6
Cheddar Cheese Wedges, Reduced Calorie (Fromageries Bel)	¾ oz	35	2
Chees'n Bacon Cheese Food (Hoffman's)	1 oz	90	6
Chees'n Onion Cheese Food (Hoffman's)	1 oz	100	7
Chees'n Salami Cheese Food (Hoffman's)	1 oz	90	6

FOOD	PORTION	CALORIES	FAT
Cheez 'N Bacon Singles Pasteurized Process Cheese	1 oz	90	7
Cheez Whiz	1 oz	80	6
Cheez Whiz, Hot Mexican	1 oz	80	6
Cheez Whiz, Mild Mexican	1 oz	80	6
Cheez Whiz, Pimento	1 oz	80	6
Cheez Whiz w/ Jalapeno Peppers	1 oz	80	6
Churney Cheese Fudge w/ Walnuts	1 oz	120	4
Churney Diet Snack, Cheddar Flavored	1 oz	70	3
Churney Diet Snack, Port Wine Flavored	1 oz	70	3
Churney Maple Walnut Cheese Fudge	1 oz	118	4
Churney Mint Cheese Fudge w/ Walnuts	1 oz	117	4
Cracker Barrel Extra Sharp Cheddar Cold Pack Cheese Food	1 oz	90	7
Cracker Barrel Port Wine Cheddar Cold Pack Cheese Food	1 oz	90	7
Cracker Barrel Sharp Cheddar Cold Pack Cheese Food	1 oz	90	7
Cracker Barrel w/ Bacon Cold Pack Cheese Food	1 oz	90	7
Deluxe Pasteurized Process American Cheese (slices)	1 oz	110	9
Deluxe Pasteurized Process American Cheese (loaf)	1 oz	110	9
Deluxe Pasteurized Process Pimento Cheese Slices	1 oz	100	8
Deluxe Pasteurized Process Swiss Cheese Slices	1 oz	90	7
Dorman's Light Lo-Chol, Low Cholesterol	1 oz	70	5
Easy Cheese American Spread	1 oz	80	6

FOOD	PORTION	CALORIES	FAT
Easy Cheese Cheddar Spread	1 oz	80	6
Easy Cheese Cheese n'Bacon Spread	1 oz	80	6
Easy Cheese Nacho Spread	1 oz	80	6
Easy Cheese Sharp Cheddar Spread	1 oz	80	6
Fineform	1 oz	70	3
Formagg American Swiss Slices	¾ oz	70	5
Formagg American White Slices	¾ oz	70	5
Formagg American Yellow Slices	¾ oz	70	5
Formagg Cheddar	1 oz	70	5
Formagg Grated Italian Pasta Topping	1 oz	100	7
Formagg Monterey Jack	1 oz	70	5
Formagg Monterey Jack Jalapeno Flavored	1 oz	70	5
Formagg Mozzarella	1 oz	70	5
Formagg Pizza Topper	1 oz	70	5
Formagg Provolone	1 oz	70	5
Formagg Ricotta	1 oz	130	5
Formagg Shredded Cheddar	1 oz	70	5
Formagg Shredded Mozzarella	1 oz	70	5
Formagg Shredded Parmesan	1 oz	70	4
Formagg Shredded Provolone	1 oz	70	5
Formagg Shredded Salad Topping	1 oz	70	5
Formagg Shredded Swiss	1 oz	70	5
Formagg Swiss	1 oz	70	5
Gruyere (M.H.Greenbaum, Inc)	1 oz	94	7
Gruyere Cheese Wedges (Fromageries Bel)	1 oz	72	6
Gruyere Cheese Wedges, Reduced Calorie (Fromageries Bel)	¾ oz	35	2

FOOD	PORTION	CALORIES	FAT
Gruyere, Hot Pepper (M.H. Greenbaum, Inc)	1 oz	93	7
Harvest Moon American Pasteurized Process Cheese	1 oz	70	4
Harvest Moon Brand Pasteurized Process Cheese (loaf)	1 oz	50	2
Hot Pepper Cheese Food (Hoffman's)	1 oz	90	7
Kraft American Pasteurized Process Cheese Spread	1 oz	80	6
Kraft American Singles, Pasteurized Process Cheese (colored)	1 oz	90	7
Kraft American Singles, Pasteurized Process Cheese (white)	1 oz	90	7
Kraft Jalapeno Pasteurized Process Cheese Spread	1 oz	80	6
Kraft Jalapeno Pepper Spread	1 oz	70	5
Kraft Jalapeno Singles Pasteurized Process Cheese	1 oz	90	7
Kraft Monterey Jack Singles Pasteurized Process Cheese	1 oz	90	7
Kraft Olives & Pimento Spread	1 oz	60	5
Kraft Pasteurized Process Cheese Food w/ Bacon	1 oz	90	7
Kraft Pasteurized Process Cheese Food w/ Garlic	1 oz	90	7
Kraft Pasteurized Process Cheese Spread w/ Bacon	1 oz	80	7
Kraft Pasteurized Process Cheese Spread w/ Garlic	1 oz	80	6
Kraft Pimento Singles, Pasteurized Process Cheese	1 oz	90	7
Kraft Pimento Spread	1 oz	70	5
Kraft Pineapple Spread	1 oz	70	5
Kraft Relish Spread	1 oz	70	5

FOOD	PORTION	CALORIES	FAT
Kraft Sharp Singles, Pasteurized Process Cheese	1 oz	100	8
Kraft Swiss Singles, Pasteurized Process Cheese	1 oz	90	7
Lactaid	1 slice (⅔ oz)	62	5
Land O'Lakes American	1 oz	110	9
Land O'Lakes American Swiss	1 oz	100	9
Land O'Lakes Golden Velvet Cheese Spread	1 oz	80	6
Land O'Lakes Jalapeno Cheese Food	1 oz	90	7
Land O'Lakes LaCheddar Cheese Food	1 oz	90	7
Land O'Lakes Onion Cheese Food	1 oz	90	7
Land O'Lakes Pepperoni Cheese Food	1 oz	90	7
Land O'Lakes Salami Cheese Food	1 oz	100	8
Laughing Cow Cheesebits (Fromageries Bel)	1	13	1
Lifetime Swiss	1 oz	60	3
Light N'Lively Singles, American Flavored Pasteurized Process Cheese	1 oz	70	4
Light N'Lively Singles, Sharp Cheddar Flavored Pasteurized Process Cheese	1 oz	70	4
Light N'Lively Singles, Swiss Flavored Pasteurized Process Cheese	1 oz	70	4
Lunch Wagon Pizza Topping made w/ Vegetable Oil	1 oz	80	6
Lunch Wagon Sandwich Slices made w/ Vegetable Oil	1 oz	80	6
Michael's Country Gourmet Spread, French Onion	1 oz	48	5
Michael's Country Gourmet Spread, Garden Vegetable	1 oz	48	5

FOOD	PORTION	CALORIES	FAT
Michael's Country Gourmet Spread, Garlic & Herbs	1 oz	48	5
Mohawk Valley Limburger Pasteurized Process Cheese Spread	1 oz	70	6
Old English Sharp Pasteurized Process American Cheese (slices)	1 oz	110	9
Old English Sharp Pasteurized Process American Cheese (loaf)	1 oz	110	9
Old English Sharp Pasteurized Process Cheese Spread	1 oz	90	7
Port Wine Cold Pack Cheese Food (Wispride)	1 oz	100	7
Sargento American Hot Pepper	1 oz	106	9
Sargento American Sharp Spread	1 oz	106	9
Sargento American w/ Pimento	1 oz	106	9
Sargento Imitation Cheddar	1 oz	85	6
Sargento Imitation Mozzarella	1 oz	80	6
Sargento Process Brick	1 oz	95	9
Sargento Process Swiss	1 oz	95	7
Sharp Cheddar Cold Pack Cheese Food (Wispride)	1 oz	100	7
Skitoast	1 oz	65	3
Smokelle Pasteurized Process Cheese Food	1 oz	100	7
Smokey Sharp (Hoffman's)	1 oz	110	9
Smokey Swiss 'N Cheddar (Hoffman's)	1 oz	110	8
Squeez-A-Snak, Garlic Flavor Pasteurized Process Cheese Spread	1 oz	90	7
Squeez-A-Snak, Hickory Smoke Flavor Pasteurized Process Cheese Spread	1 oz	80	7

FOOD	PORTION	CALORIES	FAT
Squeez-A-Snak, Pasteurized Process Cheese Spread w/ Bacon	1 oz	90	7
Squeez-A-Snak, Sharp Pasteurized Process Cheese Spread	1 oz	80	7
Super Sharp (Hoffman's)	1 oz	110	8
Swisson Rye Cheese Food (Hoffman's)	1 oz	90	7
Velveeta Hot Mexican Pasteurized Process Cheese Spread	1 oz	80	6
Velveeta Mild Mexican Pasteurized Process Cheese Spread	1 oz	80	6
Velveeta Pasteurized Process Cheese Spread	1 oz	80	6
Velveeta Pasteurized Process Cheese Spread Slices	1 oz	90	6
Velveeta Pimento Pasteurized Process Cheese Spread	1 oz	80	6
Weight Watchers Swiss Flavor	1 oz	50	2
american	1 oz	106	9
american, cheese food	1 oz	93	7
american, cheese food cold pack	1 oz	94	7
american, cheese spread	1 oz	82	6
pimento	1 oz	106	9
swiss, cheese food	1 oz	92	7

CHEESE DISHES

FOOD	PORTION	CALORIES	FAT
Mozzarella Cheese Nuggets; frzn (Banquet)	2.63 oz	233	12
fondue (home recipe)	½ cup	303	18

CHEESE SUBSTITUTE

FOOD	PORTION	CALORIES	FAT
American & Caraway Cheese Substitute (Delicia)	1 oz	80	6

FOOD	PORTION	CALORIES	FAT
American Cheese Substitute (Delicia)	1 oz	80	6
American w/ Hot Peppers Cheese Substitute (Delicia)	1 oz	80	6
Cheezola	1 oz	89	6
Cheeztwin (Borden)	1 oz	90	6
Colby Longhorn Imitation Cheese (Delicia)	1 oz	80	6
Count Down (Fisher)	1 oz	89	6
Count Down Smokey Flavor (Fisher)	1 oz	34	tr
Golden Image American Flavored Pasteurized Process Cheese	1 oz	90	6
Golden Image Imitation Colby Cheese	1 oz	110	9
Golden Image Imitation Mild Cheddar Cheese	1 oz	110	9
Hickory Smoked American Cheese Substitue (Delicia)	1 oz	80	6
Lite Line Low Cholesterol Cheese Food Substitute (Borden)	1 oz	90	7

CHERIMOYA

cherimoya	1	515	2

CHERRY

CANDIED

cherry	1 cherry	12	tr

CANNED

Cherries, sweet, in heavy syrup (White House)	½ cup	1	tr

FOOD	PORTION	CALORIES	FAT
Red Tart Pitted Cherries (White House)	3.5 oz	43	0
cherries, sour, water packed	1 cup	87	tr
maraschino	1	12	tr
sour, in heavy syrup	½ cup	116	tr
sour, in light syrup	½ cup	94	tr
sweet, in water	½ cup	57	tr
sweet, juice pack	½ cup	68	tr
FRESH cherries, sweet	10	49	1
FROZEN cherries, sour, unsweetened	1 cup	72	1
cherries, sweet, sweetened	1 cup	232	tr
JUICE Black Cherry (Smucker's)	8 oz	130	0
Mountain Cherry Pure & Light (Dole)	6 oz	87	tr

CHESTNUTS

Chinese; dried	1 oz	103	tr
Chinese; cooked	1 oz	44	tr
Chinese; roasted	1 oz	68	tr
Japanese; cooked	1 oz	16	tr
Japanese; roasted	1 oz	57	tr
cooked	1 oz	37	tr
dried; peeled	1 oz	105	1
roasted	1 oz	70	tr
roasted	1 cup	350	3

CHEWING GUM

Big Red	1 stick	10	0
Bubble Yum Sugarless, All Flavors	1 piece	20	0

FOOD	PORTION	CALORIES	FAT
Care*Free Sugarless, All Flavors	1 piece	8	0
Care*Free Sugarless Bubble Gum, All Flavors	1 piece	10	0
Extra Sugar Free	1 stick	8	0
Freedent	1 stick	10	0
Fruit Stripe, All Flavors	1 piece	10	0
Fruit Stripe Bubble Gum, All Flavors	1 piece	10	0
Hubba Bubba, Original & Fruit	1 stick	23	tr
Hubba Bubba, Strawberry, Grape & Raspberry	1 stick	23	tr
Juicy Fruit	1 stick	10	0
Wrigley's	1 stick	10	tr

CHIA SEEDS

FOOD	PORTION	CALORIES	FAT
dried	1 oz	134	7

CHICKEN
(*see also* CHICKEN DISHES, CHICKEN SUBSTITUTE, DINNER, HOT DOGS)

FOOD	PORTION	CALORIES	FAT
CANNED			
Chicken Salad (The Spreadables)	¼ can	100	6
Chunk Premium, White (Swanson)	2.5 oz	90	2
Chunk Style Mixin' (Swanson)	2.5 oz	130	8
Chunk White & Dark (Swanson)	2.5 oz	100	4
chicken w/ broth	1 can (5 oz)	234	11
chicken w/ broth	½ can (2.5 oz)	117	6
FRESH			
back, meat & skin; flour coated, fried	½ back (2.5 oz)	238	15
back, meat & skin; flour coated, fried	1.5 oz	146	9

FOOD	PORTION	CALORIES	FAT
back, meat & skin; fried	2.5 oz	238	16
back, meat & skin; fried	½ back (4.2 oz)	397	26
back, meat & skin, raw	½ back (3.5 oz)	316	28
back, meat & skin, raw	2.1 oz	188	17
back, meat & skin; roasted	1 oz	96	7
back, meat & skin; roasted	½ back (1.9 oz)	159	11
back, meat & skin; stewed	½ back (2.1 oz)	158	11
back, meat & skin; stewed	1.3 oz	93	7
back, meat only, raw	1 oz	42	2
back, meat only, raw	½ back (1.8 oz)	70	3
back, meat only; fried	½ back (2 oz)	167	9
back, meat only; fried	1.2 oz	101	5
back, meat only; fried	½ back (2 oz)	167	9
back, meat only; roasted	.7 oz	57	3
back, meat only; roasted	½ back (1.4 oz)	96	5
back, meat only; stewed	½ back (1.5 oz)	88	5
back, meat only; stewed	1 oz	45	3
breast, meat only; fried	1.8 oz	97	2
breast, meat only; fried	½ breast (3 oz)	161	4
breast, meat only, raw	½ breast (4 oz)	129	1
breast, meat only, raw	2.5 oz	78	1
breast, meat only; roasted	½ breast (3 oz)	142	3
breast, meat only; roasted	1.8 oz	86	2
breast, meat only; stewed	2 oz	86	2
breast, meat only; stewed	½ breast (3.3 oz)	144	3
breast, meat & skin; roasted	½ breast (3.4 oz)	193	8
breast, meat & skin; roasted	2 oz	115	5
breast, meat & skin; stewed	2.3 oz	121	5

FOOD	PORTION	CALORIES	FAT
breast, meat & skin; stewed	½ breast (3.9 oz)	202	8
breast, meat & skin; batter dipped, fried	½ breast (4.9 oz)	364	18
breast, meat & skin; batter dipped, fried	2.9 oz	218	11
breast, meat & skin; flour coated, fried	2.1 oz	131	5
breast, meat & skin; flour coated, fried	½ breast (3.4 oz)	218	9
breast, meat & skin, raw	3.1 oz	150	8
breast, meat & skin, raw	½ breast (5.1 oz)	250	13
broiler or fryer, meat & skin; roasted	½ chicken (10.5 oz)	715	41
broiler or fryer, meat & skin; roasted	6.2 oz	426	24
broiler or fryer, meat & skin; stewed	½ chicken (11.7 oz)	730	42
broiler or fryer, meat & skin; stewed	1 lb	437	25
capon, meat & skin, raw	½ chicken (2.1 lbs)	2257	165
capon, meat & skin, raw	10.4 oz	695	51
capon, meat & skin; roasted	6.9 oz	448	23
capon, meat & skin; roasted	½ chicken (1.4 lbs)	1457	74
capon, meat & skin, giblets & neck, raw	1 chicken (4.7 lbs)	4987	364
capon, meat & skin, giblets & neck; roasted	1 chicken (3.1 lbs)	3211	165
capon, meat & skin, giblets & neck; roasted	7.6 oz	494	25
dark meat w/ skin; batter dipped, fried	½ chicken (9.8 oz)	828	52
dark meat w/ skin; batter dipped, fried	5.9 oz	497	31

FOOD	PORTION	CALORIES	FAT
dark meat w/ skin; flour coated, fried	3.9 oz	313	19
dark meat w/ skin; flour coated, fried	½ chicken (6.5 oz)	523	31
dark meat w/ skin, raw	5.6 oz	379	29
dark meat w/ skin, raw	½ chicken (9.3 oz)	630	49
dark meat w/ skin; roasted	½ chicken (5.9 oz)	423	26
dark meat w/ skin; roasted	3.5 oz	256	16
dark meat w/ skin; stewed	3.9 oz	256	16
dark meat w/ skin; stewed	½ chicken (6.5 oz)	428	27
dark meat w/o skin; fried	1 cup	334	16
dark meat w/o skin; fried	3.2 oz	217	11
dark meat w/o skin, raw	3.8 oz	136	5
dark meat w/o skin, raw	½ chicken (6.4 oz)	227	8
dark meat w/o skin; roasted	2.8 oz	166	8
dark meat w/o skin; roasted	1 cup	286	14
dark meat w/o skin; stewed	1 cup	269	13
dark meat w/o skin; stewed	3 oz	165	8
drumstick, meat & skin; batter dipped, fried	1.5 oz	115	7
drumstick, meat & skin; batter dipped, fried	2.6 oz	193	11
drumstick, meat & skin; flour coated, fried	1 oz	71	4
drumstick, meat & skin flour coated, fried	1.7 oz	120	7
drumstick, meat & skin, raw	2.6 oz	117	6
drumstick, meat & skin, raw	1.5 oz	71	4
drumstick, meat & skin; roasted	1.8 oz	112	6
drumstick, meat & skin; roasted	1 oz	67	3

FOOD	PORTION	CALORIES	FAT
drumstick, meat & skin; stewed	2 oz	116	6
drumstick, meat & skin; stewed	1.2 oz	69	4
drumstick, meat only; fried	1.5 oz	82	3
drumstick, meat only, raw	1.3 oz	44	1
drumstick, meat only, raw	2.2 oz	74	2
drumstick, meat only; roasted	1.5 oz	76	2
drumstick, meat only; stewed	1.6 oz	78	3
drumstick, meat only; stewed	1 oz	47	2
leg, meat & skin; batter dipped, fried	5.5 oz	431	26
leg, meat & skin; batter dipped fried	3.3 oz	259	15
leg, meat & skin; flour coated, fried	3.9 oz	285	16
leg, meat & skin; flour coated, fried	2.4 oz	170	10
leg, meat & skin, raw	5.6 oz	312	20
leg, meat & skin, raw	3.5 oz	189	12
leg, meat & skin; roasted	4 oz	265	15
leg, meat & skin; roasted	2.4 oz	160	9
leg, meat & skin; stewed	4.4 oz	275	16
leg, meat & skin; stewed	2.6 oz	165	10
leg, meat only, raw	4.6 oz	156	5
leg, meat only, raw	2.7 oz	94	3
leg, meat only; fried	3.3 oz	195	9
leg, meat only; fried	2 oz	116	5
leg, meat only; roasted	3.3 oz	182	8
leg, meat only; roasted	2 oz	109	5
leg, meat only; stewed	3.5 oz	187	8
leg, meat only; stewed	2.1 oz	111	5
light meat w/ skin; batter dipped, fried	4 oz	312	17
light meat w/ skin; batter dipped, fried	½ chicken (6.6 oz)	520	29

FOOD	PORTION	CALORIES	FAT
light meat w/ skin; flour coated, fried	½ chicken (4.7 oz)	320	16
light meat w/ skin; flour coated, fried	2.7 oz	192	9
light meat w/ skin, raw	½ chicken (6.8 oz)	362	21
light meat w/ skin, raw	4.1 oz	216	13
light meat w/ skin; roasted	2.8 oz	175	9
light meat w/ skin; roasted	½ chicken (4.6 oz)	293	14
light meat w/ skin; stewed	½ chicken (5.3 oz)	302	15
light meat w/ skin; stewed	3.2 oz	181	9
light meat w/o skin; fried	2.2 oz	123	3
light meat w/o skin; fried	1 cup	268	8
light meat w/o skin, raw	½ chicken (5.2 oz)	168	2
light meat w/o skin, raw	3.1 oz	100	1
light meat w/o skin; roasted	1 cup	242	6
light meat w/o skin; roasted	2.2 oz	110	3
light meat w/o skin; stewed	2.3 oz	113	3
light meat w/o skin; stewed	1 cup	223	6
meat & skin, raw	½ chicken (16.1 oz)	990	69
meat & skin; flour coated, fried	½ chicken (11 oz)	844	47
meat & skin; flour coated; fried	1 lb	505	28
meat & skin; fried	½ chicken (16.4 oz)	1347	81
meat only; fried	1 cup	307	13
meat only; fried	5.4 oz	340	14
meat only; roasted	5.1 oz	278	11
meat only; roasted	1 cup	266	10
meat only; stewed	1 cup	248	9

FOOD	PORTION	CALORIES	FAT
meat only; stewed	5.5 oz	278	11
meat only, raw	½ chicken (11.5 oz)	392	10
neck, meat & skin; batter dipped, fried	1.8 oz	172	12
neck, meat & skin; flour coated, fried	1.3 oz	119	9
neck, meat & skin, raw	1.8 oz	148	13
neck, meat & skin; simmered	1.3 oz	95	7
neck, meat only, raw	.7 oz	31	2
neck, meat only; fried	.8 oz	50	3
neck, meat only; simmered	.6 oz	32	1
roaster, meat & skin; roasted	½ chicken (1.1 lbs)	1071	64
roaster, meat & skin; roasted	7.4 oz	469	28
skin only; roasted	from ½ chicken (2 oz)	254	23
skin only; roasted	1.2 oz	154	14
skin only; stewed	1.6 oz	160	15
skin only; stewed	from ½ chicken (2.5 oz)	261	24
skin only; flour coated, fried	1 oz	166	14
skin only; flour coated, raw	from ½ chicken (2 oz)	281	24
skin only; fried	from ½ chicken (6.7 oz)	748	55
skin only; fried	4 oz	449	33
skin only, raw	1.6 oz	164	15
skin only, raw	from ½ chicken (2.8 oz)	275	26
stewing, meat & skin; stewed	6.2 oz	507	34
stewing, meat & skin; stewed	½ chicken (9.2 oz)	744	49

FOOD	PORTION	CALORIES	FAT
thigh, meat & skin; batter dipped, fried	3 oz	238	14
thigh, meat & skin; batter dipped, fried	1.8 oz	144	9
thigh, meat & skin; flour coated, fried	2.2 oz	162	9
thigh, meat & skin; flour coated, fried	1.3 oz	99	6
thigh, meat & skin, raw	3.3 oz	199	14
thigh, meat & skin, raw	2 oz	120	9
thigh, meat & skin; roasted	2.2 oz	153	10
thigh, meat & skin; roasted	1.3 oz	91	6
thigh, meat & skin; stewed	2.4 oz	158	10
thigh, meat & skin; stewed	1.4 oz	95	6
thigh, meat only, raw	2.4 oz	82	3
thigh, meat only; fried	1.8 oz	113	5
thigh, meat only; roasted	1.8 oz	109	6
thigh, meat only; stewed	1.9 oz	107	5
whole w/ giblets & neck	1 chicken (2.3 lbs)	2223	155
whole w/ giblets & neck; batter dipped, fried	1 chicken (2.3 lbs)	2987	180
whole w/ giblets & neck; batter dipped, fried	1 lb	895	54
whole w/ giblets & neck; flour coated, fried	1 lb	577	32
whole w/ giblets & neck; flour coated, fried	1 chicken (1.6 lbs)	1928	108
whole w/ giblets & neck; roasted	1 chicken (1.5 lbs)	1598	90
whole w/ giblets & neck; roasted	1 lb	480	27
whole w/ giblets & neck; stewed	1 lb	487	28
whole w/ giblets & neck; stewed	1 chicken (1.6 lbs)	1625	93

FOOD	PORTION	CALORIES	FAT
wing, meat & skin, raw	1.7 oz	109	8
wing, meat & skin; batter dipped, fried	1.7 oz	159	11
wing, meat & skin; flour coated, fried	1.1 oz	103	7
wing, meat & skin; roasted	1.2 oz	99	7
wing, meat & skin; stewed	1.4 oz	100	7
wing, meat only; fried	.7 oz	42	2
wing, meat only, raw	1 oz	36	1
wing, meat only; roasted	.7 oz	43	2
wing, meat only; stewed	.8 oz	43	2
FROZEN, PREPARED			
Banquet Fried Chicken	6.4 oz	325	19
Banquet Fried Chicken Breast Portions	5.75 oz	218	11
Banquet Fried Chicken Thighs & Drumsticks	6.25 oz	245	14
Banquet Hot 'n Spicy Fried Chicken	6.4 oz	325	19
Banquet Hot 'n Spicy Wings	3.75 oz	135	9
Banquet Hot Bites, Breast Patties	2.63 oz	199	12
Banquet Hot Bites, Breast Tenders	2.25 oz	142	6
Banquet Hot Bites, Chicken Drum-Snackers	2.63 oz	218	14
Banquet Hot Bites, Chicken Nuggets	2.63 oz	210	14
Banquet Hot Bites, Chicken Sticks	2.63 oz	215	15
Banquet Hot Bites, Chicken w/ Cheddar	2.63 oz	247	18
Banquet Hot Bites, Hot 'n Spicy Chicken Nuggets	2.63 oz	246	18
Banquet Hot Bites, Microwave Breast Pattie & Bun	4 oz	310	14
Banquet Hot Bites, Microwave Breast Tenders	4 oz	256	10

FOOD	PORTION	CALORIES	FAT
Banquet Hot Bites, Microwave Chicken Nuggets w/ Sweet & Sour Sauce	4.5 oz	354	21
Banquet Hot Bites, Microwave Hot 'n Spicy Chicken Nuggets w/ BBQ Sauce	4.5 oz	359	21
Banquet Hot Bites, Microwave Southern Fried Breast Pattie & Biscuit	4 oz	319	14
Banquet Hot Bites, Microwave Southern Fried Breast Patties	2.63 oz	220	14
Banquet Hot Bites, Microwave Southern Fried Breast Tenders	2.25 oz	153	7
Banquet Hot Bites, Microwave Southern Fried Breast Nuggets	2.63 oz	218	14
Banquet Hot Bites, Microwave Southern Fried Chicken Breast w/ BBQ Sauce	4.5 oz	366	23
Chefwich Chicken Parmigiana Sandwich	1 (5 oz)	350	11
Country Pride Chicken Chunks	3 oz	238	15
Country Pride Chicken Patties	3 oz	245	16
Country Pride Chicken Sticks	3 oz	233	14
Country Pride Southern Fried Chicken Chunks	3 oz	276	20
Country Pride Southern Fried Chicken Patties	3 oz	232	15
Kibun Chicken Pasta Salad w/ dressing	½ pkg	220	9
Kibun Chicken Pasta Salad w/o dressing	½ pkg	150	2
MicroMagic Chicken Sandwich	1 (4.5 oz)	390	16
Swanson Chicken Duet Gourmet Nuggets, Ham & Cheese	3 oz	220	13
Swanson Chicken Duet Gourmet Nuggets, Mexican Style	3 oz	220	13

FOOD	PORTION	CALORIES	FAT
Swanson Chicken Duet Gourmet Nuggets, Pizza Style	3 oz	210	12
Swanson Chicken Duet Gourmet Nuggets, Spinach & Herb	3 oz	230	13
Swanson Chicken Nibbles	5 oz	260	18
Swanson Fried Chicken	6.5 oz	300	19
Weaver Batter Dipped Breast	3.5 oz	250	16
Weaver Batter Dipped Thighs/Drums	3.5 oz	245	16
Weaver Batter Dipped Wings	3.5 oz	270	19
Weaver Breast Fillets	3.5 oz	195	10
Weaver Breast Fillets Strips	3.5 oz	200	9
Weaver Chicken Croquetts	3.5 oz	245	15
Weaver Chicken Nuggets	4 pieces	240	14
Weaver Crispy Dutch Frye Breasts	3.5 oz	285	18
Weaver Crispy Dutch Frye Thighs/ Drums	3.5 oz	295	20
Weaver Crispy Dutch Frye Wings	3.5 oz	360	25
Weaver Crispy Light Fried Chicken	2.9 oz	160	9
Weaver Mini-Drums, Crispy	3 oz	205	11
Weaver Mini-Drums, Herbs 'n Spice	3 oz	205	11
Weaver Rondelets, Cheese	3 oz	215	13
Weaver Rondelets, Homestyle	3 oz	185	10
Weaver Rondelets, Italian	3 oz	200	11
Weaver Rondelets, Original	3 oz	185	10
Weaver Thigh Fillets Strips	3.5 oz	240	14
Weight Watchers Chicken Nuggets	4 nuggets	180	11
READY-TO-USE Bologna (Health Valley)	3.5 oz	300	30
Bologna (Weaver)	3.5 oz	240	20

FOOD	PORTION	CALORIES	FAT
Breast (Mr. Turkey)	1 slice (1 oz)	32	1
Breast, Deli Slice Browned & Roasted (Wampler Longacre)	1 oz	49	tr
Breast, Deluxe Oven Roasted (Louis Rich)	1 slice (28 g)	30	tr
Breast, Hickory Smoked (Weaver)	3.5 oz	125	4
Breast, Oven Roasted (Oscar Mayer)	1 slice (28 g)	29	tr
Breast, Oven Roasted (Weaver)	3.5 oz	120	4
Breast, Smoked (Louis Rich)	1 slice (28 g)	31	tr
Breast, Smoked (Oscar Mayer)	1 slice (28 g)	26	tr
Breast, Stuffed Cordon Bleu; not prep (Wampler Longacre)	6.5 oz	429	3
Breast, Stuffed w/ Breading; not prep (Wampler Longacre)	8 oz	472	6
Chicken (Carl Buddig)	1 oz	50	3
Cutlets, Perdue Done It!	1 oz	73	5
Diced Breast Roll (Wampler Longacre)	1 oz	49	tr
Diced White Breast (Wampler Longacre)	1 oz	38	tr
Nuggets, Breast Breaded; as prep (Wampler Longacre)	1 oz	71	1
Nuggets, White Breaded Fully Cooked (Wampler Longacre)	1 oz	71	1
Nuggets, Perdue Done It!	1 oz	73	5

FOOD	PORTION	CALORIES	FAT
Roll, Dutch Family	1 oz	61	15
Roll, Longacre	1 oz	65	17
Roll, Sliced (Wampler Longacre)	1 oz	63	1
Salad (Wampler Longacre)	1 oz	65	1
Tenders, Perdue Done It!	3 oz	201	9
White, Oven Roasted (Louis Rich)	1 slice (28 g)	39	2
White Meat Roll (Weaver)	3.5 oz	130	6
Wings, Hot & Spicy, Perdue Done It!	1 oz	59	4
chicken roll, light meat	1 slice (28 g)	45	2
chicken roll, light meat	1 (6 oz pkg)	271	13
chicken spread, canned	1 Tbsp	25	26
chicken spread, canned	1 oz	55	3
poultry salad sandwich spread	1 Tbsp	109	2
poultry salad sandwich	1 oz	238	4

CHICKEN DISHES
(*see also* CHICKEN SUBSTITUTE, DINNER)

FOOD	PORTION	CALORIES	FAT
CANNED			
Chicken & Dumplings (Swanson)	7.5 oz	220	12
Chicken A La King (Swanson)	5.25 oz	180	12
Chicken Stew (Chef Boy.ar.dee)	7 oz	140	5
Chicken Stew (Swanson)	7⅝ oz	170	7
HOME RECIPE			
chicken cacciatore	¾ cup	394	24
chicken paprikash	1½ cups	296	10

FOOD	PORTION	CALORIES	FAT
chicken & dumplings	¾ cup	256	12
chicken & noodles	¾ cup	191	6
chicken a la king	¾ cup	234	16

CHICKEN SUBSTITUTE

FOOD	PORTION	CALORIES	FAT
Chick Stiks; frzn (Worthington)	3.5 oz	232	14
Chick-Ketts; frzn (Worthington)	3.5 oz	199	9
Chik-Nuggets (Loma Linda)	5 nuggets (3 oz)	228	11
Chik-Patties (Loma Linda)	1 patty (3 oz)	226	12
Meatless Chicken (Loma Linda)	2 slices (2 oz)	93	3
Meatless Chicken Supreme Mix: not prep (Loma Linda)	¼ cup	50	tr
Meatless Fried Chicken (Loma Linda)	1 piece (2 oz)	180	14
Meatless Fried Chicken w/ Gravy (Loma Linda)	2 pieces (3 oz)	140	10
Spicy-Chik Minidrums (Loma Linda)	5 pieces (3 oz)	230	13

CHICKPEAS

FOOD	PORTION	CALORIES	FAT
CANNED			
Chick Peas (Hanover)	½ cup	100	1
Garbanzo Lite, 50% Less Salt (S&W)	½ cup	110	1
Garbanzo Premium, Large (S&W)	½ cup	110	1
chickpeas	1 cup	285	3

FOOD	PORTION	CALORIES	FAT
DRIED			
Garbanzo (Hurst Brand)	1 cup	288	4
cooked	1 cup	269	4
raw	1 cup	729	12

CHICORY

greens, raw	½ cup	21	tr

CHILI

Beef Chili w/ Beans (Chef Boy.ar.dee)	7.5 oz	330	17
Chili Beans (S&W)	½ cup	130	1
Chili Beans in Chili Gravy (Dennison's)	7.5 oz	180	1
Chili Con Carne (Health Valley)	4 oz	170	8
Chili Con Carne w/ Beans (Chef Boy.ar.dee)	7 oz	340	20
Chili Con Carne w/ Beans (Dennison's)	7.5 oz	310	15
Chili Con Carne w/o Beans (Dennison's)	7.5 oz	300	19
Chili Hot Dog Sauce w/ Beef (Chef Boy.ar.dee)	1 oz	30	1
Chili Mac (Chef Boy.ar.dee)	7 oz	230	10
Chili Makin's, Original (S&W)	½ cup	100	1
Chili with Beans (Estee)	7.5 oz	390	28
Chunky Chili w/ Beans (Dennison's)	7.5 oz	310	14
Cook-off Chili w/ Beans (Dennison's)	7.5 oz	340	19

FOOD	PORTION	CALORIES	FAT
Hot Chili Beans (Luck's)	7.5 oz	200	2
Hot Chili Con Carne w/ Beans (Chef Boy.ar.dee)	7 oz	350	21
Hot Chili Con Carne w/ Beans (Dennison's)	7.5 oz	310	16
Lentil Chili (Health Valley)	4 oz	110	5
Mild Vegetarian w/ Beans (Health Valley)	4 oz	120	6
Oscar Mayer Chili Con Carne Concentrate	1 oz	78	6
Spicy Vegetarian w/ Beans (Health Valley)	4 oz	120	6
chili w/beans	1 cup	286	14
chili w/beans (home recipe)	1 cup	399	14

CHINESE CABBAGE
(*see* CABBAGE)

CHINESE FOOD
(*see* ORIENTAL FOOD)

CHIPS
(*see also* POPCORN, PRETZELS, SNACKS)

CORN

FOOD	PORTION	CALORIES	FAT
Corn Chips (Health Valley)	1 oz	160	11
Corn Chips (Planters)	1 oz	160	10
Corn Chips (Wise)	1 oz	160	10
Corn Chips BBQ (Lance)	1 pkg (1.75 oz)	280	16
Corn Chips Plain (Lance)	1 pkg (1.75 oz)	260	17

FOOD	PORTION	CALORIES	FAT
Corn Chips w/ Cheese (Health Valley)	1 oz	160	10
Corn Crunchies (Wise)	1 oz	160	10
Corn Nacho Cheese Flavor Spirals Crispy Corn Twists (Wise)	1 oz	160	10
Corn Toasted Spirals Crispy Corn Twists (Wise)	1 oz	160	10
POTATO Eagle	1 oz	150	10
Health Valley	1 oz	160	10
Kelly's	1 oz	150	10
Lance	1 pkg (1⅛ oz)	190	15
Lay's	1 oz	150	10
Lay's Jalapeno & Cheddar Flavored	1 oz	150	9
New York Deli	1 oz	160	11
Potato, Barbecue Flavor Ripple (Wise)	1 oz	150	10
Potato, BBQ (Lance)	1 pkg (1⅛ oz)	190	12
Potato, Butter 'n Herbs (Pringle's)	1 oz	170	13
Potato, Cajun Style (Lance)	1 pkg (1 oz)	160	10
Potato Cheez-ums (Pringle's)	1 oz	170	13
Potato, Country Chips (Health Valley)	1 oz	160	10
Potato, Country Ripple (Health Valley)	1 oz	160	10
Potato Crunchies (Planters)	1.25 oz	190	11

FOOD	PORTION	CALORIES	FAT
Potato, Dip Chips (Health Valley)	1 oz	160	10
Potato, Idaho Rippled (Pringle's)	1 oz	170	12
Potato, Idaho Rippled French Onion (Pringle's)	1 oz	170	12
Potato, Idaho Rippled Taco 'n Cheddar (Pringle's)	1 oz	170	12
Potato, Light (Pringle's)	1 oz	150	8
Potato, Light B-B-Q (Pringle's)	1 oz	150	8
Potato, Natural Flavor (Wise)	1 oz	160	11
Potato, No Salt Added (Cottage Fries)	1 oz	160	11
Potato, Regular (Pringle's)	1 oz	170	13
Potato, Ripple (Lance)	1 pkg (1⅛ oz)	190	15
Potato, Rippled (Kelly's)	1 oz	150	10
Potato, Rippled (Pringle's)	1 oz	170	12
Potato, Sour Cream & Onion (Lance)	1 pkg (1⅛ oz)	190	12
Potato, Sour Cream 'n Onion (Pringle's)	1 oz	170	12
Potato, Unsalted (Kelly's)	1 oz	150	10
Ripple (Lance)	1 oz	160	13
Ruffles	1 oz	150	10
Ruffles Bar-B-Q Flavored	1 oz	150	9

FOOD	PORTION	CALORIES	FAT
Ruffles Sour Cream & Onion Artificially Flavored	1 oz	150	9
Sour Cream and Onion Ripple (Lance)	1 oz	170	11
potato	10 chips	105	7
potato	1 oz	148	10
potato sticks	1 oz pkg	148	10
TORTILLA Doritos	1 oz	140	6
Doritos, Cool Ranch Flavored	1 oz	140	7
Doritos, Nacho Cheese Flavored	1 oz	140	7
Tortilla Chips (La Famous)	1 oz	140	7
Tortilla Chips Buenitos (Health Valley)	1 oz	130	8
Tortilla Chips, Nacho Cheese Flavor Round Bravos (Wise)	1 oz	150	8
Tortilla Chips, No Salt Added (La Famous)	1 oz	140	7
Tortilla Jalapeno Cheese (Lance)	1 pkg (1⅛ oz)	160	8
Tortilla Nacho (Lance)	1 pkg (1⅛ oz)	160	8

CHITTERLINGS

pork, raw	3 oz	213	20
pork; simmered	3 oz	258	24

CHIVES

freeze-dried	1 Tbsp	1	tr
fresh, raw	1 tsp	0	tr

FOOD	PORTION	CALORIES	FAT

CHOCOLATE
(*see also* CANDY, CAROB, COCOA, ICE CREAM TOPPINGS, MILK DRINKS)

FOOD	PORTION	CALORIES	FAT
BAKING			
German Sweet (Bakers)	1 oz	144	10
Semi-Sweet Chocolate (Bakers)	1 oz	136	9
Unsweetened (Bakers)	1 oz	142	15
Unsweetened Baking Chocolate (Hershey)	1 oz	190	16
CHIPS			
Chocolate Flavored Chips (Bakers)	¼ cup	196	9
German Sweet Chocolate Chips (Bakers)	¼ cup	203	12
Milk Chocolate Chips (Hershey)	1 oz	150	8
Real Semi-Sweet Chocolate Chips (Bakers)	¼ cup	201	12
Semi-Sweet Chocolate Chips, miniature (Hershey)	¼ cup	220	12
Semi-Sweet Chocolate Chips, regular (Hershey)	¼ cup	220	12
MIX			
Hershey Instant Mix	3 Tbsp	80	1
Ovaltine; as prep w/ whole milk	8 oz	227	9
Quik Chocolate Flavor (Nestle)	2 tsp	90	1
chocolate mix; as prep w/ whole milk	9 oz	226	9
chocolate powder	2–3 heaping tsp	75	1

FOOD	PORTION	CALORIES	FAT
SYRUP			
Estee	1 Tbsp	6	0
Hershey's Chocolate Flavored	2 Tbsp	80	1
chocolate	1 cup	653	3
chocolate; as prep w/ whole milk	9 oz	232	9

CHOCOLATE MILK
(see CHOCOLATE, COCOA, MILK DRINKS)

CISCO

smoked	3 oz	151	10
smoked	1 oz	50	3

CITRON

citron	1 oz	89	tr

CLAM

CANNED			
Chopped Clams, Liquid & Solids (Doxsee)	6.5 oz	90	tr
Clam Juice (Doxsee)	3 oz	4	0
Minced & Chopped Clams (Gorton's)	½ can	70	1
Minced Clams, Liquid & Solids (Snow's)	6.5 oz	90	tr
Quahogs (American Original Foods)	4 oz	66	tr
Red Clam Sauce (Fresh Chef)	4 oz	90	4
White Clam Sauce (Fresh Chef)	4 oz	130	10
liquid only	1 cup	6	tr
liquid only	3 oz	2	tr

FOOD	PORTION	CALORIES	FAT
meat only	1 cup	236	3
meat only	3 oz	126	2
FRESH			
clam; cooked	20 sm	133	2
clam; cooked	3 oz	126	2
clam, raw	3 oz	63	1
clam, raw	9 lg	133	2
clam, raw	20 sm	133	2
FROZEN			
Breaded Clams (Van De Kamp's)	2.25 oz	210	11
Crunchy Fried Clam Strips (Gorton's)	½ pkg	310	23
Fried Clams In A Light (Mrs. Paul's)	2.5 oz	240	13
HOME RECIPE			
clam sauce	½ cup	274	22
clam; breaded & fried	3 oz	171	9
clam; breaded & fried	20 sm	379	21

COCOA
(*see also* CHOCOLATE)

FOOD	PORTION	CALORIES	FAT
MIX			
Carnation Hot Cocoa, 70 Calorie	3 tsp (21 g)	70	tr
Carnation Hot Cocoa, Milk Chocolate	1 pkg or 4 heaping tsp (1 oz)	110	1
Carnation Hot Cocoa, Natural Mint	1 pkg or 4 heaping tsp (1 oz)	110	1
Carnation Hot Cocoa, Rich Chocolate	1 pkg or 4 heaping tsp (1 oz)	110	1

FOOD	PORTION	CALORIES	FAT
Carnation Hot Cocoa, Rich Chocolate w/ Marshmallows	1 pkg or 4 heaping tsp (1 oz)	110	1
Carnation Hot Cocoa, Sugar Free Mint	1 pkg or 4 heaping tsp (15 g)	50	tr
Carnation Hot Cocoa, Sugar Free Rich Chocolate	1 pkg or 4 heaping tsp (15 g)	50	tr
Hershey's Cocoa	⅓ cup	120	4
cocoa mix	1 oz	102	1
PREPARED Hills Bros. Hot Cocoa, Sugar Free; as prep w/ water	6 oz	60	2
Hills Bros. Hot Cocoa; as prep w/ water	6 oz	110	2
hot cocoa	1 cup	218	9

COCONUT

FOOD	PORTION	CALORIES	FAT
Angel Flake, Bag (Bakers)	⅓ cup	116	8
Angel Flake, Can (Bakers)	⅓ cup	114	9
Cream of Coconut (Coco Lopez)	2 Tbsp	120	5
Premium Shred (Bakers)	⅓ cup	136	10
coconut water	1 Tbsp	3	tr
coconut water	1 cup	46	tr
cream, canned	1 Tbsp	36	3
cream, canned	1 cup	568	52
dried, creamed	1 oz	194	20
dried, sweetened; flaked	1 cup	351	24
dried, sweetened, flaked	7 oz pkg	944	64

FOOD	PORTION	CALORIES	FAT
dried, sweetened, flaked, canned	1 cup	341	24
dried, sweetened, shredded	7 oz pkg	997	71
dried, sweetened, shredded	1 cup	466	33
dried, toasted	1 oz	168	13
dried, unsweetened	1 oz	187	18
milk, canned	1 cup	445	48
milk, canned	1 Tbsp	30	3
milk, frozen	1 Tbsp	30	3
milk, frozen	1 cup	486	50
raw	1 piece	159	15

COD

FOOD	PORTION	CALORIES	FAT
CANNED			
Atlantic	3 oz	89	1
Atlantic	1 can (11 oz)	327	3
DRIED			
Atlantic	3 oz	246	2
FRESH			
Atlantic, raw	3 oz	70	1
Atlantic, raw	1 fillet (8.1 oz)	190	2
Atlantic; cooked	1 fillet (6.3 oz)	189	2
Atlantic; cooked	3 oz	89	1
Pacific, raw	1 fillet (4.1 oz)	95	1
Pacific, raw	3 oz	70	1
roe, raw	3.5 oz	130	2
FROZEN			
Au Natural Cod Fillets (Mrs. Paul's)	4 oz	90	2
Fishmarket Fresh Cod (Gorton's)	5 oz	110	1

FOOD	PORTION	CALORIES	FAT
Lightly Breaded Cod (Van De Kamp's)	1 piece	290	19
Microwave, Lightly Breaded Cod (Van De Kamp's)	5 oz	290	19
Today's Catch, Cod (Van De Kamp's)	5 oz	110	0

COFFEE
(*see also* COFFEE BEVERAGE, COFFEE SUBSTITUTE)

INSTANT			
Kava	1 tsp	2	0
powder	1 rounded tsp	4	0
powder w/ chicory	1 rounded tsp	6	0
INSTANT, DECAFFEINATED			
powder	1 rounded tsp	4	0
REGULAR			
coffee	6 oz	4	0

COFFEE BEVERAGE
(*see also* COFFEE SUBSTITUTE)

Cafe Amaretto International Coffee (General Foods)	6 oz	51	3
Cafe Francais International Coffee (General Foods)	6 oz	55	3
Cafe Francais Sugar Free International Coffee (General Foods)	6 oz	35	2
Cafe Irish Creme International Coffee (General Foods)	6 oz	55	3
Cafe Irish Creme Sugar Free International Coffee (General Foods)	6 oz	31	3
Cafe Vienna International Coffee (General Foods)	6 oz	59	2

FOOD	PORTION	CALORIES	FAT
Cafe Vienna Sugar Free International Coffee (General Foods)	6 oz	29	3
Irish Mocha Mint International Coffee (General Foods)	6 oz	51	2
Irish Mocha Mint Sugar Free International Coffee (General Foods)	6 oz	28	2
Orange Cappuccino International Coffee (General Foods)	6 oz	59	10
Orange Cappuccino Sugar Free International Coffee (General Foods)	6 oz	29	2
Suisse Mocha International Coffee (General Foods)	6 oz	53	3
Suisse Mocha Sugar Free International Coffee (General Foods)	6 oz	29	2

COFFEE SUBSTITUTE

FOOD	PORTION	CALORIES	FAT
Postum Instant; as prep	6 oz	11	tr
as prep w/ milk	6 oz	121	6
Postum Instant, Coffee Flavored; as prep	6 oz	11	tr
powder	1 tsp	9	tr

COFFEE WHITENER
(*see also* MILK SUBSTITUTE)

FOOD	PORTION	CALORIES	FAT
LIQUID			
Coffee Rich	1 Tbsp	20	2
Coffee-Mate	1 oz	31	2
Grand Union	1 Tbsp	24	2

FOOD	PORTION	CALORIES	FAT
Mocha Mix	1 Tbsp (½ oz)	19	2
non dairy; frzn	½ oz	20	2
POWDER			
Coffee-Mate	1 pkg (3 g)	16	tr
Coffee-Mate	1 tsp	10	tr
Cremora	1 tsp	12	1
nondairy	1 tsp	11	tr

COLESLAW
(see CABBAGE, SALAD)

COLLARDS

FRESH			
cooked	½ cup	13	tr
raw; chopped	1 cup	35	tr
FROZEN			
cooked	½ cup	31	tr
frzn; not prep	10 oz	93	1

COOKIE
(see also BROWNIE, CAKE, DOUGHNUT, PIE)

HOME RECIPE			
chocolate chip	1 (.4 oz)	59	4
fortune cookie	1 (½ oz)	66	4
lemon bar	1 (1 oz)	110	5
molasses	1 (1.1 oz)	138	5
oatmeal w/ raisin	1 (½ oz)	54	3
peanut butter	1 (½ oz)	61	3
pumpkin bar	1 (1.2 oz)	151	9
raspberry bar	1 (.8 oz)	76	2
sugar	1 (.4 oz)	36	2

FOOD	PORTION	CALORIES	FAT
MIX			
Chocolate Chip; as prep (Duncan Hines)	2	130	5
Golden Sugar; as prep (Duncan Hines)	2	130	6
Oatmeal Raisin; as prep (Duncan Hines)	2	130	6
Peanut Butter; as prep (Duncan Hines)	2	140	7
READY-TO-EAT			
Almond Supreme (Pepperidge Farm)	2	140	10
Almond Toast (Stella D'Oro)	1	56	1
Aloha (LU)	1	75	5
Amaranth Graham Crackers (Health Valley)	1.2 oz	110	3
Amaranth Jumbo (Health Valley)	.6 oz	70	3
Amaretti (Stella D'Oro)	1	28	5
Angel Bars (Stella D'Oro)	1	74	5
Angel Puffs (Stella D'Oro)	1	13	tr
Angel Wings (Stella D'Oro)	1	74	5
Angelica Goodies (Stella D'Oro)	1	104	4
Anginetti (Stella D'Oro)	1	30	1
Animal Crackers (FFV)	9	110	3
Animal Crackers (Sunshine)	14	120	3

FOOD	PORTION	CALORIES	FAT
Animal Crackers, Barnum's (Nabisco)	11	130	4
Anisette Sponge (Stella D'Oro)	1	52	tr
Anisette Toast (Stella D'Oro)	1	46	tr
Anisette Toast, Jumbo (Stella D'Oro)	1	109	1
Apple Newtons (Nabisco)	1	110	2
Apple Oatmeal Bar (Lance)	1 pkg (1.65 oz)	190	7
Apple Pastry, Dietetic (Stella D'Oro)	1	90	4
Apple Walnut Raisin Almost Home (Nabisco)	2	130	6
Apple-Cinnamon (Lance)	1 pkg (1 oz)	120	5
Apricot-Raspberry Fruit (Pepperidge Farm)	3	150	6
Arrowroot Biscuit National (Nabisco)	6	130	4
Baked Apple Bar (Sunbelt)	1 pkg (1.31 oz)	130	1
Banana Walnut Almost Home (Nabisco)	2	140	7
Barre Chocolat (LU)	1	65	3
Blueberry (Lance)	1 pkg (1 oz)	120	4
Blueberry Newtons (Nabisco)	1	110	2
Bonnie (Lance)	1 pkg (¾ oz)	100	4
Bordeaux (Pepperidge Farm)	3	110	5

FOOD	PORTION	CALORIES	FAT
Breakfast Treats (Stella D'Oro)	1	102	4
Brown Edge Wafers (Nabisco)	5	140	6
Brownie Chocolate Nut (Pepperidge Farm)	3	170	10
Brussels (Pepperidge Farm)	3	170	9
Brussels Mint (Pepperidge Farm)	3	200	10
Butter Flavored (Nabisco)	6	130	5
Butter Flavored (Sunshine)	4	120	5
Cappucino (Pepperidge Farm)	3	120	7
Capri (Pepperidge Farm)	2	170	9
Caramel Bars Heyday (Nabisco)	1	140	8
Caramel Patties (FFV)	2	150	7
Champagne (Pepperidge Farm)	2	110	6
Cherry Newtons (Nabisco)	1	110	2
Chessmen (Pepperidge Farm)	3	130	6
Chinese Dessert Cookies (Stella D'Oro)	1	172	9
Chip-A-Roos (Sunshine)	2	130	7
Chips Chocolat (LU)	1	85	5
Chips Deluxe (Keebler)	1	90	4

FOOD	PORTION	CALORIES	FAT
Chips'n Middles (Sunshine)	2	140	6
Choc-O-Lunch (Lance)	1⁵⁄₁₆ oz	180	6
Choc-O-Lunch (Lance)	1 oz	130	5
Choc-O-Mint (Lance)	1.25 oz	180	10
Chocolate Chip (Archway)	1	60	3
Chocolate Chip (Lance)	1 pkg (1 oz)	135	7
Chocolate Chip (Duncan Hines)	2	110	5
Chocolate Chip (Pepperidge Farm)	3	150	7
Chocolate Chip Chewy Chips Ahoy (Nabisco)	2	130	6
Chocolate Chip Fudge (Lance)	1 pkg (1 oz)	130	5
Chocolate Chip Snaps (Nabisco)	6	130	6
Chocolate Chocolate Chip (Pepperidge Farm)	3	160	8
Chocolate Chunk Pecan (Pepperidge Farm)	2	130	7
Chocolate Coated Snack Wafer (Estee)	1	120	7
Chocolate Creme Filled Wafer (Estee)	1	20	1
Chocolate Fudge Sandwich (Sunshine)	2	150	7
Chocolate Giggles (Nabisco)	2	140	6
Chocolate Grahams (Nabisco)	3	150	7

FOOD	PORTION	CALORIES	FAT
Chocolate I Screams (Nabisco)	5	150	7
Chocolate Laced Pirouettes (Pepperidge Farm)	2	110	6
Chocolate Mallomars (Nabisco)	2	130	6
Chocolate Peanut Bars, Ideal (Nabisco)	2	150	7
Chocolate Sandwich, Oreo (Nabisco)	3	140	6
Chocolate Sandwich, Oreo Big Stuf (Nabisco)	1	250	12
Chocolate Sandwich, Oreo Double Stuf (Nabisco)	2	140	7
Chocolate Snack Wafer (Estee)	1	80	4
Chocolate Snaps (Nabisco)	7	130	4
Chocolate & Marshmallow Cake, Pinwheels (Nabisco)	1	130	5
Chocolu (LU)	1	55	3
Cinnamon Crisp Graham (Keebler)	4	70	2
Cinnamon Jumbo (Health Valley)	½ oz	70	2
Coated Graham (Lance)	1⁵⁄₁₆ oz	180	9
Coconut Chips 'n More (Nabisco)	2	150	6
Coconut Macaroons (Stella D'Oro)	1	63	4
Coconut Cookies, Dietetic (Stella D'Oro)	1	50	2

FOOD	PORTION	CALORIES	FAT
Como Delight (Stella D'Oro)	1	141	7
Craquelin (LU)	1	55	3
Creme Sandwich, Baronet (Nabisco)	3	140	6
Creme Sandwich, Cameo (Nabisco)	2	140	5
Crokine (LU)	2	19	0
Cup Custard (Sunshine)	2	130	6
Date Nut Granola (Pepperidge Farm)	3	170	8
Date Pecan (Pepperidge Farm)	3	170	8
Deluxe Grahams, Fudge Covered (Keebler)	2	80	4
Devil's Food Cakes (Nabisco)	1	110	1
Egg Biscuits (Stella D'Oro)	1	43	1
Egg Biscuits, Dietetic (Stella D'Oro)	1	40	1
Egg, Jumbo (Stella D'Oro)	1	46	tr
Euphrates (LU)	2	40	2
Famous Chocolate Wafers (Nabisco)	5	130	4
Fig Bar (Keebler)	1	71	1
Fig Bar (Lance)	1.5 oz	150	2
Fig Bars (Sunshine)	2	90	2

FOOD	PORTION	CALORIES	FAT
Fig Newtons (Nabisco)	2	100	2
Fig Pastry, Dietetic (Stella D'Oro)	1	95	4
Fruit Slices (Stella D'Oro)	1	59	2
Fudge, Chips 'n More (Nabisco)	3	140	6
Fudge & Peanut Butter Chip Almost Home (Nabisco)	2	130	6
Fudge Bar (Tastykake)	1	240	8
Fudge Bars, Heyday (Nabisco)	1	140	8
Fudge Chips Chocolate (LU)	1	75	4
Fudge Chocolate Chip, Almost Home (Nabisco)	2	130	5
Fudge Chocolate Chip Raisin, Almost Home (Nabisco)	2	130	5
Fudge Covered Chocolate Sandwich, Oreo Fudge Cremes (Nabisco)	2	150	8
Fudge Cremes (Keebler)	1	60	3
Fudge Stripes (Keebler)	1	50	3
Fudge'n Nut Brownies, Almost Home (Nabisco)	1	160	7
Fudge'n Vanilla Creme Sandwiches, Almost Home (Nabisco)	1	140	6
Gaufrettes (LU)	2	85	4

FOOD	PORTION	CALORIES	FAT
Geneva (Pepperidge Farm)	3	190	11
Ginger Boys, Calcium Enriched (FFV)	6	120	3
Ginger Snaps (Sunshine)	5	100	3
Gingerman (Pepperidge Farm)	3	100	4
Gingersnaps (Archway)	1	35	1
Gingersnaps (Archway)	1	25	tr
Golden Bars (Stella D'Oro)	1	111	5
Golden Fruit Raisin Biscuits (Sunshine)	2	150	3
Graham Cinnamon (Sunshine)	4	70	3
Graham Cookies, Bugs Bunny (Nabisco)	9	120	4
Graham Honey (Sunshine)	4	60	2
Grahams, Cinnamon Honey Maid (Nabisco)	2	60	1
Grahams, Honey Maid (Nabisco)	2	60	1
Grahams, Raisin Honey Maid (Nabisco)	2	60	1
Grape Newtons (Nabisco)	1	110	3
Hazelnut (Pepperidge Farm)	3	170	8
Holiday Trinkets (Stella D'Oro)	1	37	2
Honey Graham (Health Valley)	1 oz	100	4

FOOD	PORTION	CALORIES	FAT
Honey Grahams (Keebler)	4	70	2
Hostess Assortment (Stella D'Oro)	1	41	2
Hydrox (Sunshine)	3	160	7
Iced Dutch Apple Fruit Sticks, Almost Home (Nabisco)	1	70	1
Imported Danish Cookies (Nabisco)	5	150	8
Irish Oatmeal (Pepperidge Farm)	3	150	6
Jelly Tarts (FFV)	2	110	4
Kettle Cookies (Nabisco)	4	130	5
Kichel, Dietetic (Stella D'Oro)	1	8	tr
Lady Stella Assortment (Stella D'Oro)	1	42	2
Le Petit-Beurre (LU)	1	40	1
Lemon Coolers (Sunshine)	5	140	6
Lemon Nut Crunch (Pepperidge Farm)	3	180	10
Lido (Pepperidge Farm)	2	180	11
Little Schoolboy (LU)	1	65	3
Love Cookies, Dietetic (Stella D'Oro)	1	110	6
Mallopuffs (Sunshine)	2	140	4

FOOD	PORTION	CALORIES	FAT
Malt (Lance)	1.25 oz	190	10
Margherite, Chocolate (Stella D'Oro)	1	73	3
Margherite, Vanilla (Stella D'Oro)	1	72	3
Marie-Lu (LU)	1	55	2
Marshmallow Puffs (Nabisco)	1	120	4
Marshmallow Sandwich (Nabisco)	4	120	3
Marshmallow Twirls Cakes (Nabisco)	1	130	5
Milano (Pepperidge Farm)	3	130	7
Milk Chocolate Chip (Duncan Hines)	2	110	5
Milk Chocolate Macadamia (Pepperidge Farm)	2	140	8
Milk Lunch (LU)	1	35	1
Mint Creme Chocolate Sandwich, Oreo (Nabisco)	2	140	6
Mint Milano (Pepperidge Farm)	3	120	7
Mint Sandwich (FFV)	2	160	7
Molasses (Archway)	1	100	2
Molasses Crisps (Pepperidge Farm)	3	100	4
Molasses Pantry (Nabisco)	2	130	4

FOOD	PORTION	CALORIES	FAT
Nassau (Pepperidge Farm)	2	170	10
Nilla Wafers (Nabisco)	7	130	4
Nut-O-Lunch (Lance)	1 oz	140	5
Oat Bran Animal Cookies (Health Valley)	1 oz	90	3
Oat Bran Fruit Cookies (Health Valley)	1 oz	110	4
Oat Bran Fruit Jumbos (Health Valley)	½ oz	70	2
Oat Bran Graham Crackers (Health Valley)	1.1 oz	100	3
Oat Bran Honey Jumbos (Health Valley)	½ oz	70	2
Oatmeal (Archway)	1	110	3
Oatmeal (Lance)	1 pkg (1 oz)	130	5
Oatmeal (Little Debbie)	1 pkg (2.75 oz)	340	12
Oatmeal Apple Filled (Archway)	1	90	1
Oatmeal Bakers Bonus (Nabisco)	2	130	5
Oatmeal Calcium Enriched (FFV)	5	130	5
Oatmeal Chocolate Chip, Almost Home (Nabisco)	2	130	5
Oatmeal Country Style (Sunshine)	2	110	5
Oatmeal Cremes (Keebler)	1	80	3

FOOD	PORTION	CALORIES	FAT
Oatmeal Date Filled (Archway)	1	100	2
Oatmeal Peanut Sandwich (Sunshine)	2	140	6
Oatmeal Raisin (Duncan Hines)	2	110	5
Oatmeal Raisin (Pepperidge Farm)	3	170	7
Oatmeal Raisin, Almost Home (Nabisco)	2	130	5
Oatmeal Raisin Bar (Tastykake)	1	224	8
Old Fashioned Ginger Snaps (Nabisco)	4	120	3
Old Fashioned Oatmeal (Keebler)	1	80	3
Old Fashioned Sugar, Almost Home (Nabisco)	2	130	5
Orange Milano (Pepperidge Farm)	3	230	13
Original Chips n' More (Nabisco)	2	150	8
Original Pirouettes (Pepperidge Farm)	2	110	6
Orleans (Pepperidge Farm)	3	100	5
Palmito (LU)	1	50	3
Paris (Pepperidge Farm)	2	100	5
Party Grahams Cookies n' Fudge (Nabisco)	3	140	7
Pecan Shortbread (Nabisco)	2	150	9
Peach-Apricot Pastry (Stella D'Oro)	1	96	4

FOOD	PORTION	CALORIES	FAT
Peach-Apricot Pastry, Dietetic (Stella D'Oro)	1	90	4
Peanut Bars, Heyday (Nabisco)	1	140	8
Peanut Butter & Honey Wafers (Sunbelt)	1 pkg (1.2 oz)	160	8
Peanut Butter Chocolate Chip, Almost Home (Nabisco)	2	140	6
Peanut Butter Creme Filled Wafer (Lance)	1 pkg (1.75 oz)	240	10
Peanut Butter Fudge, Almost Home (Nabisco)	2	140	7
Peanut Butter Jumbo (Health Valley)	½ oz	70	2
Peanut Butter Sandwich (FFV)	2	170	8
Peanut Butter Sandwich, Nutter Butter (Nabisco)	2	140	6
Peanut Butter Wafers (Sunshine)	3	120	6
Peanut Creme Patties, Nutter Butter (Nabisco)	4	150	8
Pecan Crunch (Archway)	1	35	1
Pecan Sandie (Keebler)	1	85	5
Pfeffernusse (Stella D'Oro)	1	34	tr
Pims (LU)	1	50	1
Pitter Patter (Keebler)	1	90	4
Prune Pastry, Dietetic (Stella D'Oro)	1	90	4

FOOD	PORTION	CALORIES	FAT
Pure Chocolate Chip Chips Chips Ahoy (Nabisco)	3	140	7
Pure Chocolate Middles (Nabisco)	2	150	8
Raisin Bran (Pepperidge Farm)	3	160	8
Raisin Oatmeal (Archway)	1	35	1
Real Chocolate Chip, Almost Home (Nabisco)	2	130	5
Regal Grahams (FFV)	2	140	7
Rich 'n Chips (Keebler)	1	80	4
Roman Egg Biscuits, Anise (Stella D'Oro)	1	138	5
Roman Egg Biscuits, Rum & Brandy (Stella D'Oro)	1	138	5
Roman Egg Biscuits, Vanilla (Stella D'Oro)	1	138	5
Royal Dainty (FFV)	2	120	6
Royal Nuggets, Dietetic (Stella D'Oro)	1	1	tr
Sandwich Cookies (Estee)	1	44–50	2–3
Sandwich Cookies, Mystic Mint (Nabisco)	2	150	8
Schoks-Chocolate (LU)	1	70	4
Select Assortment (Archway)	1	60	2
Sesame Cookies (Stella D'Oro)	1	48	2

FOOD	PORTION	CALORIES	FAT
Sesame Cookies, Dietetic (Stella D'Oro)	1	43	2
Seville (Pepperidge Farm)	2	100	5
Shortbread (Pepperidge Farm)	3	130	7
Shortbread, Lorna Doone (Nabisco)	4	140	7
Sociables (Nabisco)	6	70	3
Social Tea (Nabisco)	6	130	4
Soft'n Chewy Chocolate Chocolate Chip (Tastykake)	1	199	7
Soft'n Chewy Chocolate Chip (Tastykake)	1	188	8
Soft'n Chewy Oatmeal Raisin (Tastykake)	1	207	8
Southport (Pepperidge Farm)	2	170	10
Sprinkles (Sunshine)	2	130	3
Strawberry (Lance)	1 pkg (1 oz)	120	4
Strawberry Fruit (Pepperidge Farm)	3	160	6
Strawberry Newtons (Nabisco)	1	110	2
Strawberry Snack Wafer (Estee)	1	80	4
Striped Chocolate Chip Cookies 'n Fudge (Nabisco)	3	150	8
Striped Pure Chocolate Chip Chips Ahoy! (Nabisco)	2	150	8

FOOD	PORTION	CALORIES	FAT
Striped Shortbread Cookies 'n Fudge (Nabisco)	3	150	7
Sugar (Pepperidge Farm)	3	150	7
Sugar Wafers (Sunshine)	3	130	6
Sugar Wafers, Biscos (Nabisco)	8	150	7
Sugar Wafers, Chocolate (Tastykake)	1 pkg	367	19
Sugar Wafers, Vanilla (Tastykake)	1 pkg	366	20
Sugared Egg Biscuits (Stella D'Oro)	1	73	1
Swiss Fudge (Stella D'Oro)	1	68	3
T.C. Rounds (FFV)	2	160	8
Tahiti (Pepperidge Farm)	2	180	11
Tango (FFV)	2	160	5
Tofu Cookies (Health Valley)	1.2 oz	130	5
Trolley Cakes, Devilsfood (FFV)	2	120	2
Van-O-Lunch (Lance)	1 5/16 oz	180	7
Van-O-Lunch (Lance)	1 oz	140	4
Vanilla Creme Filled Wafer (Estee)	1	20	1
Vanilla Fig Bars (FFV)	1	60	1
Vanilla Flavored Creme Sandwiches, Cookie Break (Nabisco)	3	140	6

FOOD	PORTION	CALORIES	FAT
Vanilla Giggles (Nabisco)	2	140	6
Vanilla Shortbread (Tastykake)	1	57	3
Vanilla Snack Wafer (Estee)	1	80	4
Vanilla Wafers (FFV)	8	120	5
Vanilla Wafers (Keebler)	3	60	3
Vanilla Wafers (Sunshine)	6	130	6
Vienna Finger Sandwich (Sunshine)	2	140	6
Waffle Cremes, Biscos (Nabisco)	3	150	7
Walnut Chocolate Chip, Almost Home (Nabisco)	2	140	7
Wheat Free (Health Valley)	1.5 oz	160	6
Whole Wheat Fig Bars (FFV)	1	60	1
chocolate oatmeal	1 (½ oz)	66	4
fig bar	1 (½ oz)	49	tr
ginger snap	1 (¼ oz)	30	1
graham cracker	4	108	3
graham cracker, chocolate covered	2	123	6
lady finger	1	40	tr
macaroon	1 (½ oz)	54	2
REFRIGERATED Chocolate Chip (Pillsbury)	3	210	10
Oatmeal Raisin (Pillsbury)	3	200	8

FOOD	PORTION	CALORIES	FAT
Peanut Butter (Pillsbury)	3	200	8
Sugar (Pillsbury)	3	200	8

CORN

FOOD	PORTION	CALORIES	FAT
CANNED			
Cream Style (Libby)	½ cup	80	0
Cream Style (Owatonna)	½ cup	100	1
Cream Style, Premium Homestyle (S&W)	½ cup	105	1
Whole Kernel (Libby)	½ cup	80	1
Whole Kernel (Seneca)	½ cup	80	1
Whole Kernel in Brine (Owatonna)	½ cup	90	1
Whole Kernel Natural Pack (Libby)	½ cup	80	1
Whole Kernel Natural Pack (Seneca)	½ cup	80	1
Whole Kernel, Premium Homestyle (S&W)	½ cup	90	1
Whole Kernel Vacuum Pack (Owatonna)	½ cup	100	1
corn	½ cup	93	tr
corn, sweet	½ cup	66	1
cream style	½ cup	93	tr
FRESH			
corn sweet; cooked	1 ear (2.5 oz)	83	1
sweet kernel; raw	½ cup	66	tr

FOOD	PORTION	CALORIES	FAT
FROZEN			
Cob Corn (Ore Ida)	1 ear (5.3 oz)	180	2
Corn Cob (Birds Eye)	1 ear (4.4 oz)	120	tr
Corn Cob Little Ears (Birds Eye)	2 ears (4.6 oz)	126	1
Corn, Country Style (Budget Gourmet)	5.57 oz	140	5
Corn Fritters (Mrs. Paul's)	2	250	12
Corn On The Cob Natural Ears (Birds Eye)	1 ear (5.7 oz)	156	1
Corn, Sweet, In Butter Sauce (Budget Gourmet)	5.5 oz	190	6
Kernels; cooked (Health Valley)	5.8 oz	134	tr
White Shoepeg (Hanover)	½ cup	80	0
White Sweet (Hanover)	½ cup	80	0
Whole Kernel Tendersweet (Birds Eye)	½ cup	82	tr
Whole Kernel Cut (Birds Eye)	½ cup	82	tr
Yellow Sweet (Hanover)	½ cup	80	0
frzn; not prep	½ cup	67	tr
on-the-cob; cooked	1 ear (2.2 oz)	59	tr
on-the-cob; not prep	1 ear (4.4 oz)	123	tr
HOME RECIPE			
fritters	1 (1 oz)	62	2
scalloped	½ cup	258	7

FOOD	PORTION	CALORIES	FAT
CORN CHIPS (*see* CHIPS)			
CORNISH HEN (*see* CHICKEN)			
CORNMEAL			
Albers White	1 oz	100	0
Albers Yellow	1 oz	100	0
CORNSTARCH			
Argo	1 Tbsp	30	tr
Argo	1 cup	460	tr
Kingsford's	1 Tbsp	30	tr
Kingsford's	1 cup	460	tr
COTTAGE CHEESE			
REDUCED CALORIE			
Borden Dry Curd, .5%	½ cup	80	1
Formagg Cottage	1 oz	80	2
Friendship Lactose Reduced Lowfat	½ cup	90	1
Friendship Large Curd, Pot Style, Lowfat	½ cup	100	2
Friendship, Lowfat	½ cup	90	1
Friendship, Lowfat, No Salt Added	½ cup	90	1
Friendship 'N Fruit	6 oz	100	1
Land O'Lakes, 2% Fat	4 oz	100	2
Light n' Lively Low Fat 1%	4 oz	80	1
Lite-Line Lowfat 1½%	½ cup	90	2
lowfat, 1%	4 oz	82	1
lowfat, 1%	1 cup	164	2

FOOD	PORTION	CALORIES	FAT
lowfat, 2%	4 oz	101	2
lowfat, 2%	1 cup	203	4
REGULAR			
Borden	½ cup	120	5
Borden Unsalted	½ cup	120	5
Friendship, California Style	½ cup	120	5
Friendship w/ Pineapple	½ cup	140	4
Land O'Lakes Pot Cheese	4 oz	120	5
Sargento Pot Cheese	1 oz	26	tr
creamed	½ cup	109	5
creamed	1 cup	217	9
creamed w/ fruit	4 oz	140	4
dry curd	1 cup	123	tr

COWPEAS

CANNED			
common	1 cup	184	1
common w/ pork	½ cup	99	2
DRIED			
catjang, raw	1 cup	572	3
catjang, cooked	1 cup	200	1
common, raw	1 cup	562	2
common; cooked	1 cup	198	1
FROZEN			
cowpeas	½ cup	112	tr

CRAB

CANNED			
blue	3 oz	84	1
blue	1 cup	133	2

FOOD	PORTION	CALORIES	FAT
FRESH			
Alaska king, raw	3 oz	71	1
Alaska king, cooked	3 oz	82	1
Alaska king, raw	1 leg (6 oz)	144	1
Alaska king; cooked	1 leg (4.7 oz)	129	2
blue, raw	3 oz	74	1
blue, raw	1 crab (.7 oz)	18	tr
blue; cooked	3 oz	87	2
blue; cooked	1 cup	138	2
dungeness, raw	1 crab	140	2
dungeness, raw	3 oz	73	1
queen, raw	3 oz	76	1
FROZEN			
Crab Crisp (King & Prince)	4 oz	310	19
Crab Del Rey (King & Prince)	2 oz	102	6
Crab Del Rey (King & Prince)	3 oz	153	9
Crab Del Rey (King & Prince)	4 oz	205	12
Deviled Crab (Mrs. Paul's)	1 piece	190	8
Deviled Crab Miniatures (Mrs. Paul's)	3.5 oz	250	12
HOME RECIPE			
deviled	½ cup	182	12
imperial	½ cup	162	8
stew	1 cup	208	14
stuffed	¾ cup	129	6
READY-TO-USE			
crab cakes	1 cake (2.1 oz)	93	5

FOOD	PORTION	CALORIES	FAT
CRABAPPLE			
sliced; raw	1 cup	83	tr
CRACKER CRUMBS			
Cracker Meal (Lance)	1 oz	100	1
Cracker Meal (Nabisco)	2 Tbsp	50	0
Graham (Nabisco)	2 Tbsp	60	1
Graham (Sunshine)	1 oup	550	14
cracker meal	1 cup	538	12
CRACKERS (see also CRACKER CRUMBS)			
6 Calorie Wafer (Estee)	1	6	tr
Armenian Thin Bread (Venus)	2	100	1
Bacon Flavored Thins (Nabisco)	7	70	4
Better Blue Cheese (Nabisco)	10	70	4
Better Cheddars (Nabisco)	11	70	4
Better Cheddars, Low Salt (Nabisco)	10	70	4
Better Cheddars 'n Bacon (Nabisco)	10	70	4
Better Cheddars 'n Onion (Nabisco)	10	70	3
Better Nacho (Nabisco)	9	70	4

FOOD	PORTION	CALORIES	FAT
Better Swiss (Nabisco)	10	70	4
Bonnie (Lance)	1 3/16 oz	160	6
Captain Wafers (Lance)	2	30	1
Captain Wafers, Very Low Sodium (Lance)	2	30	1
Captain's Wafers w/ Cream Cheese & Chives (Lance)	1 5/16 oz	170	9
Cheddar American Heritage (Sunshine)	5	80	4
Cheddar Cheese Quackers (Nabisco)	28	70	3
Cheddar Crackers (Estee)	½ oz	70	4
Cheddar Thins (FFV)	7	70	2
Cheese 'n Chive Dip In A (Nabisco)	8	70	4
Cheese 'n Chives Great Crisps (Nabisco)	9	70	4
Cheese n' Crackers (Handi-Snacks)	1 pkg	130	9
Cheese Wheels (Health Valley)	1 oz	140	9
Cheese-On-Wheat (Lance)	1 5/16 oz	180	9
Cheez-It (Sunshine)	12	70	4
Chicken In A Basket (Nabisco)	7	70	4
Cinnamon Treats (Nabisco)	2	60	1

FOOD	PORTION	CALORIES	FAT
Club (Keebler)	4	60	3
Cracked Wheat (Pepperidge Farm)	4	110	4
Cracker Wheat American Classic (Nabisco)	4	70	3
Crown Pilot (Nabisco)	1	60	1
Dairy Butter American Classic (Nabisco)	4	70	3
Dark Finn Crisp Bread (Ryvita)	2	38	tr
Dark Rye Finn Crisp Bread (Ryvita)	1	26	tr
Dark w/ Caraway Seeds Finn Crisp Bread (Ryvita)	2	38	tr
Double Cheddar (FFV)	7	70	2
English Water (North Castle)	1	10	0
English Water Biscuits (Pepperidge Farm)	4	70	1
Escort (Nabisco)	3	80	4
French Onion Great Crisps (Nabisco)	7	70	4
Gold-N-Chee, Spicy (Lance)	15	70	3
Golden Sesame American Classic (Nabisco)	4	70	3
Grahams (Nabisco)	2	60	1
Ham & Cheese Crispy Wafers (FFV)	7	70	2
Harvest Wheats (Keebler)	3	70	4

FOOD	PORTION	CALORIES	FAT
Hearty Wheat (Pepperidge Farm)	4	100	4
Herb, No Salt (Health Valley)	1 oz	120	6
Hi Ho (Sunshine)	4	80	5
High Fiber Crisp Bread (Ryvita)	1	23	tr
High Fiber Snackbread (Ryvita)	1	14	tr
Holland Rusk (Nabisco)	1	60	1
Italian Great Crisps (Nabisco)	9	70	4
Krispy Saltine (Sunshine)	5	60	1
Krispy Unsalted Tops (Sunshine)	5	60	1
Lanchee (Lance)	1.25 oz	180	10
Light Rye Crisp Bread (Ryvita)	1	26	tr
Light Rye Hi-Fiber Crispbread (Finn Crisp)	1	35	1
Lunch Milk Royal (Nabisco)	1	60	2
Malted Milk Peanut Butter Sandwich (Nabisco)	2	70	3
Melba Toast, Oblong (Lance)	2	30	0
Melba Toast, Round, Garlic (Lance)	2	20	1
Melba Toast, Round, Onion (Lance)	2	20	1
Melba Toast, Round, Plain (Lance)	2	20	1

FOOD	PORTION	CALORIES	FAT
Melba Toast, Sesame (Lance)	2	25	1
Nacho Great Crisps (Nabisco)	8	70	4
Nekot (Lance)	1.5 oz	210	10
Nip-Chee (Lance)	1⁵⁄₁₆ oz	180	9
Norwegian Crispbread, Rye-Bran Style (Kavli)	2	30	tr
Norwegian Crispbread, Thick Slice (Kavli)	1	35	tr
Norwegian Crispbread, Thin Style Thin Style (Kavli)	2	40	tr
Nutty Wheat Thins (Nabisco)	7	80	5
Ocean Crisp (FFV)	1	60	1
Original Quackers (Nabisco)	28	70	3
Original Wheat Snackbread (Ryvita)	1	20	tr
Oyster (Nabisco)	37	124	3
Oyster & Soup (Sunshine)	16	60	2
Oyster Crackers (Lance)	½ oz	70	2
Oysterettes (Nabisco)	18	60	1
Parmesan American Heritage (Sunshine)	4	70	4
Party Crackers (Estee)	½ oz	40	4

FOOD	PORTION	CALORIES	FAT
Peanut Butter 'n Cheese Crackers (Handi-Snacks)	1 pkg	190	13
Peanut Butter Toasty Crackers (Little Debbie)	1 pkg (.93 oz)	140	7
Peanut Butter Toasty Crackers (Little Debbie)	1 pkg (1.4 oz)	200	12
Peanut Butter Wheat (Lance)	1⁵⁄₁₆ oz	190	10
Pepato Flavor Tuscany Toast (Tuscany)	1 oz	93	2
Pesto Flavor Tuscany Toast (Tuscany)	1 oz	96	2
Pita Crisps (Tuscany)	1 oz	90	1
Pizza Nips (Nabisco)	20	70	3
Real Bacon Great Crisps (Nabisco)	9	70	4
Real Cheddar Nips (Nabisco)	13	70	3
Ritz (Nabisco)	9	149	8
Ritz (Nabisco)	4	70	4
Ritz Cheese (Nabisco)	5	70	3
Ritz Bits (Nabisco)	22	80	5
Ritz Low Salt (Nabisco)	4	70	4
Round Toast (Planters)	1 oz	140	7
Rye Twins (Lance)	2	30	1
Rye-Chee (Lance)	1⁷⁄₁₆ oz	190	9

FOOD	PORTION	CALORIES	FAT
Rykrisp (Ralston)	4	91	tr
Saltine Low Salt (Nabisco)	5	60	2
Saltine Premium (Nabisco)	5	60	2
Saltines (Lance)	2	25	1
Saltines, Slug Pack (Lance)	4	50	1
Savory Garlic Great Crisps (Nabisco)	8	70	3
Sea Rounds (Nabisco)	1	60	2
Sesame (Health Valley)	1 oz	130	6
Sesame (Pepperidge Farm)	4	80	3
Sesame & Cheese Twigs (Nabisco)	5	70	4
Sesame American Heritage (Sunshine)	4	70	4
Sesame Bread Wafers, Meal Mates (Nabisco)	3	70	3
Sesame Crackers (Estee)	½ oz	40	4
Sesame Crisp (FFV)	2	120	3
Sesame Great Crisps (Nabisco)	9	70	4
Sesame Pita Crisps (Tuscany)	1 oz	96	2
Sesame Twins (Lance)	2	40	1
Snack Sticks, Cheese (Pepperidge Farm)	8	130	6

FOOD	PORTION	CALORIES	FAT
Snack Sticks, Original (Pepperidge Farm)	8	130	5
Snack Sticks, Pumpernickel (Pepperidge Farm)	8	130	4
Snack Sticks, Sesame (Pepperidge Farm)	8	130	5
Soda, Sultana (Nabisco)	4	60	1
Soup & Oyster Dandy (Nabisco)	20	60	1
Sour Cream & Onion Great Crisps (Nabisco)	8	70	4
Sour Cream & Onion Quackers (Nabisco)	28	70	4
Square Cheese (Planters)	1 oz	140	7
Stoned Wheat (FFV)	4	60	1
Stoned Wheat (Health Valley)	1 oz	120	6
Taco Nips (Nabisco)	14	70	4
Tam Tams (Manischewitz)	10	147	8
Tam Tams, No Salt (Manischewitz)	5	70	4
Tams Garlic (Manischewitz)	10	153	8
Tams Onion (Manischewitz)	10	150	8
Tams Wheat (Manischewitz)	10	150	8
Thin Wheat Snacks (Lance)	7	80	4
Three Cracker Assortment (Pepperidge Farm)	4	100	4

FOOD	PORTION	CALORIES	FAT
Tid-Bit Cheese (Nabisco)	16	70	4
Tiny Goldfish, Cheddar (Pepperidge Farm)	45	140	6
Tiny Goldfish, Original (Pepperidge Farm)	40	140	7
Tiny Goldfish, Parmesan Cheese (Pepperidge Farm)	45	130	6
Tiny Goldfish, Pizza (Pepperidge Farm)	45	140	7
Tiny Goldfish, Pretzel (Pepperidge Farm)	40	120	3
Toastchee (Lance)	1⅜ oz	190	10
Toasted Poppy American Classic (Nabisco)	4	70	3
Toasted Rye (Keebler)	5	80	4
Toasted Sesame (Keebler)	5	80	4
Toasted Sesame Rye Crisp Bread (Ryvita)	1	31	tr
Toasted Wheat (Keebler)	5	80	4
Toasted Wheat w/ Onion (Pepperidge Farm)	4	80	3
Toasty (Lance)	1.25 oz	180	10
Tomato & Celery Great Crisps (Nabisco)	9	70	4
Tomato-Flavor Tuscany Toast (Tuscany)	1 oz	95	2
Town House (Keebler)	9	157	9
Town House (Keebler)	5	80	5

FOOD	PORTION	CALORIES	FAT
Triscuit (Nabisco)	7	143	5
Triscuit (Nabisco)	3	60	2
Triscuit, Low Salt (Nabisco)	3	60	2
Tuc (Keebler)	3	70	4
Tuscany Toast (Tuscany)	1 oz	95	2
Uneeda Biscuit, Unsalted Tops (Nabisco)	3	60	2
Unsalted (Estee)	2	30	1
Unsalted Tops, Premium (Nabisco)	5	60	2
Vegetable Thins (Nabisco)	7	70	4
Waldorf Low Salt (Keebler)	9	130	4
Waverly (Nabisco)	4	70	3
Wheat American Heritage (Sunshine)	4	60	3
Wheat Crispy Wafers (FFV)	6	70	3
Wheat Thins (Nabisco)	8	70	3
Wheat Thins, Cheese (Nabisco)	9	70	3
Wheat Thins, Low Salt (Nabisco)	8	70	3
Wheat Twins (Lance)	2	30	1
Wheat Wafers (Sunshine)	8	80	4

FOOD	PORTION	CALORIES	FAT
Wheatswafer (Lance)	4	60	2
Wheatswafer (Lance)	2	30	1
Wheatsworth (Nabisco)	5	70	3
Zesta Saltine (Keebler)	5	60	2
Zwieback (Nabisco)	2	60	1
melba toast	1	20	tr
saltine	10	121	3
SNACK			
Cheese Crackers w/ Peanut Butter (Little Debbie)	1 pkg (.93 oz)	130	6
Cheese Crackers w/ Peanut Butter (Little Debbie)	1 pkg (1.4 oz)	190	9
Cheese Peanut Butter Sandwich (Nabisco)	2	70	3
Toasted Peanut Butter Sandwich (Nabisco)	2	70	4

CRANBERRY

FOOD	PORTION	CALORIES	FAT
CANNED			
Cranberry Sauce, Jellied, Old Fashioned (S&W)	¼ cup	90	0
Cranberry Sauce, Whole Berry Old Fashioned (S&W)	¼ cup	90	0
CranOrange (Ocean Spray)	2 oz	100	0
CranRaspberry (Ocean Spray)	2 oz	90	0
Jellied Cranberry Sauce (Ocean Spray)	2 oz	90	0

FOOD	PORTION	CALORIES	FAT
Whole Berry Sauce (Ocean Spray)	2 oz	90	0
cranberry sauce, sweetened	½ cup	209	tr
FRESH Fresh Cranberries (Ocean Spray)	¼ cup	25	0
cranberries; chopped	1 cup	54	tr
JUICE Cranberry (Smucker's)	8 oz	130	0

CRANBERRY BEANS

FOOD	PORTION	CALORIES	FAT
CANNED cranberry beans	½ cup	108	tr
DRIED cooked	½ cup	120	tr
raw	½ cup	328	1

CRAYFISH

FOOD	PORTION	CALORIES	FAT
cooked	3 oz	97	1
raw	3 oz	76	1
raw	8	24	tr

CREAM

(*see also* SOUR CREAM, SOUR CREAM SUBSTITUTE, WHIPPED TOPPING)

FOOD	PORTION	CALORIES	FAT
LIQUID Half & Half (Land O'Lakes)	1 Tbsp	20	2
Whipping Cream (Land O'Lakes)	1 Tbsp	45	5
Whipping Cream, Gourmet Heavy (Land O'Lakes)	1 Tbsp	60	6
half & half	1 Tbsp	20	2

FOOD	PORTION	CALORIES	FAT
half & half	1 cup	315	28
heavy whipping	1 Tbsp	52	6
light coffee	1 Tbsp	29	3
light whipping	1 Tbsp	44	5
medium, 25% fat	1 Tbsp	37	4
WHIPPED heavy whipping	1 cup	411	44
light whipping	1 cup	345	37

CREAM CHEESE

FOOD	PORTION	CALORIES	FAT
LIGHT REDUCED FAT			
Better Than Cream Cheese, French Onion (Tofutti)	1 oz	80	8
Better Than Cream Cheese, Herb & Chive (Tofutti)	1 oz	80	8
Better Than Cream Cheese, Plain (Tofutti)	1 oz	80	8
Formagg, Cream Cheese Style	1 oz	80	7
Philadelphia Brand Light Cream Cheese Product	1 oz	60	5
NEUFCHATEL Neufchatel (Kraft)	1 oz	80	7
neufchatel	1 oz	74	7
REGULAR Philadelphia Brand	1 oz	100	10
Philadelphia Brand w/ Chives	1 oz	90	9
Philadelphia Brand w/ Pimentos	1 oz	90	9
cream cheese	1 oz	99	10

FOOD	PORTION	CALORIES	FAT
SOFT			
Friendship	1 oz	103	10
Philadelphia Brand	1 oz	100	10
Philadelphia Brand w/ Chives & Onion	1 oz	100	9
Philadelphia Brand w/ Honey	1 oz	100	8
Philadelphia Brand w/ Olives & Pimento	1 oz	90	8
Philadelphia Brand w/ Pineapple	1 oz	90	8
Philadelphia Brand w/ Smoked Salmon	1 oz	90	8
Philadelphia Brand w/ Strawberries	1 oz	90	8
WHIPPED			
Philadelphia Brand	1 oz	100	10
Philadelphia Brand w/ Bacon & Horseradish	1 oz	90	9
Philadelphia Brand w/ Blue Cheese	1 oz	100	9
Philadelphia Brand w/ Chives	1 oz	90	9
Philadelphia Brand w/ Onions	1 oz	90	8
Philadelphia Brand w/ Pimentos	1 oz	90	8
Philadelphia Brand w/ Smoked Salmon	1 oz	100	9

CREPES

basic crepe, unfilled (home recipe)	1	75	2

CRESS
(*see also* WATERCRESS)

garden, raw	½ cup	8	tr
garden; cooked	½ cup	16	tr

FOOD	PORTION	CALORIES	FAT

CROAKER

FOOD	PORTION	CALORIES	FAT
Atlantic, raw	3 oz	89	3
Atlantic, raw	1 fillet (2.8 oz)	83	3
HOME RECIPE Atlantic; breaded & fried	1 fillet (3.1 oz)	192	11
Atlantic; breaded & fried	3 oz	188	11

CROISSANT

FOOD	PORTION	CALORIES	FAT
Colonial Wheat Croissants (Rainbo)	1	300	19
L'Original All Butter (Sara Lee)	1	170	9
L'Original All Butter, Petite Size (Sara Lee)	1	120	6
L'Original All Butter, Pre-Sliced (Sara Lee)	1	170	9
L'Original Cheese (Sara Lee)	1	170	9
Le Pastrie Cinnamon-Nut Raisin (Sara Lee)	1	350	17
Le San*wich Chicken & Broccoli (Sara Lee)	1	340	17
Le San*wich Ham & Swiss Cheese (Sara Lee)	1	340	18
Le San*wich Turkey, Bacon & Cheese (Sara Lee)	1	370	20
croissant	1	235	12

CROUTONS

FOOD	PORTION	CALORIES	FAT
Cheese & Garlic (Pepperidge Farm)	½ oz	70	3
Croutettes (Kellogg)	1 cup	144	tr

FOOD	PORTION	CALORIES	FAT
Onion & Garlic (Pepperidge Farm)	½ oz	70	3
Seasoned (Pepperidge Farm)	½ oz	70	3

CUCUMBER

raw	1	39	tr
raw; sliced	½ cup	7	tr

CURRANTS

dried, Zante	1 cup	204	tr
fresh	½ cup	36	tr

CUSK

raw	3 oz	74	1
raw	1 fillet (4.3 oz)	106	1

CUSTARD

Custard; as prep w/ skim milk (Delmark)	½ cup	97	tr
baked (home recipe)	½ cup	152	7
custard; as prep from mix	½ cup	161	5
zabaglione (home recipe)	½ cup	159	7

CUTTLEFISH

raw	3 oz	67	1

DANDELION GREENS

cooked	½ cup	17	tr
chopped, raw	½ cup	13	tr

FOOD	PORTION	CALORIES	FAT

DANISH PASTRY

fruit	1 (2.3 oz)	235	13
plain	1 (2 oz)	220	12
plain ring	1 (12 oz)	1305	71

DATES

DRIED Chopped (Dromedary)	¼ cup	130	0
Dates, California Deglet Noor	10	240	0
Dates, Diced (Bordo)	2 oz	203	1
Pitted (Dromedary)	5	100	0
chopped	1 cup	489	1

DIETING AIDS
(see NUTRITIONAL SUPPLEMENTS)

DINNER
(see also ITALIAN FOOD, MEXICAN FOOD, ORIENTAL FOOD, PASTA DINNERS, POT PIE)

FOOD	PORTION	CALORIES	FAT
FROZEN Armour BBQ Chicken	10 oz	280	8
Armour Beef Stroganoff	10 oz	320	12
Armour Boneless Beef Short Ribs	10.5 oz	390	19
Armour Chicken Fricassee	11.75 oz	340	11
Armour Chicken & Noodles	12 oz	340	13
Armour Chicken Hawaiian	10.5 oz	280	5
Armour Chicken Milan	11.5 oz	320	10
Armour Chicken w/ Wine & Mushroom Sauce	10.75 oz	350	18

FOOD	PORTION	CALORIES	FAT
Armour Classics, Lite Steak Diane	10 oz	290	9
Armour Ham Steak	11 oz	350	13
Armour Salisbury Steak	11 oz	460	25
Armour Seafood Newburg	11.5 oz	300	12
Armour Sirloin Roast	11 oz	250	8
Armour Sirloin Tips	11 oz	290	10
Armour Swedish Meatballs	12.5 oz	480	27
Armour Turkey & Dressing	11.25 oz	330	14
Armour Veal Parmigiana	10.75 oz	400	22
Armour Yankee Pot Roast	12 oz	390	17
Armour Lite Baby Bay Shrimp	10.5 oz	260	6
Armour Lite Beef Pepper Steak	10.5 oz	260	6
Armour Lite Chicken Breasts Marsala	10.5 oz	250	5
Armour Lite Chicken Breast w/ Mushroom & Tomato Sauce	10 oz	240	5
Armour Lite Chicken Burgundy	10 oz	210	2
Armour Lite Chicken Cacciatore	11 oz	250	4
Armour Lite Chicken Oriental	11 oz	250	4
Armour Lite Chicken Oriental	10 oz	230	2
Armour Lite Salisbury Steak	10 oz	270	13
Armour Lite Seafood w/ Natural Herbs	10.5 oz	220	4
Armour Lite Steak Diane	10 oz	270	9
Armour Lite Sweet & Sour Chicken	10.5 oz	240	2
Banquet All White Meat Fried Chicken Platter	9 oz	430	21
Banquet Beans & Frankfurters Dinner	10 oz	510	25
Banquet Beef Platter	10 oz	460	33
Banquet Boneless Chicken Drumsnacker Platter	7 oz	430	18

FOOD	PORTION	CALORIES	FAT
Banquet Boneless Chicken Nuggets Platter	6.4 oz	425	21
Banquet Chicken Pattie Platter	7.5 oz	370	20
Banquet Chopped Beef Dinner	11 oz	420	31
Banquet Chopped Beef Dinner	11 oz	420	31
Banquet Extra Helping Beef Dinner	16 oz	865	61
Banquet Extra Helping Chicken Nuggets Dinner w/ Barbecue Sauce	10 oz	640	36
Banquet Extra Helping Chicken Nuggets Dinner w/ Sweet & Sour Sauce	10 oz	650	33
Banquet Extra Helping Fried Chicken Dinner	16 oz	560	28
Banquet Extra Helping Fried Chicken Dinner, All White Meat	16 oz	560	28
Banquet Extra Helping Lasagne Dinner	16.5 oz	645	23
Banquet Extra Helping Salisbury Steak Dinner	18 oz	910	60
Banquet Extra Helping Salisbury Steak Dinner w/ Mushroom Gravy	18 oz	890	58
Banquet Extra Helping Turkey Dinner	19 oz	750	41
Banquet Family Favorites, Chicken & Dumplings Dinner	10 oz	420	24
Banquet Family Favorites, Macaroni & Cheese Dinner	10 oz	415	20
Banquet Family Favorites, Noodles & Chicken Dinner	10 oz	340	15
Banquet Family Favorites, Spaghetti & Meatballs Dinner	10 oz	290	9
Banquet Fish Platter	8.75 oz	445	22
Banquet Fried Chicken Dinner	10 oz	400	21
Banquet Ham Platter	10 oz	400	16
Banquet Meat Loaf Dinner	11 oz	440	27

FOOD	PORTION	CALORIES	FAT
Banquet Noodles & Julienne Beef w/ Sauce	7 oz	170	3
Banquet Onion Gravy & Beef Patties	8 oz	300	21
Banquet Pot Pies, Beef, Turkey, Chicken	7 oz	520	31–35
Banquet Salisbury Steak Dinner	11 oz	495	34
Banquet Stroganoff Sauce w/ Beef & Noodles	7 oz	190	6
Banquet Turkey Dinner	10.5 oz	385	20
Banquet Veal Parmigian Patties	8 oz	370	18
Banquet Western Dinner	11 oz	630	40
Banquet Cookin' Bag, Barbecue Sauce & Sliced Beef	4 oz	100	2
Banquet Cookin'Bag, Breaded Veal Parmigiana	4 oz	230	11
Banquet Cookin' Bag, Chicken Ala King	4 oz	110	5
Banquet Cookin' Bag, Cream Chipped Beef	4 oz	100	4
Banquet Cookin' Bag, Gravy & Salisbury Steak	5 oz	190	14
Banquet Cookin' Bag, Gravy & Sliced Beef	4 oz	100	5
Banquet Cookin' Bag, Gravy & Sliced Turkey	5 oz	100	8
Banquet Cookin' Bag, Meat Loaf	4 oz	200	14
Banquet Cookin' Bag, Mushroom Gravy & Charbroiled Beef Patty	5 oz	210	15
Banquet Cookin' Bag, Sweet & Sour Chicken	4 oz	130	2
Budget Gourmet Cheese Manicotti w/ Meat Sauce	10 oz	450	26
Budget Gourmet Chicken Cacciatore	11 oz	300	13
Budget Gourmet Chicken & Egg Noodle w/ Broccoli	10 oz	450	26

FOOD	PORTION	CALORIES	FAT
Budget Gourmet Chicken w/ Fettucini	10 oz	400	21
Budget Gourmet Italian Sausage Lasagna	10 oz	420	20
Budget Gourmet Italian Style Meatballs with Noodles & Peppers	10 oz	310	12
Budget Gourmet Linguini w/ Shrimp	10 oz	330	15
Budget Gourmet Pasta Shells and Beef	10 oz	340	14
Budget Gourmet Pepper Steak w/ Rice	10 oz	300	9
Budget Gourmet Scallops & Shrimp Mariner	11.5 oz	320	9
Budget Gourmet Seafood Newburg	10 oz	350	12
Budget Gourmet Sirloin Salisbury Steak	11.5 oz	410	22
Budget Gourmet Sirloin Tips In Burgundy Sauce	11 oz	310	11
Budget Gourmet Sirloin Tips w/ Country Style Vegetables	10 oz	310	18
Budget Gourmet Sliced Turkey Breast	11.1 oz	290	9
Budget Gourmet Slim Selects, Beef Stroganoff	8.75 oz	280	10
Budget Gourmet Slim Selects, Cheese Ravioli	10 oz	260	7
Budget Gourmet Slim Selects, Chicken Enchilada Suiza	9 oz	270	9
Budget Gourmet Slim Selects, Chicken-Au-Gratin	9.1 oz	260	11
Budget Gourmet Slim Selects, Fettucini w/ Meat Sauce	10 oz	290	10
Budget Gourmet Slim Selects, French Recipe Chicken	10 oz	260	10
Budget Gourmet Slim Selects, Glazed Turkey	9 oz	270	5
Budget Gourmet Slim Selects, Ham & Asparagus Au Gratin	9 oz	280	10

FOOD	PORTION	CALORIES	FAT
Budget Gourmet Slim Selects, Lasagne w/ Meat Sauce	10 oz	290	10
Budget Gourmet Slim Selects, Linguini w/ Scallops & Clams	9.5 oz	280	11
Budget Gourmet Slim Selects, Mandarin Chicken	10 oz	290	6
Budget Gourmet Slim Selects, Oriental Beef	10 oz	290	9
Budget Gourmet Slim Selects, Sirloin Enchilada Ranchero	9 oz	290	15
Budget Gourmet Slim Selects, Sirloin of Beef in Herb Sauce	10 oz	290	12
Budget Gourmet Slim Selects, Sirloin Salisbury Steak	9 oz	280	8
Budget Gourmet Swedish Meatballs w/ Noodles	10 oz	600	39
Budget Gourmet Sweet & Sour Chicken w/ Rice	10 oz	350	7
Budget Gourmet Teriyaki Chicken	12 oz	360	12
Budget Gourmet Three Cheese Lasagne	10 oz	400	17
Budget Gourmet Turkey A La King w/ Rice	10 oz	390	18
Budget Gourmet Veal Parmigiana	12 oz	440	20
Budget Gourmet Yankee Pot Roast	11 oz	380	21
Le Menu Beef Burgundy	7.5 oz	330	23
Le Menu Beef Sirloin Tips	11.5 oz	410	19
Le Menu Beef Stroganoff	10 oz	450	26
Le Menu Breast of Chicken Parmigiana	11.5 oz	390	19
Le Menu Chicken A La King	10.25 oz	330	13
Le Menu Chicken Cordon Bleu	11 oz	470	20
Le Menu Chicken Florentine	12.5 oz	480	24
Le Menu Chicken Kiev	8 oz	530	39

FOOD	PORTION	CALORIES	FAT
Le Menu Chopped Sirloin Beef	12.25 oz	410	19
Le Menu Ham Steak	10 oz	310	11
Le Menu Light Style, Beef A L'Orange	10 oz	290	8
Le Menu Light Style, Flounder Vin Blanc	10 oz	220	5
Le Menu Light Style, Glazed Chicken Breast	10 oz	240	5
Le Menu Light Style, Turkey Divan	10 oz	240	5
Le Menu Oriental Chicken	8.5 oz	260	6
Le Menu Pepper Steak	11.5 oz	380	14
Le Menu Sliced Breast of Turkey w/ Mushrooms	11.25 oz	460	23
Le Menu Stuffed Flounder	10.5 oz	350	18
Le Menu Sweet & Sour Chicken	11.25 oz	460	23
Le Menu Yankee Pot Roast	11 oz	360	15
Lean Cuisine Baked Rigatoni w/ Meat Sauce & Cheese	9.75 oz	260	10
Lean Cuisine Beef & Pork Cannelloni w/ Mornay Sauce	9⅝ oz	270	10
Lean Cuisine Cheese Cannelloni w/ Tomato Sauce	9⅛ oz	270	10
Lean Cuisine Chicken & Vegetables w/ Vermicelli	12.75 oz	270	7
Lean Cuisine Chicken a l'Orange w/ Almond Rice	8 oz	270	5
Lean Cuisine Fillet of Fish Divan	12⅜ oz	270	9
Lean Cuisine Fillet of Fish Florentine	9 oz	240	9
Lean Cuisine Fillet of Fish Jardiniere w/ Souffleed Potatoes	11.25 oz	280	10
Lean Cuisine Glazed Chicken w/ Vegetable Rice	8.5 oz	270	8
Lean Cuisine Herbed Lamb w/ Rice	10⅜ oz	270	8
Lean Cuisine Meatball Stew	10 oz	250	10

FOOD	PORTION	CALORIES	FAT
Lean Cuisine Oriental Beef w/ Vegetables & Rice	8⅝ oz	270	8
Lean Cuisine Salisbury Steak w/ Italian Style Sauce & Vegetables	9.5 oz	270	13
Lean Cuisine Slice Turkey Breast in Mushroom Sauce	8 oz	220	5
Lean Cuisine Spaghetti w/ Beef Mushroom Sauce	11.5 oz	280	7
Lean Cuisine Stuffed Cabbage w/ Meat in Tomato Sauce	10.75 oz	220	9
Lean Cuisine Turkey Dijon	9.5 oz	280	10
Lean Cuisine Vegetable & Pasta w/ Ham	9⅜ oz	280	13
Morton Beans & Franks Dinner	10 oz	360	14
Morton Chicken Wings w/ Corn	6.75 oz	434	25
Morton Fish & Chips	7.75 oz	386	15
Morton Fried Chicken w/ Corn	7.75 oz	472	23
Morton Salisbury Steak w/ Potatoes	7.75 oz	307	18
Morton Sliced Beef w/ Gravy	7.75 oz	248	8
Morton Southern Fried Chicken Nuggets w/ Tater Tots	6.75 oz	472	27
Morton Turkey & Dressing	9 oz	216	4
Mrs. Paul's Fish & Pasta Florentine	9.5 oz	240	9
Mrs. Paul's Fish Au Gratin	10 oz	290	8
Mrs. Paul's Fish Dijon	9.5 oz	280	15
Mrs. Paul's Fish Florentine	9 oz	210	4
Mrs. Paul's Fish Mornay	10 oz	280	14
Sensible Chef Beef Pepper Steak w/ Rice Casserole	9 oz	250	10
Sensible Chef Beef Stroganoff w/ Gravy Casserole	9 oz	240	8
Sensible Chef Beef Tips w/ Vegetable & Noodles Casserole	9 oz	250	9

FOOD	PORTION	CALORIES	FAT
Sensible Chef Chicken & Dumplings	9 oz	330	16
Sensible Chef Chicken Ala King w/ Rice	9 oz	250	8
Swanson Beans & Franks	10.5 oz	420	17
Swanson Beef	11.25 oz	350	8
Swanson Beef in Barbeque Sauce	11 oz	460	15
Swanson Chicken Drumlet	10 oz	570	33
Swanson Chicken Duet Creamy Broccoli	6 oz	310	17
Swanson Chicken Duet Creamy Green Bean	6 oz	330	18
Swanson Chicken Duet Saucy Tomato	6 oz	340	18
Swanson Chicken Duet Savory Wild Rice	6 oz	290	14
Swanson Chicken in Barbeque Sauce	11.75 oz	450	13
Swanson Chicken Nugget Platter	8.75 oz	470	25
Swanson Chopped Sirloin Beef	11 oz	380	20
Swanson Fish n' Chips	10 oz	500	20
Swanson Fish n' Fries	7.25 oz	420	21
Swanson Fish Nugget	9.5 oz	450	23
Swanson Fried Chicken	1 pkg (10.8 oz)	583	31
Swanson Fried Chicken Barbecue Flavored	10 oz	580	27
Swanson Fried Chicken Dark Meat	10 oz	580	28
Swanson Fried Chicken White Meat	10.5 oz	580	27
Swanson Hungry-Man Boneless Chicken	17.75 oz	710	27
Swanson Hungry-Man Chicken Nuggets	16 oz	600	26
Swanson Hungry-Man Chicken Parmigiana	20 oz	810	51
Swanson Hungry-Man Chopped Beef Steak	16.75 oz	590	33

FOOD	PORTION	CALORIES	FAT
Swanson Hungry-Man Fish 'n' Chips	14.75 oz	780	39
Swanson Hungry-Man Fried Chicken Breast Portion	11.75 oz	680	38
Swanson Hungry-Man Fried Chicken Dark Portion	11 oz	630	36
Swanson Hungry-Man Salisbury Steak	11.75 oz	610	38
Swanson Hungry-Man Sliced Beef	12.25 oz	330	8
Swanson Hungry-Man Turkey	13.25 oz	390	14
Swanson Hungry-Man Veal Parmigiana	18.25 oz	630	30
Swanson Hungry-Man Western Style	17.5 oz	740	34
Swanson Loin of Pork	10.75 oz	310	12
Swanson Macaroni & Cheese	12.25 oz	380	15
Swanson Macaroni & Beef	12 oz	370	15
Swanson Meat Loaf	10.75 oz	430	21
Swanson Noodle & Chicken	10.5 oz	270	9
Swanson Plump & Juicy Chicken Cutlets	3 oz	200	12
Swanson Plump & Juicy Chicken Dipsters	3 oz	220	14
Swanson Plump & Juicy Chicken Drumlets	3 oz	220	14
Swanson Plump & Juicy Chicken Nibbles	3.25 oz	300	20
Swanson Plump & Juicy Extra Crispy Fried Chicken	3 oz	250	16
Swanson Plump & Juicy Fried Chicken Assorted Pieces	3.25 oz	270	17
Swanson Plump & Juicy Fried Chicken Breast Portions	4.5 oz	360	21
Swanson Plump & Juicy Take-Out Fried	3.25 oz	270	17

FOOD	PORTION	CALORIES	FAT
Swanson Plump & Juicy Thighs & Drumsticks	3.25 oz	280	19
Swanson Polynesian Style	12 oz	360	8
Swanson Salisbury Steak	10 oz	410	32
Swanson Spaghetti & Meatballs	12.5 oz	370	15
Swanson Swedish Meatballs	9.25 oz	420	30
Swanson Sweet 'n' Sour Chicken	12 oz	390	13
Swanson Swiss Steak	10 oz	350	11
Swanson Turkey	8.75 oz	270	11
Swanson Veal Parmigiana	10 oz	280	15
Swanson Western Style	11.5 oz	440	21
Van De Kamp's Fillet of Fish Dinner	12 oz	300	10
Weight Watchers, Beef Stroganoff	9 oz	340	15
Weight Watchers, Chicken Ala King	9 oz	230	8
Weight Watchers, Chicken Patty Parmigiana	8.06 oz	280	16
Weight Watchers, Chopped Beef Steak	9 oz	280	17
Weight Watchers, Filet of Fish Au Gratin	9.25 oz	210	6
Weight Watchers, Imperial Chicken	9.25 oz	230	4
Weight Watchers, Oven Fried Fish	6.81 oz	220	12
Weight Watchers, Southern Fried Chicken Patty	6.5 oz	270	16
Weight Watchers, Stuffed Sole w/ Newburg Sauce	10.5 oz	310	9
Weight Watchers, Stuffed Turkey Breast	8.5 oz	270	10
Weight Watchers Sweet 'N Sour Chicken Tenders	10.19 oz	250	2
Weight Watchers, Veal Patty Parmigiana	8.44 oz	240	11
chicken fricassee	¾ cup	290	17

FOOD	PORTION	CALORIES	FAT
DIP			
Acapulco (Ortega)	1 oz	8	0
Avocado, Guacamole (Kraft)	2 Tbsp	50	4
Bacon & Horseradish (Kraft)	2 Tbsp	60	5
Bacon & Horseradish, Premium (Kraft)	2 Tbsp	50	5
Blue Cheese, Premium (Kraft)	2 Tbsp	45	4
Clam (Kraft)	2 Tbsp	60	4
Clam, Premium (Kraft)	2 Tbsp	45	4
Creamy Cucumber, Premium (Kraft)	2 Tbsp	50	4
Creamy Onion, Premium (Kraft)	2 Tbsp	45	4
French Onion (Kraft)	2 Tbsp	60	4
French Onion, Premium (Kraft)	2 Tbsp	45	4
Garlic (Kraft)	2 Tbsp	60	4
Green Onion (Kraft)	2 Tbsp	60	4
Jalapeno Flavored Bean (Wise)	2 Tbsp	25	0
Jalapeno Pepper (Kraft)	2 Tbsp	50	4
Jalapeno Pepper, Premium (Kraft)	2 Tbsp	60	5
Nacho Cheese, Premium (Kraft)	2 Tbsp	50	4

FOOD	PORTION	CALORIES	FAT
Picante Sauce (Wise)	2 Tbsp	12	0
Taco (Wise)	2 Tbsp	12	0

DOCK

cooked	3.5 oz	20	tr
chopped, raw	½ cup	15	tr

DOLPHINFISH

raw	1 fillet (7.2 oz)	174	1
raw	3 oz	73	1

DOUGH

Fillo Dough (Athens)	1 oz	74	tr
Plain Wiener Wrap (Pillsbury)	1	60	2

DOUGHNUT
(*see also* DUNKIN' DONUTS, WINCHELL'S)

Cake (Hostess)	1	115	7
Chocolate Covered (Hostess)	1	129	8
Chocolate Dipped (Tastykake)	1	181	10
Cinnamon (Hostess)	1	109	6
Cinnamon (Tastykake)	1	201	9
Cinnamon Apple (Earth Grains)	1	310	17
Coated, Mini (Tastykake)	1	81	5

FOOD	PORTION	CALORIES	FAT
Devil's Food (Earth Grains)	1	330	21
Donut Sticks (Little Debbie)	1 pkg (1.67 oz)	230	13
Donut Sticks (Little Debbie)	1 pkg (2.5 oz)	330	18
Glazed Old Fashioned (Earth Grains)	1	310	18
Honey Wheat, Mini (Tastykake)	1	65	3
Krunch (Hostess)	1	101	4
Old Fashioned (Hostess)	1	172	10
Plain (Tastykake)	1	172	9
Powdered Old Fashioned (Earth Grains)	1	290	19
Powdered Sugar (Hostess)	1	112	6
Powdered Sugar (Tastykake)	1	195	9
Powdered Sugar, Mini (Tastykake)	1	58	3
Premium Fudge Iced (Tastykake)	1	350	21
Premium Honey Wheat (Tastykake)	1	342	18
Premium Orange Glazed (Tastykake)	1	357	20
cake type, plain	1 (1.5 oz)	164	8
cake type, sugared	1 (1.6 oz)	184	8
jelly filled	1 (2.3 oz)	226	9
raised plain	1 (1.5 oz)	174	11

FOOD	PORTION	CALORIES	FAT

DRESSING
(*see* STUFFING/DRESSING)

DRINK MIXER
(*see also* MINERAL/BOTTLED WATER, SODA)

FOOD	PORTION	CALORIES	FAT
Bitter Lemon (Schweppes)	6 oz	78	0
Collins Mixer (Schweppes)	6 oz	70	0
Lemon Sour (Schweppes)	6 oz	75	0
Tonic Water (Schweppes)	6 oz	64	0
Tonic Water Diet (Schweppes)	6 oz	tr	0
whiskey sour mix	2 oz	55	0

DRUM

FOOD	PORTION	CALORIES	FAT
freshwater, raw	3 oz	101	4
freshwater, raw	1 fillet (6.9 oz)	236	10

DUCK

FOOD	PORTION	CALORIES	FAT
meat & skin, raw	½ duck (1.4 lbs)	2561	249
meat & skin, raw	10 oz	1159	113
meat & skin; roasted	6 oz	583	49
meat & skin; roasted	½ duck (13.4 oz)	1287	108
meat, raw	½ duck (10.6 oz)	399	18
meat, raw	4.8 oz	180	8
meat; roasted	3.5 oz	201	11
meat; roasted	½ duck (7.8 oz)	445	25

FOOD	PORTION	CALORIES	FAT
wild, breast meat, raw	½ breast (2.9 oz)	102	4
wild, meat & skin, raw	8.4 oz	505	36
wild, meat & skin, raw	9.5 oz	571	41

DUMPLING

FROZEN

Apple Dumpling (Pepperidge Farm)	3 oz	260	13

HOME RECIPE

apple	1 (10.5 oz)	566	28
dumpling	2 (1 oz)	70	1
pear	1 (10.2 oz)	540	15

EEL

FRESH

cooked	3 oz	200	13
cooked	1 fillet (5.6 oz)	375	24
raw	3 oz	156	10
raw	1 fillet (7.2 oz)	375	24

SMOKED

American smoked eel	1 .75 oz	1	25

EGG

(*see also* EGG DISHES, EGG SUBSTITUTE)

CHICKEN

Lowered Cholesterol (Full Spectrum Farms)	1 lg	60	1
fried w/ butter	1	83	6.4
hard cooked	1	79	5.6
omelet w/ butter & milk	1	95	7
poached	1	79	5.5

FOOD	PORTION	CALORIES	FAT
raw	1	79	5.6
scrambled w/ butter & milk	1	95	7
white only	1	16	tr
white only	1 cup	118	tr
yolk only	1	63	5.6
yolks	1 cup	897	80
OTHER POULTRY			
duck, raw	1	130	9.6
goose, raw	1	267	19
quail, raw	1	14	1
turkey, raw	1	135	9.4

EGG DISHES
(*see also* EGG, EGG SUBSTITUTE)

FOOD	PORTION	CALORIES	FAT
Cheese Omelet (Chefwich)	5 oz	380	17
Egg, Canadian Bacon & Cheese/ Muffin (Great Starts)	4.5 oz	310	16
Ham & Cheese Omelet (Chefwich)	5 oz	340	14
Omelets w/ Cheese Sauce (Great Starts)	7 oz	400	31
Sausage & Cheese Omelet (Chefwich)	5 oz	400	19
Sausage, Egg & Cheese/Biscuit (Great Starts)	6.25 oz	520	32
Scrambled Eggs & Sausage w/ Hashed Brown Potatoes (Great Starts)	6.25 oz	430	34
Spanish Style Omelet (Great Starts)	7.75 oz	250	17
Steak, Egg & Cheese/Muffin (Great Starts)	5.25 oz	390	23

FOOD	PORTION	CALORIES	FAT
Western Style Omelet (Chefwich)	5 oz	350	13
HOME RECIPE			
creamed	½ cup	231	17
deviled	2 halves	145	13
egg foo yong	1 (5.1 oz)	150	10
omelet; as prep from 2 eggs, butter, milk	4.5 oz	189	14
salad	½ cup	307	28

EGG SUBSTITUTE

FOOD	PORTION	CALORIES	FAT
Egg Beaters (Fleischmann's)	¼ cup	25	0
Egg Beaters w/ Cheez (Fleischmann's)	¼ cup	130	6
Egg Watchers (Tofutti)	2 oz	50	2
Eggstra (Tillie Lewis)	2 oz	433	1
Scramblers, frzn (Morningstar Farms)	3.5 oz	105	5
frozen	¼ cup	96	6.7
liquid	1.5 oz	40	1.6
liquid	1 cup	211	8.3
powder	.35 oz	44	1.3
powder	.7 oz	88	2.6

EGGNOG

FOOD	PORTION	CALORIES	FAT
Egg Nog (Borden)	4 oz	160	9
Eggnog (Land O'Lakes)	8 oz	300	15
eggnog	1 cup	342	19

FOOD	PORTION	CALORIES	FAT
eggnog	1 qt	1368	76
eggnog flavor milk; as prep w/ milk	9 oz	260	8

EGGPLANT

FRESH
cooked, cubed	½ cup	13	tr
cut up, raw	½ cup	11	tr

FROZEN
Eggplant Parmigiana (Mrs. Paul's)	5.5 oz	270	17
Fried Eggplant Sticks (Mrs. Paul's)	3.5 oz	240	12

HOME RECIPE
Baba Ghannouj	¼ cup	55	4

ELDERBERRIES

raw	1 cup	105	tr

ENDIVE

chopped, raw	½ cup	4	tr

ENGLISH MUFFIN

Best Foods Regular, Placentia	1	130	1
Pepperidge Farm, Cinnamon Raisin	1	150	2
Pepperidge Farm, Plain	1	140	2
Roman Meal	1	146	2
Shop 'n Save	1	130	1
Thomas' Honey Wheat	1	129	1
Thomas' Raisin	1	153	2
Thomas' Regular	1	130	1
Thomas' Sourdough	1	130	1

FOOD	PORTION	CALORIES	FAT
HOME RECIPE			
plain	1	158	2
cinnamon raisin	1	186	3
honey bran	1	153	3
whole wheat	1	167	tr

FALAFEL

falafel	1 pattie (½ oz)	57	3
falafel	3 patties (1.8 oz)	170	9

FAST FOOD
(*see* INDIVIDUAL NAMES IN PART II)

FAT
(*see also* BUTTER, BUTTER BLENDS, BUTTER SUBSTITUTE, MARGARINE, OIL)

Crisco	1 Tbsp	110	12
Crisco, Butter Flavor	1 Tbsp	110	12
beef fat; cooked	1 oz	193	20
beef suet, raw	1 oz	242	27
chicken fat, raw	1 oz	201	22
chicken fat, raw	from ½ chicken (1.8 oz)	327	35
duck fat	1 Tbsp	115	13
goose fat	1 Tbsp	115	13
lard	1 cup	1849	205
lard	1 Tbsp	115	13
mutton tallow, raw	1 Tbsp	116	13
pork backfat	1 oz	230	25
pork fat	1 oz	200	21
pork fat, cured; roasted	1 oz	167	18

FOOD	PORTION	CALORIES	FAT
pork fat, cured, uncooked	1 oz	164	17
shortening, lard & vegetable oil	1 Tbsp	115	13
shortening, lard & vegetable oil	1 cup	1845	205
shortening, soybean & cottonseed	1 Tbsp	113	13
shortening, soybean & cottonseed	1 cup	1812	205
shortening, soybean & palm	1 cup	1812	205
shortening, soybean & palm	1 Tbsp	113	13
tallow (beef)	1 Tbsp	115	13
tallow (beef)	1 cup	1849	205
turkey fat	1 Tbsp	115	13

FIGS

CANNED			
Kadota Figs, Whole, Fancy (S&W)	½ cup	100	0
DRIED			
cooked	½ cup	140	tr
whole	10	477	2
FRESH			
fig	1 med	50	tr

FILBERTS

dried, blanched	1 oz	191	19
dried, unblanched	1 oz	179	18
dry roasted, unblanched	1 oz	188	19
oil roasted, unblanched	1 oz	187	18

FISH

(*see also* FISH SUBSTITUTE, INDIVIDUAL NAMES)

FROZEN			
Batter-Dipped Fish & Chips (Van De Kamp's)	7 oz	440	25

FOOD	PORTION	CALORIES	FAT
Batter Dipped Fish Fillets (Mrs. Paul's)	2 fillets	390	25
Batter-Dipped Fish Fillets (Van De Kamp's)	1 fillet	180	10
Batter-Dipped Fish Kabobs (Van De Kamp's)	4 oz	240	15
Batter-Dipped Fish Sticks (Van De Kamp's)	4 sticks	220	14
Breaded Fish Fillets (Van De Kamp's)	1 fillet	180	14
Breaded Fish Nuggets (Van De Kamp's)	2 oz	130	8
Breaded Fish Sticks (Gorton's)	4 sticks	210	9
Breaded Fish Sticks (Van De Kamp's)	4 sticks	270	19
Buttered Fish Fillets (Mrs. Paul's)	2 fillets	170	9
Combination Seafood Platter (Mrs. Paul's)	9 oz	590	31
Country Seasoned Fish Fillets (Van De Kamp's)	1 fillet	195	13
Crispy Batter Dipped Fish Fillets (Gorton's)	2 fillets	300	20
Crispy Batter Dipped Fish Sticks (Gorton's)	4 sticks	220	12
Crispy Crunchy Fish Fillets (Mrs. Paul's)	2 fillets	280	16
Crispy Crunchy Fish Sticks (Mrs. Paul's)	4 sticks	200	10
Crunchy Fish Fillets (Gorton's)	2 fillets	350	26
Crunchy Fish Sticks (Gorton's)	4 sticks	220	15
Crunchy Light Batter Fish Fillets (Mrs. Paul's)	2 fillets	310	17

FOOD	PORTION	CALORIES	FAT
Crunchy Light Batter Fish Sticks (Mrs. Paul's)	4 sticks	240	13
Fish Cakes (Mrs. Paul's)	2 cakes	250	11
Fish Cakes, Thins (Mrs. Paul's)	2 cakes	290	13
Light Breaded Fish Fillets (Mrs. Paul's)	1 fillet	290	13
Light Recipe Lightly Breaded Fish Fillets (Gorton's)	1 fillet	170	7
Light Recipe, Tempura Batter Fish Fillets (Gorton's)	1 fillet	190	12
Microwave Chunky Fish Sticks (Gorton's)	6 sticks	340	22
Microwave Crunchy Fish Fillets (Gorton's)	2 fillets	350	26
Potato Crisp Fish Fillets (Gorton's)	2 fillets	340	24
Potato Crisp Fish Sticks (Gorton's)	4 sticks	260	16
Seafood Lover's Fillets Almondine (Gorton's)	1 pkg	410	33
Seafood Lover's Fillets in Herb Butter (Gorton's)	1 pkg	220	14
Seafood Lover's Seafood Stuffed Fillets (Gorton's)	1 pkg	260	13
Supreme Light Batter Fish Fillets (Mrs. Paul's)	1 fillet	210	12
Today's Catch Fish Fillets (Van De Kamp's)	5 oz	100	4
Value Pack Batter Dipped Portions (Gorton's)	1 fillet	200	13

FOOD	PORTION	CALORIES	FAT
Value Pack Fish Sticks (Gorton's)	4 sticks	210	11
breaded fillet; as prep	1 (2 oz)	155	7
sticks; as prep	1 stick (1 oz)	76	3
HOME RECIPE fish loaf; cooked	3.5 oz	124	4

FISH SUBSTITUTE

Fillets, frzn (Worthington)	3.5 oz	209	11
Ocean Fillet (Loma Linda)	1 (1.7 oz)	130	8
Ocean Fillet (Loma Linda)	1 (2 oz)	160	10
Ocean Platter; mix not prep (Loma Linda)	¼ cup	50	1
Vege-Scallops (Loma Linda)	6 pieces (2.75 oz)	70	1

FLATFISH

cooked	1 fillet (4.5 oz)	148	2
cooked	3 oz	99	1
raw	3 oz	78	1
raw	1 fillet (5.7 oz)	149	2

FLOUNDER

FROZEN Au Natural Flounder Fillets (Mrs. Paul's)	4 oz	90	2
Crispy Crunchy Flounder Fillets (Mrs. Paul's)	2 fillets	270	15
Crunchy Light Batter Flounder Fillets (Mrs. Paul's)	2 fillets	310	16

FOOD	PORTION	CALORIES	FAT
Fishmarket Fresh Flounder (Gorton's)	5 oz	110	1
Flounder Primavera (King & Prince)	9 oz	270	13
Flounder Primavera (King & Prince)	6 oz	180	9
Flounder Primavera (King & Prince)	4.5 oz	135	7
Flounder Del Rey (King & Prince)	4.5 oz	163	8
Flounder Del Rey (King & Prince)	9 oz	327	16
Light Breaded Flounder Fillets (Mrs. Paul's)	1 fillet	280	13
Stuffed Flounder (Gorton's)	1 pkg	260	14

FLOUR

FOOD	PORTION	CALORIES	FAT
All Purpose (Ballard)	1 cup	400	1
All Purpose (Pillsbury Best)	1 cup	400	1
All Purpose, Unbleached (Pillsbury Best)	1 cup	400	1
All-Purpose (Gold Medal)	1 cup	400	1
All-Purpose (Red Band)	1 cup	390	1
All-Purpose (White Deer)	1 cup	400	1
Bohemian Style, Rye and Wheat (Pillsbury Best)	1 cup	400	1
Bread (Pillsbury Best)	1 cup	400	2
Drifted Snow (General Mills)	1 cup	400	1

FOOD	PORTION	CALORIES	FAT
High Protein, Better for Bread (Gold Medal)	1 cup	400	1
La Pina (Gold Medal)	1 cup	390	1
Medium Rye (Pillsbury Best)	1 cup	400	2
Sauce 'n Blend (Pillsbury Best)	2 Tbsp	50	0
Self-Rising (Ballard)	1 cup	380	1
Self-Rising (Gold Medal)	1 cup	380	1
Self-Rising (Pillsbury Best)	1 cup	380	1
Self-Rising (Red Band)	1 cup	380	1
Softasilk (General Mills)	¼ cup	100	0
Unbleached (Gold Medal)	1 cup	400	1
White, Self-Rising (Aunt Jemima)	1 cup	479	1
Whole Wheat (Gold Medal)	1 cup	390	2
Whole Wheat (Pillsbury Best)	1 cup	400	2
Whole Wheat (Red Band)	1 cup	400	2
Whole Wheat Blend (Gold Medal)	1 cup	370	2
Wondra	1 cup	400	1
cottonseed, lowfat	1 oz	94	tr
cottonseed, partially defatted	1 Tbsp	18	tr
cottonseed, partially defatted	1 cup	337	6

FOOD	PORTION	CALORIES	FAT
peanut, defatted	1 Tbsp	13	tr
peanut, defatted	1 cup	196	tr
peanut, defatted	1 oz	92	tr
peanut, low-fat	1 oz	120	6
peanut, low-fat	1 cup	257	13
potato	½ cup	316	1
rice	1 cup	479	tr
sesame, lowfat	1 oz	95	tr

FRANKFURTER
(*see* HOT DOGS)

FRENCH BEANS

dried; cooked	1 cup	228	1
dried, raw	1 cup	631	4

FRENCH FRIES
(*see* POTATOES)

FRENCH TOAST

Cinnamon Swirl (Aunt Jemima)	2 slices	210	7
French Toast (Aunt Jemima)	2 slices	170	5
French Toast, Cinnamon Swirl (Great Starts)	6.5 oz	480	28
French Toast w/ Sausages (Great Starts)	6.5 oz	460	27
Raisin (Aunt Jemima)	2 slices	190	5
HOME RECIPE french toast	1 slice	155	7

FOOD	PORTION	CALORIES	FAT

FROGS' LEGS

FOOD	PORTION	CALORIES	FAT
frogs' leg; as prep w/ seasoned flour, fried (home recipe)	1 (.8 oz)	70	5
frogs' legs, raw	4 lg (3.5 oz)	73	tr

FROSTING
(see CAKE)

FRUCTOSE
(see also SUGAR, SUGAR SUBSTITUTE)

FOOD	PORTION	CALORIES	FAT
Fructose (Estee)	1 tsp	12	0

FRUIT DRINKS

FROZEN

FOOD	PORTION	CALORIES	FAT
Cranberry Juice Cocktail; as prep (Seneca)	6 oz	110	0
Cranberry-Apple Juice Cocktail; as prep (Seneca)	6 oz	110	0
Grape-Cranberry Juice Cocktail; as prep (Seneca)	6 oz	110	0
Raspberry Cranberry Juice Cocktail; as prep (Seneca)	6 oz	110	0
White Grape Juice; as prep (Seneca)	6 oz	110	0
cranberry juice cocktail; as prep	6 oz	102	0
fruit punch; as prep w/ water	1 cup	113	tr
lemonade; as prep w/ water	1 cup	100	tr
limeade; as prep w/ water	1 cup	102	tr

MIX

FOOD	PORTION	CALORIES	FAT
Berry Blend; as prep (Crystal Light)	8 oz	3	0

FOOD	PORTION	CALORIES	FAT
Black Cherry; as prep (Kool-Aid)	8 oz	98	0
Cherry Sugar Free; as prep (Kool-Aid)	8 oz	3	0
Citrus Blend; as prep (Crystal Light)	8 oz	3	tr
Grape; as prep (Crystal Light)	8 oz	3	0
Grape; as prep (Kool-Aid)	8 oz	98	0
Lemon-Lime; as prep (Crystal Light)	8 oz	4	0
Lemon-Lime Sugar; as prep (Country Time)	8 oz	5	0
Lemon-Lime Sweetened; as prep (Country Time)	8 oz	82	tr
Lemonade Sugar Free; as prep (Kool-Aid)	8 oz	4	tr
Lemonade Sugar Free; as prep (Country Time)	8 oz	5	0
Lemonade Sugar Sweetened; as prep (Kool-Aid)	8 oz	78	tr
Lemonade, Sweetened; as prep (Country Time)	8 oz	82	tr
Lemonade; as prep (Crystal Light)	8 oz	5	0
Lemonade; as prep (Kool-Aid)	8 oz	99	tr
Lemonade Flavor Flavor Crystals; as prep (Wyler's)	8 oz	92	2
Mountain Berry Punch, Sugar Sweetened; as prep (Kool-Aid)	8 oz	78	tr
Orange; as prep (Crystal Light)	8 oz	4	tr

FOOD	PORTION	CALORIES	FAT
Orange; as prep (Kool-Aid)	8 oz	98	0
Rainbow Punch; as prep (Kool-Aid)	8 oz	98	0
Raspberry Sugar Sweetened; as prep (Kool-Aid)	8 oz	79	tr
Sunshine Punch; as prep (Kool-Aid)	8 oz	99	0
Tang Orange; as prep (General Foods)	8 oz	87	tr
Tang Orange, Sugar Free; as prep (General Foods)	8 oz	5	tr
Tropical Punch, Sugar Free; as prep (Kool-Aid)	8 oz	3	tr
Tropical Punch, Sugar Sweetened; as prep (Kool-Aid)	8 oz	84	tr
Wild Strawberry Artificial Flavor Crystal; as prep (Wyler's)	8 oz	80	tr
fruit punch; as prep w/ water	9 oz	97	0
lemonade powder; as prep w/ water	9 oz	113	tr
READY-TO-USE Any flavor (Land O'Lakes)	8 oz	120	0
Apple (Juice Works)	6 oz	100	0
Apple (SIPPS)	8.45 oz	130	0
Apple Cranberry (Mott's)	10 oz	176	0
Apple Cranberry (Mott's)	9.5 oz	167	0
Apple Raspberry (Mott's)	9.5 oz	150	0

FOOD	PORTION	CALORIES	FAT
Apple Raspberry (Mott's)	10 oz	158	0
Appleberry (Juice Works)	6 oz	100	0
Black Cherry Cooler (Health Valley)	13 oz	144	1
Cherry (Juice Works)	6 oz	100	0
Cran-Blueberry (Ocean Spray)	6 oz	120	0
Cran-Grape (Ocean Spray)	6 oz	130	0
Cran-Orange (Ocean Spray)	6 oz	100	0
Cran-Raspberry (Ocean Spray)	6 oz	110	0
Cran-Raspberry, Low Calorie (Ocean Spray)	6 oz	40	0
Cran-Tastic (Ocean Spray)	6 oz	110	0
Cranapple (Ocean Spray)	6 oz	130	0
Cranapple, Low Calorie (Ocean Spray)	6 oz	40	0
Cranberry Apple Cooler (Health Valley)	13 oz	144	1
Cranberry Juice Cocktail (Ocean Spray)	6 oz	110	0
Cranberry Juice Cocktail (Seneca)	6 oz	110	0
Cranberry Juice Cocktail, Low Calorie (Ocean Spray)	6 oz	40	0
Cranberry-Apple Juice Cocktail (Seneca)	6 oz	110	0
Cranicot (Ocean Spray)	6 oz	110	0

FOOD	PORTION	CALORIES	FAT
Fruit Juicy Red (Hawaiian Punch)	6 oz	90	0
Fruit Punch (Bama)	8.45 oz	130	0
Fruit Punch (Mott's)	9.5 oz	150	0
Fruit Punch (Mott's)	10 oz	170	0
Fruit Punch (SIPPS)	8.45 oz	130	0
Grape (Bama)	8.45 oz	120	0
Grape (Hawaiian Punch)	6 oz	90	0
Grape (Juice Works)	6 oz	100	0
Grape (SIPPS)	8.45 oz	130	0
Grape Apple (Mott's)	10 oz	167	0
Grape Apple (Mott's)	9.5 oz	158	0
Island Fruit Cocktail (Hawaiian Punch)	6 oz	90	0
Lemon Lime Cooler (SIPPS)	8.45 oz	130	0
Lemonade (SIPPS)	8.45 oz	85	0
Lemonade (Shasta)	12 oz	146	0
Lite Fruit Juicy Red (Hawaiian Punch)	6 oz	60	0
Mauna La'i Hawaiian Guava Fruit Drink (Ocean Spray)	6 oz	100	0

FOOD	PORTION	CALORIES	FAT
Mauna La'i Hawaiian Guava Passion Fruit Drink (Ocean Spray)	6 oz	100	0
Mixed Berry (SIPPS)	8.45 oz	130	0
Orange (Bama)	8.45 oz	120	0
Orange (Hawaiian Punch)	6 oz	100	0
Orange (Juice Works)	6 oz	90	0
Orange (SIPPS)	8.45 oz	130	0
Orange Fruit Juice Blend (Mott's)	10 oz	144	0
Pineapple Grapefruit Juice Cocktail (Ocean Spray)	6 oz	110	0
Pink Grapefruit Juice Cocktail (Ocean Spray)	6 oz	80	0
Raspberry Cranberry Juice Cocktail (Seneca)	6 oz	110	0
Strawberry (Juice Works)	6 oz	100	0
Sunny Delight Florida Citrus Punch (Sundor)	6 oz	90	0
Sunshine Punch (SIPPS)	8.45 oz	130	0
Tropical Fruit (Hawaiian Punch)	6 oz	90	0
Very Berry (Hawaiian Punch)	6 oz	90	0
Wild Cherry (SIPPS)	8.45 oz	130	0
Wild Cherry Cooler (Health Valley)	13 oz	144	1

FOOD	PORTION	CALORIES	FAT
Wild Fruit (Hawaiian Punch)	6 oz	90	0
cranberry apricot	6 oz	118	0
cranberry apple	6 oz	123	0
cranberry grape	6 oz	103	tr
cranberry juice cocktail	6 oz	108	tr
fruit punch	6 oz	87	tr
grape	6 oz	94	0
orange	6 oz	94	0
orange & apricot	1 cup	128	tr
pineapple & grapefruit	1 cup	117	tr
pineapple & orange	1 cup	125	0

FRUIT, MIXED
(see also INDIVIDUAL NAMES)

FOOD	PORTION	CALORIES	FAT
CANNED			
Fruit Cocktail, Heavy Syrup (S&W)	½ cup	90	0
Fruit Cocktail, Natural Lite (S&W)	½ cup	60	0
Fruit Cocktail Natural Style (S&W)	½ cup	90	0
Fruit Salad, Chilled (Kraft)	½ cup	50	0
Mixed Fruit, Chunky Natural Style (S&W)	½ cup	90	0
fruit cocktail in heavy syrup	½ cup	93	tr
fruit cocktail in juice	½ cup	56	tr
fruit cocktail in water	½ cup	40	tr
fruit salad in heavy syrup	½ cup	94	tr
fruit salad in juice	½ cup	62	tr
fruit salad, tropical, in heavy syrup	½ cup	110	tr

FOOD	PORTION	CALORIES	FAT
DRIED			
Fruit 'n Nut Mix (Planters)	1 oz	150	9
mixed	11 oz pkg	712	1
FROZEN			
Mixed Fruit in Syrup (Birds Eye)	½ cup	123	tr
JUICE			
Apple Citrus (Tree Top)	6 oz	90	0
Apple Citrus, frzn; as prep (Tree Top)	6 oz	90	0
Apple Cranberry (Mott's)	6 oz	83	0
Apple Cranberry (Mott's)	9.5 oz	147	0
Apple Cranberry (Mott's)	8.45 oz	136	0
Apple Cranberry (Tree Top)	6 oz	100	0
Apple Cranberry, frzn; as prep (Tree Top)	6 oz	100	0
Apple Grape (Mott's)	6 oz	86	0
Apple Grape (Mott's)	8.45 oz	128	0
Apple Grape (Mott's)	9.5 oz	139	0
Apple Grape (Tree Top)	6 oz	100	0
Apple Grape, frzn; as prep (Tree Top)	6 oz	100	0
Apple Pear (Tree Top)	6 oz	90	0
Apple Pear, frzn; as prep (Tree Top)	6 oz	90	0

FOOD	PORTION	CALORIES	FAT
Apple Raspberry (Mott's)	6 oz	83	0
Apple Raspberry (Mott's)	8.45 oz	124	0
Apple Raspberry (Tree Top)	6 oz	80	0
Apple Raspberry, frzn; as prep (Tree Top)	6 oz	80	0
Apricot Pineapple Nectar (S&W)	6 oz	120	0
Orange Banana (Chiquita)	6 oz	90	0
Orange Banana (Smucker's)	8 oz	120	0
Orange Fruit Juice Blend (Mott's)	9.5 oz	139	0
Orange-Grapefruit Juice, 100% Pure Unsweetened (Kraft)	6 oz	80	0
Orange-Pineapple Juice, 100% Pure Unsweetened (Kraft)	6 oz	80	0
Pineapple Pink Grapefruit (Dole)	6 oz	101	tr
Pineapple-Orange Banana (Dole)	6 oz	90	tr
orange-grapefruit	1 cup	107	tr

FRUIT SNACKS

FOOD	PORTION	CALORIES	FAT
Del Monte Sierra Trail Mix	.9 oz	130	7
Del Monte Tropical Fruit Mix	9 oz	90	1
Flavor Tree Cherry Fruit Nibbles & Chocolate	1.05 oz	135	5
Flavor Tree Cherry Fruit People	1 oz	111	2
Flavor Tree Fruit Bears	1.05 oz	117	2

FOOD	PORTION	CALORIES	FAT
Flavor Tree Fruit Circus	1.05 oz	117	2
Flavor Tree Fruit Nibbles	½ pkg	118	2
Flavor Tree Fruit Nibbles, Cherry & Yogurt	½ pkg	133	4
Flavor Tree Fruit Nibbles, Orange & Yogurt	½ pkg	133	4
Flavor Tree Fruit Nibbles, Strawberry	½ pkg	135	5
Flavor Tree Fruit People	1 oz	111	1
Flavor Tree Lemon Fruit People	1 oz	111	2
Flavor Tree Orange Fruit People	1 oz	111	2
Flavor Tree Stawberry Fruit Roll	1 roll	67	tr
Flavor Tree Strawberry Fruit People	1 oz	111	2
Sunkist Fun Fruit Alphabets	9 oz	100	1
Sunkist Fun Fruit Animals	9 oz	100	1
Sunkist Fun Fruit Berry Bunch	9 oz	100	1
Sunkist Fun Fruits Cherry	9 oz	100	1
Sunkist Fun Fruits Creme Supremes, Cherry/Chocolate Coated	½ pkg	135	5
Sunkist Fun Fruits Creme Supremes, Cherry/Yogurt Coated	.9 oz	113	4
Sunkist Fun Fruit Dinosaurs, Strawberry	.9 oz.	100	1
Sunkist Fun Fruit Fantastic Fruit Punch	9 oz	100	1
Sunkist Fun Fruits Grape	9 oz	100	1
Sunkist Fun Fruits Numbers	9 oz	100	1
Sunkist Fun Fruits Orange	9 oz	100	1
Sunkist Fun Fruit Raspberry	.9 oz	100	1
Sunkist Fun Fruits Strawberry	9 oz	100	1
Sunkist Fun Fruit Tropical Fruit	9 oz	100	1

GARBANZO
(*see* CHICKPEAS)

FOOD	PORTION	CALORIES	FAT

GARLIC

raw	1 clove	4	tr

GEFILTEFISH

sweet recipe	1 piece (1.5 oz)	35	1

GELATIN

DRINKS

Orange Flavored Drinking Gelatin w/ Nutrasweet (Knox)	1 envelope	39	tr

MIX

All Flavors; as prep (Royal)	½ cup	80	0
All Flavors, Sugar Free; as prep (Royal)	½ cup	6	0
Apricot; as prep (Jell-O)	½ cup	80	tr
Black Cherry; as prep (Jell-O)	½ cup	81	tr
Black Raspberry; as prep (Jell-O)	½ cup	81	tr
Blackberry; as prep (Jell-O)	½ cup	81	tr
Cherry; as prep (Jell-O)	½ cup	81	tr
Cherry, Sugar Free (Diamond Crystal)	½ cup	8	tr
Cherry, Sugar Free; as prep (Jell-O)	1 pop	9	tr
Cherry w/ Nutrasweet; as prep (D-Zerta)	½ cup	8	tr
Concord Grape; as prep (Jell-O)	½ cup	81	tr

FOOD	PORTION	CALORIES	FAT
Gelatin Desserts; as prep (Estee)	½ cup	8	0
Hawaiian Pineapple Sugar Free; as prep (Jell-O)	1 pop	8	tr
Lemon; as prep (Jell-O)	½ cup	81	tr
Lemon Sugar Free; as prep (Jell-O)	1 pop	8	tr
Lemon Sugar Free (Diamond Crystal)	½ cup	8	tr
Lemon w/ Nutrasweet; as prep (D-Zerta)	½ cup	8	tr
Lime; as prep (Jell-O)	½ cup	81	tr
Lime, Sugar Free; as prep (Jell-O)	1 pop	8	tr
Lime Sugar Free (Diamond Crystal)	½ cup	8	tr
Lime w/ Nutrasweet; as prep (D-Zerta)	½ cup	9	tr
Mixed Fruit; as prep (Jell-O)	½ cup	81	tr
Mixed Fruit, Sugar Free; as prep as prep (Jell-O)	1 pop	8	tr
Orange; as prep (Jell-O)	½ cup	81	tr
Orange Pineapple; as prep (Jell-O)	½ cup	81	tr
Orange Sugar Free; as prep (Jell-O)	1 pop	8	tr
Orange Sugar Free (Diamond Crystal)	½ cup	8	tr
Orange w/ Nutrasweet; as prep (D-Zerta)	½ cup	8	tr

FOOD	PORTION	CALORIES	FAT
Peach; as prep (Jell-O)	½ cup	81	tr
Peach, Sugar Free; as prep (Jell-O)	1 pop	8	tr
Raspberry; as prep (Jell-O)	½ cup	81	tr
Raspberry Sugar Free; as prep (Jell-O)	1 pop	8	tr
Raspberry Sugar Free (Diamond Crystal)	½ cup	8	tr
Raspberry w/ Nutrasweet; as prep (D-Zerta)	½ cup	8	tr
Strawberry; as prep (Jell-O)	½ cup	81	tr
Strawberry Banana, Sugar Free; as prep (Jell-O)	1 pop	8	tr
Strawberry Banana; as prep (Jell-O)	½ cup	81	tr
Strawberry Sugar Free; as prep (Jell-O)	1 pop	8	tr
Strawberry Sugar Free (Diamond Crystal)	½ cup	8	tr
Strawberry w/ Nutrasweet; as prep (D-Zerta)	½ cup	8	tr
Triple Berry Sugar Free; as prep (Jell-O)	1 pop	8	tr
Wild Strawberry; as prep (Jell-O)	½ cup	81	tr
dry, unsweetened	1 Tbsp	23	tr

GIBLETS

FOOD	PORTION	CALORIES	FAT
capon, raw	4 oz	150	6
capon; simmered	1 cup	238	8
chicken; simmered	1 cup	228	7

FOOD	PORTION	CALORIES	FAT
chicken; flour coated, fried	1 cup	402	19
chicken, raw	2.6 oz	93	3
duck; simmered	1 cup	238	8
turkey, raw	8.6 oz	314	10
turkey; simmered	1 cup	243	7

GINKGO NUTS

canned	1 oz	32	tr
dried	1 oz	99	tr

GIZZARD

chicken; simmered	1 cup	222	5
chicken, raw	1.3 oz	41	2
turkey, raw	4 oz	133	4
turkey; simmered	1 cup	236	6

GOOSE

FRESH

meat & skin, raw	½ goose (2.9 lbs)	4893	443
meat & skin, raw	11.2 oz	1187	108
meat & skin; roasted	6.6 oz	574	41
meat & skin; roasted	½ goose (1.7 lbs)	2362	170
meat, raw	½ goose (2.3 lbs)	1237	55
meat, raw	6.5 oz	299	13
meat; roasted	5 oz	340	18
meat; roasted	½ goose (1.3 lbs)	1406	75

FOOD	PORTION	CALORIES	FAT

GOOSEBERRIES

FOOD	PORTION	CALORIES	FAT
canned in light syrup	½ cup	93	tr
fresh, raw	1 cup	67	tr

GRANOLA
(*see also* CEREAL)

BARS

FOOD	PORTION	CALORIES	FAT
Kudos Chocolate Chip	1.2 oz	180	9
Kudos Nutty Fudge	1.3 oz	190	11
Kudos Peanut Butter	1.3 oz	190	11
New Trail, Chocolate Chip	1	190	9
New Trail, Chocolate Covered Cocoa Creme	1	200	12
New Trail, Chocolate Covered Honey Graham	1	200	12
New Trail, Chocolate Covered Peanut Butter	1	200	11
New Trail, Peanut Butter	1	190	9
New Trail, Peanut Butter & Chocolate Chip	1	180	9
Quaker Chewy Chocolate Chip	1	130	5
Quaker Chewy Chocolate, Graham & Marshmallow	1	130	4
Quaker Chewy Chunky Nut & Raisin	1	130	6
Quaker Chewy Cinnamon & Raisin	1	130	5
Quaker Chewy Honey & Oats	1	130	4
Quaker Chewy Peanut Butter	1	140	6
Quaker Chewy Peanut Butter & Chocolate Chip	1	130	5
Quaker Dipps, Caramel Nut	1	150	6
Quaker Dipps, Chocolate Chip	1	140	6
Quaker Dipps, Honey & Oats	1	140	6

FOOD	PORTION	CALORIES	FAT
Quaker Dipps, Mint Chocolate Chip	1	140	6
Quaker Dipps, Peanut Butter	1	150	7
Quaker Dipps, Raisin & Almond	1	140	6
Quaker Dipps, Rocky Road	1	140	7
Sunbelt Chewy Granola, Chocolate Chip	1 bar (1.25 oz)	150	7
Sunbelt Chewy Granola, Oats & Honey	1 bar (1 oz)	130	5
Sunbelt Chewy Granola w/ Almonds	1 bar (1 oz)	120	6
Sunbelt Chewy Granola w/ Chocolate Chips	1 bar (1.75 oz)	220	9
Sunbelt Chewy Granola w/ Raisins	1 bar (1.25 oz)	150	6
Sunbelt Fudge Dipped Chewy Granola Chocolate Chip	1 bar (1.63 oz)	220	11
Sunbelt Fudge Dipped Chewy Granola Oats & Honey	1 bar (1.38 oz)	190	10
Sunbelt Fudge Dipped Chewy Granola w/ Peanuts	1 bar (1.5 oz)	200	12
Sunbelt Fudge Dipped Chewy Granola w/ Peanuts	1 bar (2.25 oz)	300	18
Sunbelt Granola Cereal, Fruit & Nut	1 bar (1 oz)	120	5
CEREAL Cinnamon & Raisin (Nature Valley)	⅓ cup	120	4
Coconut & Honey (Nature Valley)	⅓ cup	150	7
Erewhon Date Nut	1 oz	130	6
Erewhon Honey Almond	1 oz	130	6
Erewhon Maple	1 oz	130	5
Erewhon Spiced Apple	1 oz	130	6
Erewhon Sunflower Crunch	1 oz	130	4
Erewhon w/ Bran	1 oz	130	6

FOOD	PORTION	CALORIES	FAT
Fruit & Nut (Nature Valley)	⅓ cup + ½ cup milk	170	5
Health Valley Real Granola	1 oz	120	3
Post Hearty Granola	¼ cup	127	4
Post Hearty Granola	¼ cup + ½ cup milk	203	8
Post Hearty Granola w/ Raisins	¼ cup	123	4
Toasted Oat Mixture (Nature Valley)	⅓ cup	130	5

GRAPES

CANNED			
Thompson Seedless Premium (S&W)	½ cup	100	0
grapes in heavy syrup	½ cup	94	tr
FRESH			
grapes	10	36	tr
JUICE			
Concord, Unsweetened (S&W)	6 oz	100	0
Grape (Seneca)	6 oz	115	0
Grape (Tree Top)	6 oz	120	0
Grape, frzn; as prep (Seneca)	6 oz	100	0
Grape 100% Pure (Sippin' Pak)	8.45 oz	130	0
Natural Grape, frzn; as prep (Seneca)	6 oz	115	0
frzn, sweetened; as prep	1 cup	128	tr
frzn, sweetened; not prep	6 oz container	386	tr
grape	1 cup	155	tr

FOOD	PORTION	CALORIES	FAT
GRAPEFRUIT			
CANNED			
Sections, Chilled, Unsweetened (Kraft)	½ cup	50	0
Sections, in Light Syrup (S&W)	½ cup	80	0
Sections, Natural Style (S&W)	½ cup	40	0
in juice	½ cup	46	tr
in light syrup	½ cup	76	tr
in water	½ cup	44	tr
FRESH			
Pink (Ocean Spray)	½ med	50	0
Ruby Red (Chiquita)	½ fruit	40	0
White (Ocean Spray)	½ med	45	0
grapefruit	½ fruit	38	tr
JUICE			
Grapefruit (Mott's)	9.5 oz	118	0
Grapefruit (Mott's)	10 oz	124	0
Grapefruit Juice (Ocean Spray)	6 oz	70	0
Grapefruit Juice, 100% Pure Unsweetened (Kraft)	6 oz	70	0
Pink Premium Grapefruit Juice (Ocean Spray)	6 oz	60	0
Unsweetened (S&W)	6 oz	80	0
fresh	1 cup	96	tr

FOOD	PORTION	CALORIES	FAT
frzn; unsweetened	1 cup	93	tr
frzn; as prep	1 cup	102	tr
frzn; not prep	6 oz container	302	tr

GRAVY
(*see also* SAUCE)

FOOD	PORTION	CALORIES	FAT
CANNED			
Au Jus (Franco-American)	2 oz	5	0
Beef (Franco-American)	2 oz	25	1
Brown w/ Onions (Franco-American)	2 oz	25	1
Chicken (Franco-American)	2 oz	50	4
Chicken Giblet (Franco-American)	2 oz	30	2
Mushroom (Franco-American)	2 oz	25	1
Pork (Franco-American)	2 oz	40	3
Turkey (Franco-American)	2 oz	30	2
au jus	1 cup	38	tr
au jus	1 can (10.5 oz)	48	1
beef	1 can (10.2 oz)	155	7
beef	1 cup	124	5
chicken	1 cup	189	14
chicken	1 can (10.5 oz)	236	17
mushroom	1 can (10.5 oz)	150	8
mushroom	1 cup	120	6
turkey	1 cup	122	5
turkey	1 can (10.5 oz)	152	6

FOOD	PORTION	CALORIES	FAT
DRY			
Brown; as prep (Pillsbury)	¼ cup	15	0
Brown Gravy Mix; as prep (Estee)	¼ cup	14	0
Chicken (Diamond Crystal)	2 oz	30	1
Chicken; as prep (Pillsbury)	¼ cup	25	1
Chicken and Herb Gravy Mix; as prep (Estee)	¼ cup	20	tr
Home Style; as prep (Pillsbury)	¼ cup	15	0
au jus; as prep w/ water	1 cup	19	1
au jus; not prep	1 pkg (.8 oz)	79	3
brown; as prep w/ water	1 cup	9	tr
brown; not prep	1 pkg (.9 oz)	85	2
chicken; as prep w/ water	1 cup	83	2
chicken; not prep	1 pkg (.8 oz)	83	2
mushroom; as prep w/ water	1 cup	70	1
mushroom; not prep	1 pkg (.7 oz)	70	1
onion; as prep w/ water	1 cup	80	1
onion; not prep	1 pkg (.8 oz)	77	1
pork; as prep w/ water	1 cup	76	2
pork; not prep	1 pkg (.7 oz)	76	2
turkey; as prep w/ water	1 cup	87	2
turkey; not prep	1 pkg (.9 oz)	87	2

GREAT NORTHERN BEANS

FOOD	PORTION	CALORIES	FAT
CANNED			
Great Northern Beans (Hanover)	½ cup	110	0

FOOD	PORTION	CALORIES	FAT
Great Northern Beans, Seasoned w/ Pork (Luck's)	7.25 oz	220	5
great northern	1 cup	300	1
DRIED Great Northern (Hurst Brand)	1 cup	277	1
cooked	1 cup	210	1
raw	1 cup	621	2

GREEN BEANS

FOOD	PORTION	CALORIES	FAT
CANNED Cut Green Beans (Owatonna)	½ cup	20	0
Cut Premium Blue Lake (S&W)	½ cup	20	0
Cuts (Libby)	½ cup	20	0
Cuts (Seneca)	½ cup	20	0
Cuts Natural Pack (Libby)	½ cup	20	1
Cuts Natural Pack (Seneca)	½ cup	20	0
Dilled (S&W)	½ cup	60	0
French (Libby)	½ cup	20	0
French (Seneca)	½ cup	20	0
French Natural Pack (Libby)	½ cup	20	1
French Natural Pack (Seneca)	½ cup	20	0

FOOD	PORTION	CALORIES	FAT
French Style (Owatonna)	½ cup	20	0
French Style Premium Blue Lake (S&W)	½ cup	20	0
Whole (Libby)	½ cup	20	0
Whole (Seneca)	½ cup	20	0
Whole Fancy Stringless (S&W)	½ cup	20	0
Whole Vertical Pack (S&W)	½ cup	20	0
FROZEN Bavarian Style Beans & Spaetzle & Spaetzle (Birds Eye)	½ cup	98	5
Cut Beans (Southland)	3 oz	25	0
Cut Green Beans (Hanover)	½ cup	20	0
French (Southland)	3 oz	25	0
French; cooked (Health Valley)	4.7 oz	36	tr
French Green Beans w/ Toasted Almonds (Birds Eye)	½ cup	52	2
French Style Blue Lake (Hanover)	½ cup	25	0
Green Beans, Cut (Birds Eye)	½ cup	25	tr
Green Beans, French (Birds Eye)	½ cup	26	tr
Green Beans, Italian (Birds Eye)	½ cup	31	tr

FOOD	PORTION	CALORIES	FAT
Green Beans, Whole (Birds Eye)	½ cup	30	tr
Italian Cut (Hanover)	½ cup	35	0
Whole (Birds Eye)	½ cup	23	tr
Whole Blue Lake (Hanover)	½ cup	30	0

GROUNDCHERRIES

groundcherries	½ cup	37	tr

GROUPER

cooked	1 fillet (7.1 oz)	238	3
cooked	3 oz	100	1
raw	3 oz	78	1
raw	1 fillet (9.1 oz)	238	3

GUAVA

guava	1	45	tr
guava sauce (home recipe)	½ cup	43	tr

GUINEA HEN

meat & skin, raw	½ hen (12.1 oz)	545	22
meat, raw	½ hen (9.3 oz)	292	7

HADDOCK

FRESH

cooked	1 fillet (5.3 oz)	168	1
cooked	3 oz	95	1
raw	3 oz	74	1

FOOD	PORTION	CALORIES	FAT
raw	1 fillet (6.8 oz)	168	1
roe, raw	3.5 oz	130	2
FROZEN			
Au Natural Haddock Fillets (Mrs. Paul's)	4 oz	80	1
Batter-Dipped Haddock (Van De Kamp's)	2 pieces	240	12
Breaded Haddock Fillets (Van De Kamp's)	1 fillet	180	13
Crispy Crunchy Haddock Fillets (Mrs. Paul's)	2 fillets	250	12
Crunchy Light Batter Haddock Fillets (Mrs. Paul's)	2 fillets	330	17
Filet of Haddock w/ Lemon Butter Sauce (Gorton's)	1 pkg	250	13
Fishmarket Fresh Haddock (Gorton's)	5 oz	110	1
Light Breaded Haddock Fillets (Mrs. Paul's)	1 fillet	290	13
Lightly Breaded Haddock (Van De Kamp's)	5 oz	300	19
Microwave Lightly Breaded Haddock (Van De Kamp's)	5 oz	300	19
Today's Catch, Haddock (Van De Kamp's)	5 oz	110	0
SMOKED			
smoked	3 oz	99	1
smoked	1 oz	33	tr

HALIBUT

FRESH			
Atlantic & Pacific, raw	½ fillet (7.2 oz)	223	5
Atlantic & Pacific, raw	3 oz	93	2

FOOD	PORTION	CALORIES	FAT
Atlantic & Pacific; cooked	3 oz	119	2
Atlantic & Pacific; cooked	½ fillet (5.6 oz)	223	5
Greenland, raw	½ fillet (7.2 oz)	380	28
Greenland, raw	3 oz	158	12
FROZEN			
Batter-Dipped Halibut (Van De Kamp's)	3 pieces	260	16
Lightly Breaded Halibut (Van De Kamp's)	4 oz	220	11
Microwave Lightly Breaded Halibut (Van De Kamp's)	4 oz	220	11

HAM

(see also HAM DISHES, LUNCHEON MEAT/COLD CUTS, PORK, TURKEY)

FOOD	PORTION	CALORIES	FAT
Armour Golden Star, Boneless	1 oz	33	1
Armour Golden Star, Canned	1 oz	32	tr
Armour Lower Salt, Boneless	1 oz	34	1
Armour Lower Salt, 93% Fat Free	1 oz	35	1
Armour Star, Boneless	1 oz	41	2
Armour Star, Canned	1 oz	34	1
Armour Star, Speedy Cut	1 oz	44	3
Armour 1877, Boneless	1 oz	42	2
Carl Buddig	1 oz	50	3
Krakus Polish Cooked	3.5 oz	193	12
Oscar Mayer Baked; cooked	1 slice (21 g)	21	tr
Oscar Mayer Boiled w/ Natural Juices	1 slice (21 g)	23	tr
Oscar Mayer Breakfast Ham, Water Added	1 slice (43 g)	52	2
Oscar Mayer, Chopped w/ Natural Juices	1 slice (28 g)	55	4
Oscar Mayer, Cracked Black Pepper	1 slice (21 g)	24	tr

FOOD	PORTION	CALORIES	FAT
Oscar Mayer Ham & Cheese Loaf	1 slice (28 g)	76	6
Oscar Mayer Ham & Cheese Spread	1 oz	67	5
Oscar Mayer Ham Salad Spread w/ Natural Juices	1 oz	59	4
Oscar Mayer Honey w/ Natural Juices	1 slice (21 g)	26	1
Oscar Mayer Jubilee Boneless	1 oz	46	3
Oscar Mayer Jubilee, Canned w/ Natural Juices	1 oz	31	1
Oscar Mayer Jubilee Slice w/ Water Added	1 oz	29	1
Oscar Mayer Jubilee Steak w/ Water Added	1 slice (2 oz)	59	2
Oscar Mayer Smoked; cooked	1 slice (21 g)	23	tr
The Spreadables, Ham Salad	¼ can	100	6
center slice, lean only, raw	4 oz	220	9
chopped	1 slice (21 g)	48	4
chopped	1 oz	65	5
chopped, canned	1 slice (21 g)	50	4
chopped, canned	1 oz	68	5
ham (13% fat), canned; roasted	3 oz	192	13
ham (13% fat), canned; unheated	1 oz	54	4
ham patties; uncooked	1 patty (2.3 oz)	206	18
ham salad spread	1 Tbsp	32	2
ham salad spread	1 oz	61	4
ham, boneless (11% fat); roasted	3 oz	151	8
ham, boneless, extra lean; roasted	3 oz	140	7
ham, boneless, extra lean; unheated	1 slice (1 oz)	46	2
ham, center slice, lean & fat; unheated	4 oz	229	15
ham, extra lean, canned; roasted	3 oz	142	7
ham, extra lean, canned; unheated	1 oz	41	2

FOOD	PORTION	CALORIES	FAT
minced	1 slice (21 g)	55	4
minced	1 oz	75	6
patties; grilled	1 patty (2 oz)	203	18
sliced, extra lean (5% fat)	1 slice (28 g)	37	1
sliced, regular (11% fat)	1 slice (28 g)	52	3
steak, boneless, extra lean; unheated	1 oz	35	1
whole, lean only; roasted	3 oz	133	5
whole, lean & fat; roasted	3 oz	207	14

HAM DISHES

HOME RECIPE			
croquettes	1 (3.1 oz)	217	14
salad	½ cup	287	23

HAZELNUTS

dried, blanched	1 oz	191	19
dried, unblanched	1 oz	179	18
dry roasted, unblanched	1 oz	188	19
oil roasted, unblanched	1 oz	187	18

HEART

beef, raw	4 oz	132	4
beef; simmered	3 oz	148	5
chicken, raw	6.1 g	9	1
chicken; simmered	1 cup	268	11
pork, raw	1 heart (7.9 oz)	267	10
pork; braised	1 heart (4.3 oz)	191	7
turkey, raw	1 oz	41	2
turkey; simmered	1 cup	257	9

FOOD	PORTION	CALORIES	FAT

HERBAL TEA
   (*see* TEA/HERBAL TEA)

HERBS/SPICES

DRIED

FOOD	PORTION	CALORIES	FAT
Bar-B-Q Shaker (Diamond Crystal)	½ tsp	4	0
Chef Seasoning (.45 oz) (Diamond Crystal)	1 pkg	2	0
Chef Shaker (Diamond Crystal)	½ tsp	4	0
French Shaker (Diamond Crystal)	½ tsp	4	0
Italian Shaker (Diamond Crystal)	½ tsp	4	0
Mexican Shaker (Diamond Crystal)	½ tsp	4	0
allspice; ground	1 tsp	5	tr
anise seed	1 tsp	7	tr
basil; ground	1 tsp	4	tr
bay leaf; crumbled	1 tsp	2	tr
caraway seed	1 tsp	7	tr
cardamom; ground	1 tsp	6	tr
cayenne	1 tsp	6	tr
celery seed	1 tsp	8	tr
chervil	1 tsp	1	tr
chili powder	1 tsp	8	tr
chives; freeze-dried	1 Tbsp	1	tr
cinnamon; ground	1 tsp	6	tr
cloves; ground	1 tsp	7	tr
coriander leaf	1 tsp	2	tr
coriander leaf; dried	1 tsp	2	tr

FOOD	PORTION	CALORIES	FAT
coriander seed	1 tsp	5	tr
cumin seed	1 tsp	8	tr
curry powder	1 tsp	6	tr
dill seed	1 tsp	6	tr
dill weed; dried	1 tsp	3	tr
fennel seed	1 tsp	7	tr
fenugreek seed	1 tsp	12	tr
garlic powder	1 tsp	9	tr
ginger; ground	1 tsp	6	tr
mace; ground	1 tsp	8	tr
marjoram; dried	1 tsp	2	tr
mustard seed, yellow	1 tsp	15	1
nutmeg; ground	1 tsp	12	1
onion powder	1 tsp	7	tr
oregano; ground	1 tsp	5	tr
paprika	1 tsp	6	tr
parsley	1 Tbsp	1	tr
parsley; dried	1 tsp	1	tr
parsley; freeze-dried	1 Tbsp	1	tr
pepper, black	1 tsp	5	tr
pepper, red	1 tsp	6	tr
pepper, white	1 tsp	7	tr
poppy seed	1 tsp	15	1
poultry seasoning	1 tsp	5	tr
pumpkin pie spice	1 tsp	6	tr
rosemary; dried	1 tsp	4	tr
saffron	1 tsp	2	tr
sage; ground	1 tsp	2	tr
savory; ground	1 tsp	4	tr
tarragon; ground	1 tsp	5	tr

FOOD	PORTION	CALORIES	FAT
thyme; ground	1 tsp	4	tr
turmeric; ground	1 tsp	8	tr
FRESH			
coriander	¼ cup	4	tr
ginger root	5 slices	8	tr
ginger root	½ oz	7	tr
parsley, raw; chopped	½ cup	10	tr

HERRING

CANNED			
w/ tomato sauce	1.9 oz	97	6
FRESH			
Atlantic, raw	3 oz	134	8
Atlantic, raw	1 fillet (6.5 oz)	291	17
Atlantic; cooked	1 fillet (5 oz)	290	17
Atlantic; cooked	3 oz	172	10
Pacific, raw	1 fillet (6.5 oz)	359	26
Pacific, raw	3 oz	166	12
roe, raw	3.5 oz	130	2
READY-TO-USE			
Atlantic, kippered	1 fillet (1.4 oz)	87	5
Atlantic, pickled	½ oz	39	3
kippered, fillet	1 sm piece (.7 oz)	42	3
kippered, fillet	1 med piece (1.4 oz)	84	5

HICKORY NUTS

dried	1 oz	187	18

HONEYDEW

Honey Dew (Chiquita)	1 cup	70	0
cubed	1 cup	60	tr

FOOD	PORTION	CALORIES	FAT

HORSERADISH

FOOD	PORTION	CALORIES	FAT
Gold's Hot	1 Tbsp	4	1
Gold's Red	1 Tbsp	4	1
Gold's White	1 Tbsp	4	1
Kraft Cream Style Prepared	1 Tbsp	8	0
Kraft Horseradish Mustard	1 Tbsp	4	0
Kraft Horseradish Sauce	1 Tbsp	50	5
Kraft Prepared	1 Tbsp	4	0
Sauceworks Horseradish Sauce	1 Tbsp	50	5

HOTCAKES
(see PANCAKES)

HOT DOGS
(see also MEAT SUBSTITUTE, SAUSAGE, SAUSAGE SUBSTITUTE)

CHICKEN

FOOD	PORTION	CALORIES	FAT
Health Valley Weiners	3.5 oz	290	26
Wampler Longacre	1 (1.6 oz)	115	3
Wampler Longacre	1 (2 oz)	144	5
Weaver	1 (1.6 oz)	115	10
chicken	1 (1.5 oz)	116	9

MEAT

FOOD	PORTION	CALORIES	FAT
Armour Lower Salt, Jumbo Beef	1	170	15
Armour Star, Jumbo Beef	1	190	18
Chefwich Chili Dog	5 oz	380	15
Health Valley Beef Weiners	3.5 oz	288	25
Hebrew National Frankfurters	1 (1.6 oz)	140	13
Hebrew National Frankfurters	1 (1.8 oz)	160	15
Hebrew National Frankfurters, Deli	1 (2.3 oz)	200	19
Oscar Mayer Bacon & Cheddar Cheese	1 (1.6 oz)	143	13

FOOD	PORTION	CALORIES	FAT
Oscar Mayer Beef Franks	1 (1.6 oz)	144	13
Oscar Mayer Beef w/ Cheddar Franks	1 (1.6 oz)	130	11
Oscar Mayer Bun-Length Franks	1 (2 oz)	186	17
Oscar Mayer Bun-Length Wieners	1 (2 oz)	181	17
Oscar Mayer Cheese Hot Dogs	1 (1.6 oz)	145	13
Oscar Mayer German Brand Frankfurters	1 (2.7 oz)	230	21
Oscar Mayer Wieners	1 (1.6 oz)	144	13
Oscar Mayer Wieners, Little	1 (.3 oz)	28	3
beef	1 (1.75 oz)	184	17
beef	1 (1.5 oz)	142	13
beef	1 (1.9 oz)	180	16
beef & pork	1 (1.75 oz)	183	17
pork, cheesefurter smokie	1 (1.5 oz)	141	12
TURKEY			
Bil Mar Foods Cheese Franks	1 (1.6 oz)	109	9
Health Valley Weiners	3.5 oz	238	20
Louis Rich Cheese Franks	1 (1.6 oz)	108	9
Louis Rich Franks	1 (1.6 oz)	103	9
Mr. Turkey Franks	1 (1.6 oz)	106	9
Mr. Turkey Franks	1 (½ oz)	79	7
Mr. Turkey Franks	1 (2 oz)	132	11
Wampler Longacre	1 (1.6 oz)	102	3
turkey	1 (1.5 oz)	102	8

HUMMUS

HOME RECIPE			
hummus	⅓ cup	140	7
hummus	1 cup	420	21

FOOD	PORTION	CALORIES	FAT

HYACINTH BEANS

DRIED
cooked	1 cup	228	1
raw	1 cup	723	4

ICE CREAM AND FROZEN DESSERT
   (*see also* ICE CREAM, NON-DAIRY)

Banana, Fruit & Cream (Chiquita)	1 bar	80	2
Berry Blend Pops (Crystal Light)	1 bar	14	tr
Berry Punch (Jell-O)	1 pop	31	tr
Blueberry Fruit and Juice Bars (Dole)	1 bar	90	1
Blueberry Fruit & Cream (Chiquita)	1 bar	80	1
Bubble Crazy (Good Humor)	3 oz	74	1
Bubble O Bill (Good Humor)	3.5 oz	149	8
Buttered Pecan (Lady Borden)	½ cup	180	12
Cherry (Jell-O)	1 pop	32	tr
Cherry Cola Kick (Good Humor)	4.5 oz	106	1
Cherry & Ice Cream Swirl (Chiquita)	1 bar	80	3
Cherry Fresh Lites (Dole)	1 bar	25	tr
Cherry Fruit & Juice Bars (Chiquita)	1 bar (2 oz)	50	0
Cherry Fruit & Yogurt Bars (Dole)	4 oz	80	tr

FOOD	PORTION	CALORIES	FAT
Cherry Fruit Bars (Jell-O)	1 bar (1.8 oz)	39	tr
Cherry Italian Ice (Good Humor)	6 oz	138	tr
Cherry Vanilla, Coffee, Peach or Strawberry Ice Cream Breyers	½ cup	135	35–50
Cherry/Orange Ice Stripes (Good Humor)	1.5 oz	35	0
Chip Candy Crunch (Good Humor)	3 oz	347	24
Chocolate (Ben & Jerry's)	4 oz	290	18
Chocolate Ice Milk (Borden)	½ cup	100	2
Chocolate Creamy Lites Bar (Carnation)	1 bar	50	2
Chocolate Eclair (Good Humor)	3 oz	187	10
Chocolate Flavor Coated Vanilla Ice Cream (Good Humor)	3 oz	198	14
Chocolate Fudge Cake (Good Humor)	6.3 oz	214	15
Chocolate Fudge Heaven Sundae Bar (Carnation)	1 bar	150	9
Chocolate Malt (Good Humor)	3 oz	187	13
Chocolate Malted Bars (Carnation)	1 bar	70	3
Chocolate Swirl (Borden)	½ cup	130	6
Chocolate/Banana Fruit & Juice Bars (Dole)	1 bar	175	9

FOOD	PORTION	CALORIES	FAT
Chocolate/Strawberry Fruit & Cream Bars (Dole)	1 bar	140	8
Chocolate/Vanilla Cool 'n Creamy Bars (Crystal Light)	1 bar	55	2
Coconut Bar (Good Humor)	3 oz	207	14
Combo Cup, Vanilla/Chocolate (Good Humor)	6 oz	201	9
Cookies 'n Cream, Chocolate (Oreo)	3 oz	140	8
Cookies 'n Cream, Mint (Oreo)	3 oz	140	8
Cookies 'n Cream on a Stick (Oreo)	1 bar	220	15
Cookies 'n Cream Sandwich (Oreo)	1	240	11
Cookies 'n Cream Snackwich (Oreo)	1	60	3
Cookies 'n Cream, Vanilla (Oreo)	3 oz	140	8
Deluxe Sundae (Good Humor)	6 oz	300	11
Double Chocolate Fudge Cool 'n Creamy Bars (Crystal Light)	1 bar	55	2
Dutch Chocolate (American Glace)	4 oz	48	0
Dutch Chocolate, Olde Fashioned Recipe (Borden)	½ cup	130	6
Fat Frog (Good Humor)	3 oz	154	9
French Vanilla (Ben & Jerry's)	4 oz	267	17

FOOD	PORTION	CALORIES	FAT
Fruit Flavored Sherbet (Land O'Lakes)	4 oz	130	2
Fruit Punch Fruit Slush (Wyler's)	4 oz	140	0
Fruit Punch Pops (Crystal Light)	1 bar	14	tr
Fruit Punch Suntops (Dole)	1 bar	40	tr
Fudge Bar (Good Humor)	2.5 oz	127	tr
Full O'Chocolate (Good Humor)	3 oz	245	18
Grape (Jell-O)	1 pop	31	tr
Grape SunTops (Dole)	1 bar	40	tr
Grape/Lemon Ice Stripes (Good Humor)	1.5 oz	35	0
Grape/Lemon Italian Ice (Good Humor)	6 oz	138	tr
Ice Cream Sandwich, Chocolate Chip Cookie, Chocolate (Good Humor)	4 oz	268	11
Ice Cream Sandwich, Chocolate Chip Cookie Vanilla (Good Humor)	4 oz	246	11
Ice Cream Sandwich, Vanilla (Good Humor)	2.5 oz	162	5
Jumbo Jet Star (Good Humor)	4.5 oz	85	tr
King Cone (Good Humor)	5.5 oz	315	19
Lemon Calippo (Good Humor)	4.5 oz	112	tr
Lemon Fresh Lites (Dole)	1 bar	25	tr

FOOD	PORTION	CALORIES	FAT
Lemon White Italian Ice (Good Humor)	6 oz	138	tr
Lemon/Cherry w/ Gummy Dinosaur Colossal Fossil (Good Humor)	3 oz	75	tr
Lemon/Grape w/ Gummy Dinosaur Colossal Fossil (Good Humor)	3 oz	75	tr
Lemon/Lime Swirl (Jell-O)	1 pop	33	tr
Lemonade SunTops (Dole)	1 bar	40	tr
Life Savers Pops, All Flavors (Nabisco)	1	40	0
Mandarin Orange Sorbet (Dole)	4 oz	110	tr
Mixed Berry (Jell-O)	1 pop	31	tr
Mixed Berry Bars (Jell-O)	1 bar (1.8 oz)	42	tr
Mixed Berry & Ice Cream Swirl (Chiquita)	1 bar	80	3
Orange (Jell-O)	1 pop	31	tr
Orange Bars (Jell-O)	1 bar (1.8 oz)	42	tr
Orange Calippo (Good Humor)	4.5 oz	110	tr
Orange & Ice Cream Swirl (Chiquita)	1 bar	80	3
Orange Pops (Crystal Light)	1 bar	13	tr
Orange Sherbet (Borden)	½ cup	110	1
Orange Sherbet, Push-Up (Good Humor)	3 oz	56	tr

FOOD	PORTION	CALORIES	FAT
Orange/Pineapple Swirl (Jell-O)	1 pop	31	tr
Orange/Raspberry Italian Ice (Good Humor)	6 oz	138	tr
Orange/Vanilla Cool 'n Creamy Bars (Crystal Light)	1 bar	31	tr
Original Cheesecake Bar (Carnation)	1 bar	120	6
Passion-fruit (Vitari)	4 oz	80	0
Peach (Vitari)	4 oz	80	0
Peach Fruit & Cream (Chiquita)	1 bar	80	1
Peach Fruit & Juice Bars (Dole)	1 bar	90	1
Peach Sorbet (Dole)	4 oz	120	tr
Pina Colada Fruit 'n Juice Bars (Dole)	1 bar	90	tr
Pineapple Fruit 'n Juice Bars (Dole)	1 bar	70	tr
Pineapple Sorbet (Dole)	4 oz	120	tr
Pineapple Orange Fresh Lites (Dole)	1 bar	25	tr
Pineapple Pops (Crystal Light)	1 bar	13	tr
Pink Lemonade Pops (Crystal Light)	1 bar	14	tr
Raspberry (Jell-O)	1 pop	29	tr
Raspberry & Ice Cream Swirl (Chiquita)	1 bar	80	3
Raspberry, Banana, Fruit & Juice Bars (Chiquita)	1 bar (2 oz)	50	0

FOOD	PORTION	CALORIES	FAT
Raspberry Bars (Jell-O)	1 bar (1.8 oz)	41	tr
Raspberry Berry Swirl Bars (Carnation)	1 bar	70	3
Raspberry Fresh Lites (Dole)	1 bar	25	tr
Raspberry Fruit & Cream (Chiquita)	1 bar	80	1
Raspberry Fruit & Juice Bars (Chiquita)	1 bar	50	0
Raspberry Fruit & Yogurt Bars (Dole)	4 oz	70	tr
Raspberry Fruit 'n Juice Bars (Dole)	1 bar	70	tr
Raspberry Peach Bars (Jell-O)	1 bar (1.8 oz)	40	tr
Raspberry/Peach Swirl (Jell-O)	1 pop	29	tr
Raspberry Pops (Crystal Light)	1 bar	14	tr
Raspberry Sorbet (Dole)	4 oz	110	tr
Scribbler (Good Humor)	3 oz	120	1
Shark Bar (Good Humor)	3 oz	63	tr
Skinny Dip	4 oz	36	0
Strawberries and Cream (Good Humor)	3 oz	96	2
Strawberries 'n Cream Olde Fashioned Recipe (Borden)	½ cup	130	5
Strawberry (Borden)	½ cup	130	6
Strawberry (Jell-O)	1 pop	31	tr

FOOD	PORTION	CALORIES	FAT
Strawberry & Ice Cream Swirl (Chiquita)	1 bar	80	3
Strawberry Banana (Jell-O)	1 pop	31	tr
Strawberry Banana Bars (Jell-O)	1 bar (1.8 oz)	39	tr
Strawberry Banana Fruit & Cream (Chiquita)	1 bar	80	2
Strawberry Banana Fruit & Juice Bars (Chiquita)	1 bar (2 oz)	50	0
Strawberry Banana Swirl (Jell-O)	1 pop	31	tr
Strawberry Bars (Jell-O)	1 bar (1.8 oz)	41	tr
Strawberry Berry Swirl Bar (Carnation)	1 bar	70	3
Strawberry Cheesecake Bars (Carnation)	1 bar	125	6
Strawberry Creamy Lites Bar (Carnation)	1 bar	50	2
Strawberry Finger Bar (Good Humor)	2.5 oz	49	tr
Strawberry Fruit & Cream (Chiquita)	1 bar	80	1
Strawberry Fruit & Juice Bars (Chiquita)	1 bar (2 oz)	50	0
Strawberry Fruit & Yogurt Bars (Dole)	4 oz	70	tr
Strawberry Fruit 'n Juice Bars (Dole)	1 bar	70	tr
Strawberry Ice Milk (Borden)	½ cup	90	2
Strawberry Pops (Crystal Light)	1 bar	13	tr
Strawberry Shortcake (Good Humor)	3 oz	186	12

FOOD	PORTION	CALORIES	FAT
Strawberry Sorbet (Dole)	4 oz	110	tr
Strawberry Tropical Mix (Jell-O)	1 bar (1.8 oz)	40	tr
Supreme (Good Humor)	3.5 oz	342	23
Tahitian Vanilla (American Glace)	4 oz	48	0
Tasti D-Lite	4 oz	40	1
Toasted Almond (Good Humor)	3 oz	193	10
Tropical Orange SunTops (Dole)	1 bar	40	tr
Twister (Good Humor)	3 oz	131	7
Vanilla (Eagle Brand)	½ cup	150	9
Vanilla Caramel Nut, Heaven Bars (Carnation)	1 bar	225	15
Vanilla Cup (Good Humor)	3 oz	98	5
Vanilla Fosters Freeze	1 oz	43	1
Vanilla Fudge Heaven Sundae Bars (Carnation)	1 bar	150	9
Vanilla Fudge Nut (Carnation)	1 bar	222	15
Vanilla Ice Cream (Land O'Lakes)	4 oz	140	7
Vanilla Ice Milk (Land O'Lakes)	4 oz	90	3
Vanilla Ice Milk (Borden)	½ cup	90	2
Vanilla Olde Fashioned Recipe (Borden)	½ cup	130	7

FOOD	PORTION	CALORIES	FAT
Viennetta Petites, Chocolate Mint (Good Humor)	5 oz	236	14
Viennetta Petites, Vanilla (Good Humor)	5 oz	236	14
Viennetta Regular, Chocolate (Good Humor)	5 oz	225	14
Viennetta Regular, Vanilla (Good Humor)	5 oz	225	14
Watermelon Italian Ice (Good Humor)	6 oz	138	tr
Whammy (Good Humor)	1.6 oz	95	7
Wild Cherry Pops (Crystal Light)	1 bar	13	tr
orange sherbet	⅔ cup	181	3
orange sherbet	1 cup	270	4
orange sherbet (home recipe)	½ cup	120	2
vanilla French, soft serve	1 cup	377	23
vanilla ice milk	1 cup	184	6
vanilla ice milk, soft serve	1 cup	223	5
vanilla, 10% fat	1 cup	269	14
vanilla, 16% fat	1 cup	349	24

ICE CREAM CONES & CUPS

FOOD	PORTION	CALORIES	FAT
Comet Cups	1	20	0
Comet Sugar Cone	1	40	0

ICE CREAM, NON-DAIRY

FOOD	PORTION	CALORIES	FAT
Mocha Mix Chocolate Chip	½ cup	160	9
Mocha Mix Dutch Chocolate	½ cup	135	8
Mocha Mix Mocha Almond Fudge	½ cup	150	8
Mocha Mix Neapolitan	½ cup	130	7
Mocha Mix Strawberry Swirl	½ cup	140	7

FOOD	PORTION	CALORIES	FAT
Mocha Mix Toasted Almond	½ cup	150	9
Mocha Mix Vanilla	½ cup	138	7
Mocha Mix Vanilla, Chocolate Chocolate Almond	½ cup	150	9
Tofulite	4 oz	150	7
Tofutti Cappuccino Love Drops	4 oz	230	12
Tofutti Chocolate Cuties	4 oz	140	5
Tofutti Chocolate Love Drops	4 oz	220	13
Tofutti Chocolate Supreme	4 oz	210	13
Tofutti Lite, lite Applejack Vanilla Twirl	4 oz	90	tr
Tofutti Lite, lite Cappuccino Vanilla Twirl	4 oz	90	tr
Tofutti Lite, lite Chocolate Vanilla Twirl	4 oz	90	tr
Tofutti Lite, lite Chocolate Strawberry Twirl	4 oz	90	tr
Tofutti Lite, lite Strawberry Twirl	4 oz	90	tr
Tofutti Lite, lite Vanilla, Chocolate, Strawberry Twirl	4 oz	90	tr
Tofutti Soft Serve, Lite Hi-Lite Chocolate	4 oz	100	1
Tofutti Soft Serve, Hi-Lite Vanilla	4 oz	90	1
Tofutti Soft Serve, Regular	4 oz	158	8
Tofutti Vanilla	4 oz	200	11
Tofutti Vanilla Almond Bark	4 oz	230	14
Tofutti Vanilla Cuties	4 oz	130	5
Tofutti Vanilla Love Drops	4 oz	220	12
Tofutti Wildberry	4 oz	210	12

ICE CREAM TOPPINGS
(see also SYRUP)

FOOD	PORTION	CALORIES	FAT
Butterscotch Artificially Flavored Topping (Kraft)	1 Tbsp	60	1

FOOD	PORTION	CALORIES	FAT
Butterscotch Flavored Topping Topping (Smucker's)	2 Tbsp	140	1
Caramel Topping (Kraft)	1 Tbsp	60	0
Caramel Flavored Topping (Smucker's)	2 Tbsp	140	1
Cherry (Smucker's)	1 Tbsp	53	tr
Chocolate Caramel Topping (Kraft)	1 Tbsp	60	0
Chocolate Flavored Syrup Toping (Smucker's)	2 Tbsp	130	0
Chocolate Fudge Magic Shell (Smucker's)	2 Tbsp	190	15
Chocolate Fudge Topping (Hershey)	2 Tbsp	100	4
Chocolate Fudge Topping (Smucker's)	2 Tbsp	130	1
Chocolate Magic Shell (Smucker's)	2 Tbsp	190	15
Chocolate Nut Magic Shell (Smucker's)	2 Tbsp	200	16
Chocolate Topping (Kraft)	1 Tbsp	60	0
Hot Caramel Topping (Smucker's)	2 Tbsp	150	4
Hot Fudge Topping (Kraft)	1 Tbsp	70	0
Hot Fudge Topping (Smucker's)	2 Tbsp	110	4
Marshmallow (Smucker's)	1 Tbsp	68	tr
Marshmallow Creme (Kraft)	1 Tbsp	90	0
Peanut Butter Magic Caramel (Smucker's)	2 Tbsp	150	2

FOOD	PORTION	CALORIES	FAT
Pecans in Syrup (Smucker's)	2 Tbsp	130	1
Pineapple (Smucker's)	2 Tbsp	130	0
Pineapple (Smucker's)	1 Tbsp	54	tr
Pineapple Topping (Kraft)	1 Tbsp	50	0
Red Raspberry Topping (Kraft)	1 Tbsp	50	0
Strawberry (Smucker's)	2 Tbsp	120	0
Strawberry (Smucker's)	1 Tbsp	44	tr
Strawberry Topping (Kraft)	1 Tbsp	50	0
Swiss Milk Chocolate Fudge Topping (Smucker's)	2 Tbsp	140	1
Walnuts in Syrup (Smucker's)	2 Tbsp	130	1
Walnut Topping (Kraft)	1 Tbsp	90	5
butterscotch sauce (home recipe)	2 Tbsp	151	6
chocolate sauce (home recipe)	2 Tbsp	108	3
hard sauce (home recipe)	2 Tbsp	142	6

ICING
(see CAKE)

INSTANT BREAKFAST
(see BREAKFAST DRINKS)

FOOD	PORTION	CALORIES	FAT

ITALIAN FOOD
(*see also* DINNER, PASTA, PASTA DINNERS, PASTA SALAD)

FROZEN

Italian Style International Recipe (Birds Eye)	½ cup	101	5
Italian Style International Rice (Birds Eye)	½ cup	119	tr

JAM/JELLY/PRESERVES

ALL FRUIT

All Flavors, Simply Fruit Spread (Smucker's)	1 tsp	16	0
Blueberry Fruit Spread (Pritikin Foods)	1 tsp	14	0
Peach Fruit Spread (Pritikin Foods)	1 tsp	14	0
Red Raspberry Fruit Spread (Pritikin Foods)	1 tsp	14	0
Strawberry Fruit Spread (Pritikin Foods)	1 tsp	14	0

REDUCED CALORIE

All Flavors, Imitation Jelly Single Service (Smucker's)	⅜ oz pkg	2	0
All Flavors, Jellies, Single Service (Smucker's)	½ oz pkg	38	0
All Flavors, Low Sugar Spreads (Smucker's)	1 tsp	8	0
All Flavors, Preserves, Single Service (Smucker's)	½ oz pkg	38	0
All Flavors, Slenderella Low Calorie Imitation Jam (Smucker's)	1 tsp	8	0

FOOD	PORTION	CALORIES	FAT
All Flavors, Slenderella Low Calorie Imitation Jelly (Smucker's)	1 tsp	8	0
Grape Jelly Reduced Calorie (Kraft)	1 tsp	5	0
Grape, Imitation Jelly (Smucker's)	1 tsp	2	0
Jellies, All Flavors (Estee)	1 tsp	2	0
Preserves, All Flavors (Estee)	1 tsp	2	0
Preserves, All Flavors (Louis Sherry)	1 tsp	2	0
Strawberry Imitation Jelly (Smucker's)	1 tsp	2	0
Strawberry Preserves, Reduced Calorie (Kraft)	1 tsp	8	0
REGULAR Apple Butter (BAMA)	2 tsp	25	0
Apple Butter (White House)	1 oz	50	0
Apple Butter, Natural (Smucker's)	1 tsp	12	0
Apple Jelly (BAMA)	2 tsp	30	0
Cider Apple Butter (Smucker's)	1 tsp	12	0
Grape Jelly (BAMA)	2 tsp	30	0
Jam, All Flavors (Smucker's)	1 tsp	18	0
Jam, All Flavors (Kraft)	1 tsp	18	0
Jelly, All Flavors (Home Brands)	2 tsp	35	0

FOOD	PORTION	CALORIES	FAT
Jelly, All Flavos (Kraft)	1 tsp	16	0
Orange Marmalade (Smucker's)	1 tsp	18	0
Peach Butter (Smucker's)	1 tsp	15	0
Peach Preserves (BAMA)	2 tsp	30	0
Preserves, All Flavors (Home Brands)	2 tsp	35	0
Preserves, All Flavors (Smucker's)	1 tsp	18	0
Preserves, All Flavors (Kraft)	1 tsp	16	0
Red Plum Jam (BAMA)	2 tsp	30	0
Strawberry Preserves (BAMA)	2 tsp	30	0

JAPANESE FOOD
(see ORIENTAL FOOD)

JELLY
(see JAM/JELLY/PRESERVES)

KALE

FOOD	PORTION	CALORIES	FAT
FRESH			
chopped; cooked	½ cup	21	tr
chopped, raw	½ cup	21	tr
FROZEN			
chopped; cooked	½ cup	20	tr
frzn; not prep	10 oz pkg	79	1

FOOD	PORTION	CALORIES	FAT
KIDNEY			
beef, raw	4 oz	212	3
beef; simmered	3 oz	122	3
pork, raw	3 oz	84	3
pork; braised	3 oz	128	4
KIDNEY BEANS			
CANNED			
Dark Red (Ranch Style)	7.5 oz	170	1
Dark Red (Trappey's)	½ cup	90	0
Dark Red Kidney Beans (Hanover)	½ cup	110	0
Dark Red Lite, 50% Less Salt (S&W)	½ cup	120	1
Dark Red Premium (S&W)	½ cup	120	1
Jalapeno Light Red (Trappey's)	½ cup	90	0
Light Red (Trappey's)	½ cup	90	0
Red w/ Chili Gravy (Trappey's)	½ cup	100	1
Light Red Kidney Beans in Sauce (Hanover)	½ cup	120	0
Red Kidney Baked Beans (B&M)	⅞ cup	290	7
Red Kidney Beans Seasoned w/ Pork (Luck's)	7.5 oz	220	6
Red w/ Chili Gravy (Trappey's)	½ cup	100	1
Special Cook Red Kidney Beans (Luck's)	7.5 oz	190	4

FOOD	PORTION	CALORIES	FAT
kidney	1 cup	208	1
red	1 cup	216	1
DRIED			
Kidney (Hurst Brand)	1 cup	254	1
California red, raw	1 cup	609	tr
California red; cooked	1 cup	219	tr
cooked	1 cup	225	1
raw	1 cup	613	2
red, raw	1 cup	619	2
red, royal, raw	1 cup	605	1
red, royal; cooked	1 cup	218	tr
red; cooked	1 cup	225	1
SPROUTS			
cooked	1 lb	152	3
raw	½ cup	27	tr

KIWIFRUIT

California kiwifruit	2	90	1
kiwifruit	1	46	tr

KOHLRABI

sliced, raw	½ cup	19	tr
sliced; cooked	½ cup	24	tr

KUMQUATS

kumquats	1	12	tr

LAMB
(see also LAMB DISHES)

FRESH			
chopped, lean & fat; cooked	½ cup	195	13

FOOD	PORTION	CALORIES	FAT
ground, lean & fat; cooked	½ cup	153	10
leg, w/o bone, lean & fat; roasted	3 oz	237	16
leg, w/o bone, lean only; roasted	3 oz	158	6
loin chop w/ bone, lean & fat; broiled	1 (2.5 oz)	255	21
loin chop w/ bone, lean only; broiled	1 (1.7 oz)	92	4
patty, lean & fat; cooked	3 oz	229	16
rib chop w/ bone, lean & fat; cooked	1 (2.4 oz)	273	24
rib chop w/ bone, lean only; cooked	1 (1.5 oz)	91	5
shoulder, lean & fat; roasted	3 oz	287	23
shoulder shank, lean & fat; cooked	3.2 oz	306	25
shoulder w/o bone, lean only; roasted	3 oz	174	9
shoulder w/o bone, lean & fat; roasted	3 oz	287	23

LAMB DISHES

curry	¾ cup	345	17
stew	¾ cup	124	5
lamb & potato casserole	¾ cup	277	17

LAMB'S-QUARTERS

chopped; cooked	½ cup	29	1

LECITHIN
(*see* SOY)

LEEKS

DRIED

freeze dried	1 Tbsp	1	0

FRESH

chopped; cooked	¼ cup	8	tr

FOOD	PORTION	CALORIES	FAT
raw	1 (4.4 oz)	76	tr
chopped, raw	¼ cup	16	tr

LEMON

CANDIED
lemon peel	1 oz	90	tr

FRESH
peel	1 Tbsp	0	tr

HOME RECIPE
lemon sauce	2 Tbsp	57	1

JUICE
Lemon (Seneca)	1 Tbsp	6	0
Realemon (Borden)	1 oz	6	0
fresh	1 Tbsp	4	0
frzn	1 Tbsp	3	0
lemon	1 Tbsp	3	0

LEMONADE
(*see* FRUIT DRINKS)

LEMON EXTRACT

Virginia Dare	1 tsp	22	0

LENTILS

CANNED
Lentils; cooked (Hurst Brand)	1 cup	258	tr
Zesty Lentil Pilaf (Health Valley)	4 oz	110	3

FOOD	PORTION	CALORIES	FAT
DRIED			
cooked	1 cup	231	1
raw	1 cup	649	2
SPROUTS			
sprouts	½ cup	40	tr

LETTUCE

butterhead	2 leaves	2	tr
iceberg	1 leaf	3	tr
looseleaf; shredded	½ cup	5	tr
romaine; shredded	½ cup	4	tr

LIMA BEANS

CANNED			
Giant Lima Beans Seasoned w/ Pork (Luck's)	7.5 oz	230	7
Lima Beans (Libby)	½ cup	80	0
Lima Beans (Seneca)	½ cup	80	0
Lima Beans w/ Ham (Dennison's)	7.5 oz	250	7
Small Fancy (S&W)	½ cup	80	0
Small Green Limas, Seasoned w/ Pork (Luck's)	7.5 oz	220	7
large	1 cup	191	tr
lima beans	½ cup	93	tr
DRIED			
Baby Lima (Hurst Brand)	1 cup	262	1
baby, raw	1 cup	677	2

FOOD	PORTION	CALORIES	FAT
baby; cooked	1 cup	229	1
cooked	½ cup	104	tr
large, raw	1 cup	602	1
large; cooked	1 cup	217	1
FROZEN Baby (Birds Eye)	½ cup	127	tr
Baby Lima Beans (Hanover)	½ cup	110	0
Fordhook (Birds Eye)	½ cup	100	tr
Fordhook Lima Beans (Hanover)	½ cup	100	0
Thin; cooked (Health Valley)	6.3 oz	188	tr
lima beans	½ cup	94	tr
lima beans	½ cup	85	tr

LIME

FOOD	PORTION	CALORIES	FAT
Realime juice (Borden)	1 oz	6	0
lime juice	1 Tbsp	3	tr

LINGCOD

FOOD	PORTION	CALORIES	FAT
raw	3 oz	72	1
raw	½ fillet (6.8 oz)	164	2

LIQUOR/LIQUEUR
(*see also* BEER, ALE AND MALT LIQUOR, DRINK MIXER, WINE, WINE COOLER)

FOOD	PORTION	CALORIES	FAT
anisette	⅔ oz	74	0
apricot brandy	⅔ oz	64	0
benedictine	⅔ oz	69	0

FOOD	PORTION	CALORIES	FAT
bloody mary	1 cocktail (5 oz)	116	tr
bourbon & soda	1 cocktail (4 oz)	105	0
coffee liqueur	1.5 oz	174	tr
coffee w/ cream liqueur	1.5 oz	154	7
creme de menthe	1.5 oz	186	tr
creme de menthe	⅔ oz	67	0
curacao liqueuer	⅔ oz	54	0
daiquiri	2.5 oz	87	0
gin	1.5 oz	110	0
gin & tonic	1 cocktail (7.5 oz)	171	0
highball	8 oz	166	0
manhattan	2.5 oz	116	0
martini	1 cocktail (2.5 oz)	156	0
mint julep	10 oz	210	0
old-fashioned	2.5 oz	127	0
pina colada	1 cocktail (4.5 oz)	262	3
rum	1.5 oz	97	0
screwdriver	1 cocktail (7 oz)	174	tr
sloe gin fizz	2.5 oz	132	0
tequila sunrise	1 cocktail (5.5 oz)	189	tr
tom collins	1 cocktail (7.5 oz)	121	0
vodka	1.5 oz	97	0
whiskey	1.5 oz	105	0
whiskey sour	1 cocktail (3 oz)	123	tr
whiskey sour mix; as prep	1 oz	48	0

FOOD	PORTION	CALORIES	FAT

LIVER
(*see also* PATE)

FOOD	PORTION	CALORIES	FAT
beef, raw	4 oz	161	4
beef; braised	3 oz	137	4
beef; pan-fried	3 oz	184	7
chicken, raw	1.1 oz	40	1
duck, raw	1.5 oz	60	2
goose, raw	3.3 oz	125	4
pork, raw	3 oz	151	4
pork; braised	3 oz	141	4
turkey, raw	3.6 oz	140	4
turkey; simmered	1 cup	237	8

LOBSTER

FRESH

FOOD	PORTION	CALORIES	FAT
northern, raw	3 oz	77	1
northern, raw	1 lobster (5.3 oz)	136	1
northern; cooked	1 cup	142	1
northern; cooked	3 oz	83	1
spiny, raw	3 oz	95	1
spiny, raw	1 lobster (7.3 oz)	233	3

FROZEN

FOOD	PORTION	CALORIES	FAT
Gulfstream Tails (King & Prince)	6 oz	170	1
Gulfstream Tails (King & Prince)	7 oz	199	2
Gulfstream Tails (King & Prince)	8 oz	227	2

HOME RECIPE

FOOD	PORTION	CALORIES	FAT
newburg	1 cup	485	27

FOOD	PORTION	CALORIES	FAT

LOGANBERRIES

loganberries	1 cup	80	tr

LOQUATS

loquats	1	5	tr

LOTUS ROOT

sliced; cooked	10 slices	59	tr
sliced, raw	10 slices	45	tr

LOTUS SEEDS

dried	1 oz	94	tr

LOX
(*see* SALMON)

LUNCHEON MEATS/COLD CUTS
(*see also* CHICKEN, HAM, MEAT SUBSTITUTE, TURKEY)

Armour Beef Bologna, Lower Salt	1 oz	90	8
Armour Bologna, Lower Salt	1 oz	90	8
Armour Salami, Lower Salt	1 oz	80	7
Carl Buddig Beef	1 oz	40	2
Carl Buddig Corned Beef	1 oz	40	2
Carl Buddig Pastrami	1 oz	40	2
Health Valley Bologna, Beef	3.5 oz	310	30
Health Valley Pork Breakfast, Sliced	3.5 oz	560	60
Health Valley Salami	3.5 oz	400	35
Health Valley Salami, Midget	1 oz	57	4
Hebrew National Bologna, Midget	1 oz	60	5
Oscar Mayer Bar-B-Q Loaf	1 slice (28 g)	48	3
Oscar Mayer Bologna	1 slice (28 g)	90	8

FOOD	PORTION	CALORIES	FAT
Oscar Mayer Bologna, Beef	1 slice (28 g)	90	8
Oscar Mayer Bologna, Beef, Garlic Flavored	1 slice (28 g)	89	8
Oscar Mayer Bologna, Beef Lebanon	1 link (23 g)	49	3
Oscar Mayer Bologna w/ Cheese	1 slice (23 g)	74	7
Oscar Mayer Braunschweiger German Brand	1 oz	94	9
Oscar Mayer Braunschweiger, Sliced	1 slice (28 g)	96	9
Oscar Mayer Braunschweiger, Tube	1 oz	96	9
Oscar Mayer Corned Beef	1 slice (17 g)	16	tr
Oscar Mayer Cotto Salami	1 slice (23 g)	54	4
Oscar Mayer Cotto Salami, Beef	1 slice (23 g)	46	3
Oscar Mayer Genoa Salami, Beef	1 slice (9 g)	34	3
Oscar Mayer Hard Salami	1 slice (9 g)	34	3
Oscar Mayer Head Cheese	1 slice (28 g)	55	4
Oscar Mayer Honey Loaf	1 slice (28 g)	35	1
Oscar Mayer Jalapeno	1 slice (28 g)	72	6
Oscar Mayer Liver Cheese Pork Fat Wrap	1 slice (38 g)	116	10
Oscar Mayer Luncheon Meat	1 slice (28 g)	98	9
Oscar Mayer Luxury Loaf	1 slice (28 g)	38	1
Oscar Mayer New England Brand Sausage	1 slice (23 g)	31	2
Oscar Mayer Old Fashioned Loaf	1 slice (28 g)	64	4
Oscar Mayer Olive Loaf	1 slice (28 g)	62	4
Oscar Mayer Pastrami	1 slice (17 g)	16	tr
Oscar Mayer Peppered Loaf	1 slice (28 g)	43	2
Oscar Mayer Pickle & Pimento Loaf	1 slice (28 g)	63	4
Oscar Mayer Picnic Loaf	1 slice (28 g)	62	4
Oscar Mayer Salami For Beer	1 slice (23 g)	55	5
Oscar Mayer Salami For Beer Beef	1 slice (23 g)	66	6

FOOD	PORTION	CALORIES	FAT
Oscar Mayer Sandwich Spread	1 oz	67	5
Oscar Mayer Smoked Beef	1 slice (14 g)	14	tr
Oscar Mayer Summer Sausage Thuringer Cervelat	1 slice (23 g)	73	7
Oscar Mayer Summer Sausage Thuringer Cervelat Beef	1 slice (23 g)	72	6
barbecue loaf, beef	1 slice (23 g)	40	2
beerwurst	1 slice (23 g)	75	7
beerwurst, beef	1 slice (6 g)	19	2
beerwurst, pork	1 slice (6 g)	14	1
beerwurst, pork	1 slice (23 g)	55	4
berliner, pork & beef	1 slice (23 g)	53	4
blood sausage	1 slice (25 g)	95	9
bologna, beef	1 slice (23 g)	72	7
bologna, beef & pork	1 slice (23 g)	73	7
bologna, lebanon beef	1 slice (23 g)	52	3
bologna, pork	1 slice (23 g)	57	5
braunschweiger	1 oz	102	9
braunschweiger, pork	1 slice (18 g)	65	6
corned beef loaf	1 slice (28 g)	46	2
dried beef	1 oz	47	1
dried beef	5 slices (21 g)	35	tr
dutch brand loaf, pork & beef	1 slice (28 g)	68	5
ham & cheese loaf	1 slice (28 g)	147	11
headcheese, pork	1 slice (28 g)	60	4
honey loaf, pork & beef	1 slice (28 g)	36	1
honey roll sausage	1 slice (23 g)	42	2
liver cheese, pork	1 slice (38 g)	115	10
liver cheese, pork	1 oz	86	7
liverwurst	1 oz	93	8
liverwurst, pork	1 slice (18 g)	59	5

FOOD	PORTION	CALORIES	FAT
luncheon meat, beef	1 slice (28 g)	87	7
luncheon meat, beef	1 slice (1 oz)	87	7
luncheon meat, beef, thin slice	5 slices (21 g)	26	tr
luncheon meat, pork & beef	1 slice (28 g)	200	18
luncheon meat, pork, canned	1 slice (21 g)	70	6
luncheon meat, pork, canned	1 oz	95	9
luncheon sausage, pork & beef	1 slice (23 g)	60	5
luxury loaf, pork	1 slice (28 g)	40	5
mortadella, beef & pork	1 slice (15 g)	47	4
mother's loaf, pork	1 slice (21 g)	59	5
new england brand sausage, pork & beef	1 slice (23 g)	37	2
olive loaf, pork	1 slice (28 g)	67	5
pastrami, beef	1 slice (1 oz)	99	8
peppered loaf, pork & beef	1 slice (28 g)	42	2
pepperoni, pork & beef	1 sausage (9 oz)	1248	110
pickle & pimento loaf, pork	1 slice (28 g)	74	6
picnic loaf, pork & beef	1 slice (28 g)	66	5
salami, cooked, beef	1 slice (23 g)	58	5
salami, cooked, beef & pork	1 slice (23 g)	57	5
salami, hard, pork	1 slice (10 g)	41	4
salami, hard, pork	1 pkg (4 oz)	460	38
salami, hard, pork & beef	1 slice (10 g)	42	3
salami, hard, pork & beef	1 pkg (4 oz)	472	39
sandwich spread, pork & beef	1 Tbsp	35	3
sandwich spread, pork & beef	1 oz	67	5
smoked chopped beef	1 slice (1 oz)	38	1
summer sausage, thuringer cervelat	1 slice (23 g)	80	7

FOOD	PORTION	CALORIES	FAT
LUPINS			
cooked	1 cup	197	5
dried, raw	1 cup	668	17
LYCHEES			
lychees	1	6	tr
MACADAMIA NUTS			
dried	1 oz	199	21
oil roasted	1 oz	204	22
MACKEREL			
CANNED			
jack	1 can (12.7 oz)	563	23
jack	1 cup	296	12
FRESH			
Atlantic, raw	3 oz	174	12
Atlantic, raw	1 fillet (3.9 oz)	229	16
Atlantic; cooked	1 fillet (3.1 oz)	231	16
Atlantic; cooked	3 oz	223	15
Spanish, raw	3 oz	118	5
Spanish, raw	1 fillet (6.6 oz)	260	12
Spanish; cooked	1 fillet (5.1 oz)	230	9
Spanish; cooked	3 oz	134	5
king, raw	½ fillet (6.9 oz)	207	2
king, raw	3 oz	89	2

MACARONI
(*see* PASTA)

FOOD	PORTION	CALORIES	FAT

MALTED MILK

LIQUID

chocolate	1 cup	233	9
natural flavor	1 cup	236	10

POWDER

Carnation, Chocolate	3 heaping tsp (21 g)	79	tr
Carnation, Original	3 heaping tsp (21 g)	90	2
Kraft Malted Milk, Chocolate, Instant: as prep w/ whole milk	3 tsp + 1 cup milk	240	9
Kraft Malted Milk, Natural, Instant; as prep w/ whole milk	3 tsp + 1 cup milk	240	10
chocolate	¾ oz	83	1
natural flavor	¾ oz	86	2

MANGO

mango	1	135	1

MARGARINE

REDUCED CALORIE

Blue Bonnet Diet	1 Tbsp	50	6
Fleischmann's Diet	1 Tbsp	50	6
Fleischmann's Diet w/ Lite Salt	1 Tbsp	50	6
Kraft Spread	1 Tbsp	50	6
Kraft Spread (stick)	1 Tbsp	60	7
Mazola Diet	1 Tbsp	50	6
Mazola Diet	1 cup	815	92
Mazola Light Corn Oil Spread	1 Tbsp	50	6
Mazola Light Corn Oil Spread	1 cup	835	94
Parkay Diet Soft	1 Tbsp	50	6

FOOD	PORTION	CALORIES	FAT
Parkay Light Corn Oil Spread	1 Tbsp	70	8
Parkay Spread	1 Tbsp	60	7
Weight Watchers	1 Tbsp	50	6
corn	1 tsp	17	2
corn	1 cup	801	90
soybean	1 cup	801	90
soybean	1 tsp	17	2
soybean & cottonseed	1 tsp	17	2
soybean & cottonseed	1 cup	801	90
soybean & palm	1 cup	801	90
soybean & palm	1 tsp	17	2
REGULAR Blue Bonnet	1 Tbsp	100	11
Fleischmann's	1 Tbsp	100	11
Fleischmann's Light Corn Oil Stick	1 Tbsp	80	8
Fleischmann's Sweet Unsalted	1 Tbsp	100	11
Krona	1 Tbsp	100	11
Land O'Lakes, Premium Corn Oil Stick	1 Tbsp	100	11
Land O'Lakes, Regular Stick	1 Tbsp	100	11
Mazola	1 Tbsp	100	11
Mazola	1 cup	1650	184
Mazola, Unsalted	1 Tbsp	100	11
Mazola, Unsalted	1 cup	1635	183
Mother's	1 Tbsp	100	11
Mother's, Unsalted	1 Tbsp	100	11
Nucoa	1 Tbsp	100	11
Nucoa	1 cup	1630	184
Parkay	1 Tbsp	100	11
Promise	1 Tbsp	90	10

FOOD	PORTION	CALORIES	FAT
Shedd's Spread Country Crock Classic Quarters	1 Tbsp	80	9
coconut, safflower, palm	1 tsp	34	4
coconut, safflower, palm	1 stick	815	91
corn	1 stick	815	91
corn	1 tsp	34	4
corn, soybean & cottonseed	1 stick	815	91
corn, soybean & cottonseed	1 tsp	34	4
corn, soybean & cottonseed, unsalted	1 tsp	34	4
corn, soybean & cottonseed, unsalted	1 stick	809	91
soybean & palm	1 tsp	34	4
soybean & palm	1 stick	815	91
soybean, hydrogenated	1 stick	815	91
soybean, hydrogenated	1 tsp	34	4
sunflower, soybean & cottonseed	1 stick	815	91
sunflower, soybean & cottonseed	1 tsp	34	4
SOFT			
Blue Bonnet Light Tasty Spread	1 Tbsp	60	7
Blue Bonnet Soft	1 Tbsp	100	11
Blue Bonnet Spread	1 Tbsp	80	8
Blue Bonnet Spread Stick (70% fat)	1 Tbsp	90	10
Blue Bonnet Spread Stick (75% fat)	1 Tbsp	90	11
Fleischmann's	1 Tbsp	100	11
Fleischmann's Light Corn Oil Spread	1 Tbsp	80	8
Fleischmann's Sweet Unsalted	1 Tbsp	100	11
I Can't Believe It's Not Butter! (Lever)	1 Tbsp	90	10
Land O'Lakes Regular Soft Tub	1 Tbsp	100	11
Mother's Salted	1 Tbsp	100	11

FOOD	PORTION	CALORIES	FAT
Mother's, Unsalted	1 Tbsp	100	11
Nucoa	1 Tbsp	90	10
Nucoa	1 cup	1415	160
Parkay Corn Oil, Soft	1 Tbsp	100	11
Parkay Soft	1 Tbsp	100	11
Promise	1 Tbsp	90	10
Shedd's Spread Country Crock	1 Tbsp	80	7
corn	1 tsp	34	4
corn	1 cup	1626	183
safflower	1 tsp	34	4
safflower	1 cup	1626	183
safflower, cottonseed & peanut	1 cup	1626	183
safflower, cottonseed & peanut	1 tsp	34	4
soybean, salted	1 tsp	34	4
soybean, salted	1 cup	1626	183
soybean, unsalted	1 cup	1626	182
soybean, unsalted	1 tsp	34	4
soybean & cottonseed	1 cup	1626	183
soybean & cottonseed	1 tsp	34	4
soybean & cottonseed, unsalted	1 tsp	34	4
soybean & cottonseed, unsalted	1 cup	1626	182
soybean & palm	1 cup	1626	183
soybean & palm	1 tsp	34	4
soybean & safflower	1 tsp	34	4
soybean & safflower	1 cup	1626	183
sunflower & peanut	1 cup	1626	183
sunflower & peanut	1 tsp	34	4
SQUEEZE			
Fleischmann's	1 Tbsp	100	11
Parkay Squeeze	1 Tbsp	100	11
soybean & cottonseed	1 tsp	34	4

FOOD	PORTION	CALORIES	FAT
WHIPPED			
Blue Bonnet Soft Whipped	1 Tbsp	70	7
Blue Bonnet Whipped Stick	1 Tbsp	70	7
Fleischmann's Lightly Salted	1 Tbsp	70	7
Fleischmann's Unsalted	1 Tbsp	70	7
Miracle Brand	1 Tbsp	60	7
Miracle Brand Stick	1 Tbsp	70	7
Parkay	1 Tbsp	60	7
Parkay Stick	1 Tbsp	60	7

MARSHMALLOW

FOOD	PORTION	CALORIES	FAT
Campfire (Borden)	2 lg	40	0
Campfire, Miniature (Borden)	24	40	0
Funmallows (Kraft)	1	25	0
Funmallows, Miniatures (Kraft)	10	18	0
Jet-Puffed (Kraft)	1	25	0
Miniature (Kraft)	10	18	0
miniature	1	2	tr

MATZO

FOOD	PORTION	CALORIES	FAT
American Matzo Crackers (Manischewitz)	1 cup	115	2
Daily Thin Tea (Manischewitz)	1	103	tr
Dietetic Thins (Manischewitz)	1	91	tr
Egg n' Onion (Manischewitz)	1	112	tr

FOOD	PORTION	CALORIES	FAT
Matzo Cracker, Miniatures (Manischewitz)	10–20	90	tr
Matzo Farfel (Manischewitz)	1 cup	280	tr
Matzo Meal (Manischewitz)	1 cup	514	1
Passover (Manischewitz)	1	129	tr
Passover Egg (Manischewitz)	1	132	2
Passover Egg Matzo Crackers (Manischewitz)	10	108	2
Unsalted (Manischewitz)	1	110	tr
Wheat Matzo Crackers (Manischewitz)	10	90	1
Whole Wheat w/ Bran (Manischewitz)	1	110	1

MAYONNAISE

(*see also* MAYONNAISE-TYPE SALAD DRESSING, RELISH)

FOOD	PORTION	CALORIES	FAT
REDUCED CALORIE			
Best Foods Light	1 Tbsp	50	5
Best Foods Light	1 cup	760	78
Diamond Crystal	1 Tbsp	50	5
Estee	1 Tbsp	100	10
Hellman's Light	1 Tbsp	50	5
Hellman's Light	1 cup	760	78
Kraft Light Reduced Calorie	1 Tbsp	45	5
imitation	1 cup	232	12
imitation	1 Tbsp	15	1
soybean	1 Tbsp	34	3
soybean	1 cup	556	46

FOOD	PORTION	CALORIES	FAT
REGULAR			
Best Foods Real	1 Tbsp	100	11
Best Foods Real	1 cup	1570	175
Hellman's Real	1 Tbsp	100	11
Kraft Real Mayonnaise	1 Tbsp	100	12
Kraft Sandwich Spread	1 Tbsp	50	5
Mother's	1 Tbsp	100	11
mayonnaise	2 Tbsp	196	22
sandwich spread	1 Tbsp	60	5
soybean	1 Tbsp	99	11
soybean	1 cup	1577	175

MAYONNAISE-TYPE SALAD DRESSING
(*see also* MAYONNAISE, RELISH)

FOOD	PORTION	CALORIES	FAT
Bright Day Dressing	1 Tbsp	60	6
Miracle Whip Salad Dressing	1 Tbsp	70	7
Weight Watchers Reduced Calorie Dressing	1 Tbsp	40	4
home recipe	1 Tbsp	25	2
home recipe	1 cup	400	24
mayonnaise type salad dressing	1 cup	916	78
mayonnaise type salad dressing	2 Tbsp	114	10
soybean, w/o cholesterol	1 cup	1084	107
soybean w/o cholesterol	1 Tbsp	68	7

MEAT SUBSTITUTE
.(*see also* CHICKEN SUBSTITUTE, SAUSAGE SUBSTITUTE, TURKEY SUBSTITUTE)

FOOD	PORTION	CALORIES	FAT
Bolono; frzn (Worthington)	3.5 oz	138	5

FOOD	PORTION	CALORIES	FAT
Corn Dogs (Loma Linda)	1 (2.5 oz)	250	19
Dinner Cuts (Loma Linda)	2 (3.5 oz)	110	1
Dinner Cuts, No Salt Added (Loma Linda)	2 (3.5 oz)	110	1
Fripats; frzn (Worthington)	3.5 oz	294	19
Griddle Steaks (Loma Linda)	1 (1.7 oz)	160	11
Griddle Steaks (Loma Linda)	1 (2 oz)	190	13
Leanies; frzn (Worthington)	3.5 oz	252	17
Meatless Big Franks (Loma Linda)	1 (1.8 oz)	100	5
Meatless Bologna (Loma Linda)	2 slices (2 oz)	150	9
Meatless Redi-slice Burger Loma Linda)	½ slice (2.4 oz)	130	6
Meatless Roast Beef (Loma Linda)	2 slices (2 oz)	107	3
Meatless Salami (Loma Linda)	2 slices (2 oz)	98	2
Meatless Salami; frzn (Worthington)	3.5 oz	198	11
Meatless Savory Meatballs (Loma Linda)	7 meatballs (2.5 oz)	190	8
Meatless Sizzle Burger (Loma Linda)	1 (2.5 oz)	210	11
Meatless Sizzle Franks (Loma Linda)	2 (2.4 oz)	170	13
Meatless Swiss Steak w/ Gravy (Loma Linda)	1 steak (2.6 oz)	140	8
Meatless Vita-Burger Chunks (Loma Linda)	¼ cup	70	tr

FOOD	PORTION	CALORIES	FAT
Meatless Vita-Burger Granules (Loma Linda)	3 Tbsp	70	tr
Nuteena (Loma Linda)	½ slice (2.4 oz)	160	12
Okara Pattie; frzn (Natural Touch)	3.5 oz	208	16
Olive Loaf (Loma Linda)	2 slices (2 oz)	119	6
Patties; frzn (Morningstar Farms)	3.5 oz	240	17
Patty Mix (Loma Linda)	¼ cup	50	1
Prime Stakes, canned (Worthington)	3.5 oz	182	12
Prosage Chub; frzn (Worthington)	3.5 oz	245	17
Prosage Links; frzn (Worthington)	3.5 oz	280	20
Prosage Patties; frzn (Worthington)	3.5 oz	279	18
Proteena (Loma Linda)	½ slice (2.5 oz)	140	6
Saucettes, canned (Worthington)	3.5 oz	210	14
Savory Dinner Loaf; mix not prep (Loma Linda)	¼ cup	50	1
Stakelets; frzn (Worthington)	3.5 oz	178	12
Stew Pac (Loma Linda)	2 oz	70	2
Tastee Cuts (Loma Linda)	2 pieces (2.5 oz)	70	1
Tender Bits (Loma Linda)	4 pieces (2 oz)	80	3

FOOD	PORTION	CALORIES	FAT
Tender Rounds w/ Gravy (Loma Linda)	6 pieces (2.6 oz)	120	4
Tofu Pups (Lightlife)	1 (1.5 oz)	92	5
Vege-Burger (Loma Linda)	½ cup	110	1
Vege-Burger NSA (Loma Linda)	½ cup	140	2
Vegelona (Loma Linda)	½ slice	100	1
Wham; frzn (Worthington)	3.5 oz	184	11
simulated sausage	1 link (25 g)	64	11
simulated sausage	1 patty (38 g)	97	7

MELON
(*see also* INDIVIDUAL NAMES)

FRESH Cantalene (Chiquita)	1 cup	60	0
Honey Mist (Chiquita)	1 cup	80	0
FROZEN melon balls	1 cup	55	tr

MEXICAN FOOD
(*see also* CHIPS, DINNER, SNACKS)

CANNED Enchilada Sauce, Hot (Ortega)	1 oz	12	0
Enchilada Sauce, Mild (Ortega)	1 oz	12	0
Green Chiles (Ortega)	1 oz	10	0

FOOD	PORTION	CALORIES	FAT
Green Chili Salsa, Hot (Ortega)	1 oz	10	0
Green Chili Salsa, Medium (Ortega)	1 oz	8	0
Green Chili Salsa, Mild (Ortega)	1 oz	8	0
Hot Enchilada Sauce (El Molino)	2 Tbsp	16	1
Hot Peppers (Ortega)	1 oz	8	0
Jalapeno Peppers (Ortega)	1 oz	10	0
Jalapeno Sliced (Trappey's)	1 oz	6	0
Jalapeno Whole (Trappey's)	2 med peppers	8	0
Mexican Jalapeno Peppers (Vlasic)	1 oz	8	0
Mexican Sauce (Pritikin Foods)	4 oz	50	1
Mexican Style Stewed Tomatoes (S&W)	½ cup	40	0
Mild Green Chili Sauce (El Molino)	2 Tbsp	10	0
Picante Salsa (Ortega)	1 oz	10	0
Picante Sauce (Estee)	2 Tbsp	8	0
Ranchera Salsa (Ortega)	1 oz	12	0
Red Taco Sauce, Mild (El Molino)	2 Tbsp	10	0
Taco Salsa, Hot (Ortega)	1 oz	10	0
Taco Salsa, Mild (Ortega)	1 oz	10	0

FOOD	PORTION	CALORIES	FAT
Taco Sauce (Estee)	2 Tbsp	14	0
Taco Sauce, Hot (Ortega)	1 oz	12	0
Taco Sauce, Mild (Ortega)	1 oz	12	0
Tamalitos in Chili Gravy (Dennison's)	7.5 oz	310	16
Tomatoes & Jalapenos (Ortega)	1 oz	8	0
Western Style Taco Sauce (Ortega)	1 oz	8	0
refried beans	½ cup	134	1
tomatoes w/ green chilis	½ cup	18	tr
FRESH Taco/Tostada Shells (Ortega)	1	50	2
chili peppers, hot, raw	1 pepper	18	tr
chili peppers, hot, raw; chopped,	½ cup	30	tr
tamale	1 (3.9 oz)	155	8
tortilla; baked	1 (.7 oz)	43	tr
tortilla; steamed	1 (.7 oz)	43	tr
FROZEN 3 Beef Enchiladas (El Charrito)	11 oz	560	31
3 Cheese Enchiladas (El Charrito)	11 oz	470	20
3 Chicken Enchiladas (El Charrito)	11 oz	440	13
4 Beef Enchiladas, Mexican Holiday (Van De Kamp's)	8.5 oz	340	15
4 Cheese Enchiladas, Mexican Holiday (Van De Kamp's)	8.5 oz	370	20

FOOD	PORTION	CALORIES	FAT
4 Grande Beef Enchiladas (El Charrito)	16.5 oz	890	47
6 Beef Enchiladas (El Charrito)	16.25 oz	880	49
6 Beef & Cheese Enchiladas (El Charrito)	16.25 oz	880	42
6 Cheese Enchiladas (El Charrito)	16.25 oz	780	30
Beef Enchilada Mexican Holiday (Van De Kamp's)	7.5 oz	250	15
Beef Enchilada Dinner (El Charrito)	13.75 oz	620	31
Beef Enchiladas Suiza (Weight Watchers)	9.12 oz	310	13
Beef & Bean Burrito (Van De Kamp's)	5 oz	320	9
Beef & Bean Burritos (Patio)	5 oz	361	16
Beef & Bean Green Chili (Patio)	5 oz	330	12
Beef & Cheese Burrito (Van De Kamp's)	5 oz	320	11
Beef & Red Bean Chili Burritos (Patio)	5 oz	333	13
Beef Enchilada Dinner (Patio)	13.25 oz	514	24
Beef Enchilada Dinner Mexican Holiday (Van De Kamp's)	12 oz	390	15
Beef Enchiladas (Swanson)	13.75 oz	480	24
Beef Fajitas (Weight Watchers)	6.75 oz	270	7
Beef Tostada Supreme Mexican Classic (Van De Kamp's)	8.5 oz	530	30

FOOD	PORTION	CALORIES	FAT
Beef/Cheese Enchilada w/ Rice & Beans Mexican Classic (Van De Kamp's)	14.75 oz	540	20
Beefsteak Burrito (Weight Watchers)	7.62 oz	330	12
Burrito Dinner (Patio)	12 oz	517	16
Burrito Grande, B & B (El Charrito)	6 oz	430	16
Burrito Grande, Green Chili B & B (El Charrito)	6 oz	410	14
Burrito Grande, Jalapeno (El Charrito)	6 oz	410	15
Burrito Grande, Red Chili B & B (El Charrito)	6 oz	410	15
Burrito, Green Chili B & B (El Charrito)	5 oz	370	16
Burrito, Red Chili B & B (El Charrito)	5 oz	380	18
Burrito, Red Hot B & B (El Charrito)	5 oz	540	18
Burrito, Red Hot, Beef (El Charrito)	5 oz	340	17
Cheese Enchilada Dinner (El Charrito)	13.75 oz	570	24
Cheese Enchilada Dinner (Patio)	12.25 oz	378	9
Cheese Enchilada Mexican Holiday (Van De Kamp's)	7.5 oz	270	15
Cheese Enchilada Dinner, Mexican Holiday (Van De Kamp's)	12 oz	450	20
Cheese Enchilada Ranchero, Mexican Holiday (Van De Kamp's)	5.5 oz	250	15
Cheese Enchilada w/ Rice & Beans, Mexican Classic (Van De Kamp's)	14.75 oz	620	30

FOOD	PORTION	CALORIES	FAT
Cheese Enchiladas Ranchero (Weight Watchers)	8.87 oz	370	22
Chicken Burrito (Weight Watchers)	7.62 oz	330	14
Chicken Enchilada, Mexican Holiday (Van De Kamp's)	7.5 oz	250	10
Chicken Enchilada Dinner (El Charrito)	13.75 oz	510	17
Chicken Enchilada Suiza, Mexican Classic (Van De Kamp's)	5.5 oz	220	10
Chicken Enchiladas Suiza (Weight Watchers)	9.37 oz	360	17
Chicken Fajitas (Weight Watchers)	6.75 oz	260	6
Chicken Suiza w/ Rice & Beans, Mexican Classic (Van De Kamp's)	14.75 oz	550	20
Crispy Fried Burrito, Mexican Classic (Van De Kamp's)	6 oz	365	15
Fiesta Dinner (Patio)	12.25 oz	461	20
Grande Beef Enchilada Dinner (El Charrito)	21 oz	950	49
Grande Burrito w/ Rice & Corn, Mexican Classic (Van De Kamp's)	14.75 oz	530	20
Grande Mexican Style Dinner (El Charrito)	20 oz	850	47
Grande Satillo Dinner (El Charrito)	20.75 oz	820	34
Green Chile Beef/Bean Burrito (Van De Kamp's)	5 oz	330	11
Hungry Man Mexican Style (Swanson)	20.25 oz	750	39
Mexican Dinner (Patio)	13.25	533	24

FOOD	PORTION	CALORIES	FAT
Mexican Style Combination (Swanson)	14.25 oz	500	25
Mexican Style Dinner (El Charrito)	14.25 oz	690	35
Mexican Style Dinner, Mexican Holiday (Van De Kamp's)	11.5 oz	420	20
Queso Dinner (El Charrito)	13.25 oz	490	16
Ranchera Dinner (Patio)	13 oz	468	21
Red Chile Beef/Bean Burrito (Van De Kamp's)	5 oz	320	12
Red Hot Burritos (Patio)	5 oz	352	15
Satillo Dinner (El Charrito)	13.5 oz	570	24
Shredded Beef Enchilada, Mexican Classic (Van De Kamp's)	5.5 oz	180	10
Shredded Beef Enchilada w/ Rice & Corn, Mexican Classic (Van De Kamp's)	14.75 oz	490	15
Shredded Beef Taquitos w/ Guacamole, Mexican Classic (Van De Kamp's)	8 oz	490	25
Sirloin Burrito Grande, Mexican Classic (Van De Kamp's)	11 oz	440	15
Tortillas, Corn (El Charrito)	2	95	1
Tortillas, Flour (El Charrito)	2	170	4
HOME RECIPE burrito	1 (8 oz)	332	20
enchiladas, eggplant	1	142	5

FOOD	PORTION	CALORIES	FAT
taco salad	1 cup	292	20
tacos verde, blanco y rojo	1 (5.6 oz)	296	22
MIX			
Taco Meat Seasoning, Mild (Ortega)	1 oz	90	1
Taco Meat Seasoning, Mild; as prep w/ ground beef (Ortega)	3 oz	180	12
Tortilla, Corn Masa Harina; not prep (Quaker)	1 cup	421	5
Tortilla, Wheat Masa Trigo; not prep (Quaker)	1 cup	458	12

MILK

(*see also* CHOCOLATE, COCOA, MILK DRINKS)

FOOD	PORTION	CALORIES	FAT
CANNED			
Carnation Evaporated	½ cup	170	10
Carnation Evaporated, Lowfat	½ cup	110	3
Carnation Evaporated, Skimmed	½ cup	100	tr
Carnation Sweetened, Condensed	1 oz	123	3
Carnation Sweetened, Condensed	⅓ cup	318	9
Eagle Sweetened, Condensed	⅓ cup	320	9
Pet 99 Evaporated, Skimmed	½ cup	100	0
Pet Evaporated	½ cup	170	10
condensed, sweetened	1 oz	123	3
evaporated	1 oz	42	2
evaporated, skim	1 oz	25	tr
DRIED			
Carnation Nonfat Dry; as prep w/ water	8 oz	80	tr
Carnation Nonfat Dry; as prep w/ water	1 qt	320	tr
Flash Instant Nonfat; as prep	8 oz	80	tr

FOOD	PORTION	CALORIES	FAT
buttermilk, sweet cream	1 Tbsp	25	tr
instantized	1 cup	244	tr
nonfat	¼ cup	109	tr
whey, sweet	1 cup	512	1.6
whole	¼ cup	159	9
LIQUID, LOWFAT			
1%, nonfat milk solids added	1 cup	104	9
1%, protein fortified	1 cup	119	3
1%	1 cup	102	3
2%, protein fortified	1 cup	137	5
2%	1 cup	121	5
Borden Lowfat Buttermilk, 1½%	1 cup	120	4
Borden Lowfat Hi-Protein, 2%	1 cup	120	5
Borden Lowfat w/ Acidophilus Culture, 1%	1 cup	100	2
Friendship Buttermilk	8 oz	120	4
Lactaid	8 oz	102	0
Land O'Lakes, 1%	8 oz	100	3
Land O'Lakes, 2%	8 oz	120	5
Viva Lowfat, 2%	1 cup	120	5
buttermilk	1 cup	99	2
whey, sweet	1 cup	66	1
LIQUID, REGULAR Borden	1 cup	150	8
Borden Hi-Calcium	1 cup	150	8
Land O'Lakes	8 oz	150	8
filled milk	1 cup	154	8
goat milk	1 cup	168	10
human milk	1 oz	21	1.4
imitation milk	1 cup	150	8

FOOD	PORTION	CALORIES	FAT
indian buffalo	1 cup	236	17
sheep milk	1 cup	264	17
whole, 3.3% fat	1 cup	150	8
whole, low sodium	1 cup	149	8
LIQUID, SKIM			
Borden	1 cup	90	1
Borden Slim-Line Protein Fortified	1 cup	100	1
Land O'Lakes	8 oz	90	tr
skim	1 cup	86	tr
skim, nonfat milk solids added	1 cup	90	1
skim, protein fortified	1 cup	100	1

MILK DRINKS
(*see also* BREAKFAST DRINKS, CHOCOLATE, COCOA)

FOOD	PORTION	CALORIES	FAT
Chocolate Milk (Land O'Lakes)	8 oz	210	8
Chocolate Milk (Meadow Gold)	1 cup	210	8
Chocolate Milk, 1% (Land O'Lakes)	8 oz	160	3
Chocolate Milk, 2% Low Fat (Hershey)	1 cup	190	5
Chocolate Skim Milk (Land O'Lakes)	8 oz	140	tr
Dutch Brand Chocolate, Lowfat (Borden)	1 cup	180	5
chocolate, lowfat, 1%	1 cup	158	2.5
chocolate, lowfat, 2%	1 cup	179	5
chocolate, whole	1 cup	208	8
strawberry flavor mix; as prep w/ whole milk	9 oz	234	8

FOOD	PORTION	CALORIES	FAT
MILK SUBSTITUTE			
(*see also* COFFEE WHITENERS)			
Vitamite (Deihl)	8 oz	100	5
MILKFISH			
raw	3 oz	126	6
MILKSHAKE			
Chocolate (Frostee)	1 cup	200	8
Chocolate (Micro Magic)	11.5 oz	440	14
Strawberry (Frostee)	1 cup	180	7
Strawberry (Micro Magic)	11.5 oz	440	13
Vanilla (Micro Magic)	11.5 oz	490	19
chocolate, fast food	10 oz	360	11
chocolate thick shake	10.6 oz	356	8.1
strawberry, fast food	10 oz	319	8
vanilla, fast food	10 oz	314	8
vanilla thick shake	11 oz	350	9.5
MINERAL/BOTTLED WATER			
Artesia	7 oz	0	0
Artesia Almund	7 oz	0	0
Artesia Cranberi	7 oz	0	0
Artesia Lemin	7 oz	0	0
Artesia Orange	7 oz	0	0
Crystal Geyser Sparkling Mineral Water	6 oz	0	0

FOOD	PORTION	CALORIES	FAT
Crystal Geyser Sparkling Mineral Water, Cherry Chocolate	6 oz	0	0
Crystal Geyser Sparkling Mineral Water, Lemon	6 oz	0	0
Crystal Geyser Sparkling Mineral Water, Lime	6 oz	0	0
Crystal Geyser Sparkling Mineral Water, Natural Wild Cherry w/ Vitafort	6 oz	0	0
Crystal Geyser Sparkling Mineral Water, Orange	6 oz	0	0
Diamond Spring Water	1 qt (liter)	0	0
Glenpatrick Spring Pure Irish Water	8 oz	0	0
Mountain Valley Water	1 qt (liter)	0	0
Perrier	6.5 oz	0	0
Poland Spring	1 cup	0	0
Schweppes Vichy	6 oz	0	0

MISO

FOOD	PORTION	CALORIES	FAT
miso	½ cup	284	8

MOCHA

FOOD	PORTION	CALORIES	FAT
Bavarian Mint Mocha; as prep (Hills Bros.)	6 oz	50	1
Bavarian Mint Mocha Sugar Free; as prep (Hills Bros.)	6 oz	35	1
Cafe Mocha; as prep (Hills Bros.)	6 oz	50	1
Cafe Mocha; as prep (MJB Co.)	6 oz	50	1
Cherry Mocha; as prep (MJB Co.)	6 oz	50	1
Fudge Mocha Sugar Free; as prep (MJB Co.)	6 oz	40	2

FOOD	PORTION	CALORIES	FAT
Mint Mocha; as prep (MJB Co.)	6 oz	50	1
Mint Mocha Sugar Free; as prep (MJB Co.)	6 oz	35	1
Swiss Mocha; as prep (Hills Bros.)	6 oz	40	2
Vanilla Mocha Sugar Free; as prep (MJB Co.)	6 oz	40	2

MOLASSES

Brer Rabbit, Dark	1 Tbsp	60	0
Brer Rabbit, Light	1 Tbsp	60	0
Grandma's Gold Label	1 Tbsp	70	0
Grandma's Green Label	1 Tbsp	70	0
blackstrap	1 Tbsp	43	0
molasses	1 Tbsp	46	0

MONKFISH

raw	3 oz	64	1

MOTHBEANS

dried; cooked	1 cup	207	1
raw	1 cup	673	3

MOUSSE

FROZEN

Chocolate Mousse (Weight Watchers)	1	170	6
Light Classics, Chocolate (Sara Lee)	1 slice (60.9 g)	200	14
Light Classics, Strawberry (Sara Lee)	1 slice (53.8 g)	180	11
Raspberry Mousse (Weight Watchers)	1	160	6

FOOD	PORTION	CALORIES	FAT
HOME RECIPE			
crab	¼ cup	364	20
orange	½ cup	87	5
MIX			
Black Forest Mousse, Tiarra Dessert; as prep (Duncan Hines)	1/12 cake	260	13
Cherries & Cream Mousse, Tiarra Dessert; as prep (Duncan Hines)	1/12 cake	250	11
Chocolate Amaretto Mousse, Tiarra Dessert; as prep (Duncan Hines)	1/12 cake	270	16
Chocolate Mousse, No Bake Dessert (Jell-O)	1 pkg (3.5 oz)	415	14
Chocolate Mousse, No Bake Dessert; as prep (Jell-O)	½ cup	141	5
Chocolate Mousse, Tiarra Dessert; as prep (Duncan Hines)	1/12 cake	270	16
Chocolate Fudge Mousse, No Bake Dessert (Jell-O)	1 pkg (3.5 oz)	406	14
Chocolate Fudge Mousse, No Bake Dessert; as prep (Jell-O)	½ cup	138	6

MUFFIN

FOOD	PORTION	CALORIES	FAT
FROZEN			
Apple Cinnamon Spicy Hearty Fruit Muffins (Sara Lee)	1	220	8
Banana Nut Bran Hearty Fruit Fruit Muffins (Sara Lee)	1	230	9

FOOD	PORTION	CALORIES	FAT
Blueberry (Pepperidge Farm)	1	170	6
Blueberry Hearty Fruit Muffins (Sara Lee)	1	200	8
Bran With Raisins (Pepperidge Farm)	1	170	6
Carrot Walnut (Pepperidge Farm)	1	200	6
Chocolate Chip (Pepperidge Farm)	1	210	8
Cinnamon Swirl (Pepperidge Farm)	1	190	6
Corn (Pepperidge Farm)	1	180	7
Golden Corn Hearty Fruit Muffins (Sara Lee)	1	250	13
Oatmeal 'N Fruit Hearty Fruit Muffins (Sara Lee)	1	230	9
Raisin Bran Hearty Fruit Muffins (Sara Lee)	1	220	7
HOME RECIPE			
apple	1 (1.6 oz)	137	7
blueberry	1 (1.9 oz)	147	7
bran	1 (1.9 oz)	104	4
corn	1 (1.6 oz)	169	9
orange	1 (1.6 oz)	137	6
plain	1 (1.6 oz)	158	8
whole wheat	1 (1.6 oz)	123	3
MIX			
Blueberry, Bakery Style; as prep (Duncan Hines)	1	190	6
Bran & Honey, Bakery Style; as prep (Duncan Hines)	1	120	4

FOOD	PORTION	CALORIES	FAT
Bran & Honey Nut, Bakery Style; as prep (Duncan Hines)	1	200	7
Cinnamon Swirl, Bakery Style; as prep (Duncan Hines)	1	200	7
Corn Muffin; as prep (Dromedary)	1	120	4
Cranberry Orange Nut, Bakery Style; as prep (Duncan Hines)	1	200	8
Pecan Nut, Bakery Style; as prep (Duncan Hines)	1	220	11
Wild Blueberry; as prep (Duncan Hines)	1	110	3
READY-TO-USE			
Oat Bran Almond/Date (Health Valley)	2 oz	170	6
Oat Bran Blueberry (Health Valley)	2 oz	140	4
Oat Bran Raisin (Health Valley)	2 oz	140	3

MULLET

striped, raw	3 oz	99	3
striped, raw	1 fillet (4.2 oz)	139	5
striped; cooked	1 fillet (3.3 oz)	139	5
striped; cooked	3 oz	127	4

MUNG BEANS

DRIED			
cooked	1 cup	213	1
mung beans long rice	1 cup	492	tr
raw	1 cup	719	2

FOOD	PORTION	CALORIES	FAT
SPROUTS			
cooked	½ cup	13	tr
raw	½ cup	16	tr
stir fried	½ cup	31	tr

MUSHROOM

FOOD	PORTION	CALORIES	FAT
CANNED			
Mushrooms (Libby)	¼ cup	35	0
Mushrooms (Seneca)	¼ cup	35	0
mushrooms	½ cup	19	tr
DRIED			
shitake	4	44	tr
FRESH			
raw	1	5	tr
raw; sliced	½ cup	9	tr
shitake; cooked	4	40	tr
sliced; cooked	½ cup	21	tr
FROZEN			
Mushroom Vegetable Crisp (Ore Ida)	2⅔ oz	130	7

MUSSEL

FOOD	PORTION	CALORIES	FAT
blue, raw	3 oz	73	2
blue, raw	1 cup	129	3
blue; cooked	3 oz	147	4

MUSTARD

FOOD	PORTION	CALORIES	FAT
Grey Poupon Dijon	1 Tbsp	18	1
Gulden's Diablo	1 tsp	8	0
Gulden's Mild	1 tsp	6	0

FOOD	PORTION	CALORIES	FAT
Gulden's Spicy Brown	1 tsp	8	0
Kosciusko	1 Tbsp	11	1
Kraft Horseradish Mustard	1 Tbsp	4	0
Kraft Pure Prepared	1 Tbsp	4	0
La Choy Chinese Hot Mustard	1 tsp	8	tr
Plochman's Dijon Mustard	1 Tbsp	11	1
Plochman's Spicy Brown Mustard	1 Tbsp	11	1
Plochman's Stone Ground Mustard	1 Tbsp	11	1
Plochman's Yellow Mustard	1 Tbsp	11	1
Sauceworks Hot Mustard Sauce	1 Tbsp	35	2

MUSTARD GREENS

FOOD	PORTION	CALORIES	FAT
FRESH			
chopped; cooked	½ cup	11	tr
chopped, raw	½ cup	7	tr
FROZEN			
chopped; cooked	½ cup	14	tr
frzn; not prep	½ cup	15	tr

NATTO

FOOD	PORTION	CALORIES	FAT
natto	½ cup	187	10

NAVY BEANS

FOOD	PORTION	CALORIES	FAT
CANNED			
Navy Beans (Hanover)	½ cup	100	0
Navy Beans Seasoned w/ Pork (Luck's)	7.5 oz	230	7
Ole Fashion Navies (Ranch Style)	7.5 oz	160	2
navy	1 cup	296	1

FOOD	PORTION	CALORIES	FAT
DRIED			
Navy	1 cup	277	1
(Hurst Brand)			
cooked	1 cup	259	1
raw	1 cup	697	3
SPROUTS			
cooked	3.5 oz	78	1
raw	½ cup	35	tr

NECTARINE

nectarine	1	67	1

NEUFCHATEL CHEESE
(*see* CREAM CHEESE)

NON-DAIRY CREAMER
(*see* COFFEE WHITENERS)

NON-DAIRY WHIPPED TOPPING
(*see* WHIPPED TOPPING)

NOODLES
(*see also* PASTA DINNERS)

FOOD	PORTION	CALORIES	FAT
CANNED			
chow mein noodles	½ cup	228	5
DRY			
Chow Mein Noodles	½ cup	150	8
(La Choy)			
Egg Noodles	2 oz	221	3
(Creamette)			
Egg Noodles	2 oz	220	3
(Skinner)			
Egg Noodles, Enriched	2 oz	211	2
(Ronzoni)			

FOOD	PORTION	CALORIES	FAT
Egg Noodles; uncooked (Mueller's)	2 oz	220	3
Fine, Medium, Wide & Extra Wide (P&R)	2 oz	220	3
Noodles & Sauce, Alfredo; as prep (Lipton)	¼ pkg	146	4
Noodles & Sauce, Beef; as prep (Lipton)	¼ pkg	128	2
Noodles & Sauce, Butter; as prep (Lipton)	¼ pkg	148	4
Noodles & Sauce, Butter & Herb; as prep (Lipton)	¼ pkg	140	3
Noodles & Sauce, Cheese; as prep (Lipton)	¼ pkg	141	2
Noodles & Sauce, Chicken Flavor; as prep (Lipton)	¼ pkg	130	2
Noodles & Sauce, Parmesan; as prep (Lipton)	¼ pkg	143	4
Noodles & Sauce, Sour Cream and Chive; as prep (Lipton)	¼ pkg	144	3
Noodles & Sauce, Stroganoff; as prep (Lipton)	¼ pkg	131	3
Ramen Noodles w/ Beef Flavoring; as prep (La Choy)	½ pkg	190	7
Ramen Noodles w/ Chicken Flavoring; as prep (La Choy)	½ pkg	190	7
Ramen Noodles w/ Oriental Flavoring; as prep (La Choy)	½ pkg	190	7
Rice Noodles (La Choy)	½ cup	130	5

FOOD	PORTION	CALORIES	FAT
Spinach Egg Noodles (Ronzoni)	2 oz	209	2
Spinach Egg Noodles, Light 'N Fluffy (Skinner)	2 oz	220	3
egg noodles	½ cup	100	1

NOODLE DISHES

noodle pudding (home recipe)	½ cup	132	7

NUTRITIONAL SUPPLEMENTS
(*see also* BREAKFAST BAR, BREAKFAST DRINKS)

DIET

FOOD	PORTION	CALORIES	FAT
Figurines, Chocolate (Pillsbury)	1 bar	100	5
Figurines, Chocolate Caramel (Pillsbury)	1 bar	100	6
Figurines, Chocolate Peanut Butter (Pillsbury)	1 bar	100	6
Figurines, S'Mores (Pillsbury)	1 bar	100	5
Figurines, Vanilla (Pillsbury)	1 bar	100	5
Slender Chocolate (Carnation)	10 oz	220	
Slender Chocolate Fudge (Carnation)	10 oz	220	4
Slender Chocolate Malt (Carnation)	10 oz	220	4
Slender Milk Chocolate (Carnation)	10 oz	220	.
Slender Vanilla (Carnation)	10 oz	220	
Slender Bars, Chocolate (Carnation)	2 bars	270	1
Slender Bars, Chocolate Chip (Carnation)	2 bars	270	.

FOOD	PORTION	CALORIES	FAT
Slender Bars, Chocolate Peanut Butter (Carnation)	2 bars	270	15
Slender Bars, Vanilla (Carnation)	2 bars	270	15
Slender Instant Chocolate (Carnation)	1 pkg (1.06 oz)	110	1
Slender Instant Chocolate; as prep w/ 2% milk (Carnation)	1 pkg + 6 oz milk	200	5
Slender Instant Dutch Chocolate (Carnation)	1 pkg (1.06 oz)	110	1
Slender Instant Dutch Chocolate; as prep w/ 2% milk (Carnation)	1 pkg + 6 oz milk	200	5
Slender Instant French Vanilla (Carnation)	1 pkg (1.04 oz)	110	tr
Slender Instant French Vanilla; as prep w/ 2% milk (Carnation)	1 pkg + 6 oz milk	200	4
REGULAR			
Ensure, Black Walnut (Ross)	8 oz	254	9
Ensure, Coffee (Ross)	8 oz	254	9
Ensure, Eggnog (Ross)	8 oz	254	9
Ensure, Strawberry (Ross)	8 oz	254	9
Ensure, Vanilla (Ross)	8 oz	254	9
Ensure Plus, Coffee (Ross)	8 oz	355	13
Ensure Plus, Eggnog (Ross)	8 oz	355	13
Ensure Plus, Strawberry (Ross)	8 oz	355	13

FOOD	PORTION	CALORIES	FAT
Ensure Plus, Vanilla (Ross)	8 oz	355	13
Isocal (Mead Johnson)	8 oz	250	11
Isocal HCN (Mead Johnson)	8 oz	473	22
Lonalac (Mead Johnson)	1 oz	20	1
Malsovit Mealwafers	2	152	8
Meal On The Go Food Bar	1 (3 oz)	340	9
Nutri-Care, Strawberry	1 pkg (1.13 oz)	120	1
Nutri-Care, Strawberry as prep w/ 1 cup whole milk	1 pkg (1.13 oz)	280	9
Nutri-Care, Strawberry; as prep w/ 1 cup 2% milk	1 pkg (1.13 oz)	260	5
Sustacal (Mead Johnson)	8 oz	240	6
Sustacal HC (Mead Johnson)	8 oz	360	14
Sustacal Pudding (Mead Johnson)	5 oz	240	10

NUTS, MIXED
(*see also* INDIVIDUAL NAMES)

FOOD	PORTION	CALORIES	FAT
Cashews & Peanuts, Honey Roasted (Planters)	1 oz	170	12
Mixed Nuts Deluxe, Oil Roasted (Planters)	1 oz	180	17
Mixed Nuts, Dry Roasted (Planters)	1 oz	170	15
Mixed Nuts, Dry Roasted, Unsalted (Planters)	1 oz	170	15
Mixed Nuts, Oil Roasted (Planters)	1 oz	180	16
Mixed Nuts, Oil Roasted, Unsalted (Planters)	1 oz	180	16

FOOD	PORTION	CALORIES	FAT
Mixed Nuts w/ Peanuts (Guy's)	1 oz	180	16
Nut Topping (Planters)	1 oz	180	16
Tasty Mix (Guy's)	1 oz	130	7
Tavern Nuts (Planters)	1 oz	170	15
mixed, dry roasted w/ peanuts	1 oz	169	15
mixed, oil roasted w/ peanuts	1 oz	175	16
mixed, oil roasted, w/o peanuts	1 oz	175	16

OCTOBER BEANS

FOOD	PORTION	CALORIES	FAT
October Beans, Seasoned w/ Pork (Luck's)	7.25 oz	230	6

OCTOPUS

FOOD	PORTION	CALORIES	FAT
raw	3 oz	70	1

OIL
 (see also FAT)

FOOD	PORTION	CALORIES	FAT
Bertolli Classico	1 Tbsp	120	14
Bertolli Extra Light	1 Tbsp	120	14
Bertolli Extra Virgin	1 Tbsp	120	14
Crisco	1 Tbsp	120	14
Crisco Corn Oil	1 Tbsp	120	14
Italica	1 Tbsp	120	9
Mazola	1 Tbsp	120	14
Mazola	1 cup	1955	221
Mazola No Stick	2.5-second spray	6	1
Planters Peanut	1 Tbsp	120	14
Planters Popcorn	1 Tbsp	120	14

FOOD	PORTION	CALORIES	FAT
Pompeian	1 Tbsp	130	14
Puritan	1 Tbsp	120	14
almond	1 cup	1927	218
almond	1 Tbsp	120	14
apricot kernel	1 cup	1927	218
apricot kernel	1 Tbsp	120	14
cocoa butter	1 Tbsp	120	14
coconut	1 Tbsp	120	14
corn	1 cup	1927	218
corn	1 Tbsp	120	14
cottonseed	1 cup	1927	218
cottonseed	1 Tbsp	120	14
grapeseed	1 Tbsp	120	14
hazelnut	1 cup	1927	218
hazelnut	1 Tbsp	120	14
olive	1 Tbsp	119	14
olive	1 cup	1909	216
palm	1 cup	1927	218
palm	1 Tbsp	120	14
palm kernel	1 Tbsp	120	14
palm kernel	1 cup	1927	218
palm, Babassu	1 Tbsp	120	14
peanut	1 cup	1909	216
peanut	1 Tbsp	119	14
poppyseed	1 Tbsp	120	14
rapeseed	1 Tbsp	120	14
rapeseed	1 cup	1927	218
rice bran	1 Tbsp	120	14
safflower	1 Tbsp	120	14
safflower	1 cup	1927	218

FOOD	PORTION	CALORIES	FAT
sesame	1 Tbsp	120	14
soybean	1 Tbsp	120	14
soybean	1 cup	1927	218
soybean & cottonseed	1 Tbsp	120	14
soybean & cottonseed	1 cup	1927	218
soybean, hydrogenated	1 cup	1927	218
soybean, hydrogenated	1 Tbsp	120	14
sunflower	1 Tbsp	120	14
sunflower	1 cup	1927	218
walnut	1 cup	1927	218
walnut	1 Tbsp	120	14
wheat germ	1 Tbsp	120	14

OKRA

FOOD	PORTION	CALORIES	FAT
CANNED			
Okra Cut (Trappey's)	½ cup	25	0
FRESH			
raw	8 pods	36	tr
sliced, raw	½ cup	19	tr
sliced; cooked	½ cup	25	tr
FROZEN			
Cut Okra (Hanover)	½ cup	25	0
Okra Vegetable Crisp (Ore Ida)	3 oz	160	9
Whole Okra (Hanover)	½ cup	35	0
frzn; not prep	10 oz pkg	85	tr
okra sliced; cooked	½ cup	34	tr
okra; cooked	10 oz pkg	94	1

FOOD	PORTION	CALORIES	FAT

OLIVES

FOOD	PORTION	CALORIES	FAT
Ripe Extra Large (S&W)	1 oz	47	5
Ripe Large (S&W)	1 oz	47	5
Ripe Pitted, Extra Large (S&W)	1 oz	47	5
Ripe Pitted, Jumbo (S&W)	1 oz	47	5
Ripe Pitted, Large (S&W)	1 oz	47	5
Spanish Green (Tee Pee)	2 oz	98	10

ONION

FOOD	PORTION	CALORIES	FAT
CANNED			
Lightly Spiced Cocktail Onions (Vlasic)	1 oz	4	0
Whole Small (S&W)	½ cup	35	0
onions; chopped	½ cup	21	tr
DRIED			
onions	1 Tbsp	16	tr
FRESH			
chopped; cooked	½ cup	29	tr
chopped, raw	1 Tbsp	3	tr
FROZEN			
Chopped (Ore Ida)	2 oz	20	tr
Chopped (Southland)	2 oz	15	0
Crispy Onion Rings (Mrs. Paul's)	2.5 oz	180	10

FOOD	PORTION	CALORIES	FAT
Onions, Small, Whole (Birds Eye)	½ cup	40	tr
Onions Small w/ Cream Sauce (Birds Eye)	½ cup	100	6
Rings (Ore Ida)	2 oz	140	7
chopped; cooked	1 Tbsp	4	tr
chopped; cooked	½ cup	30	tr
chopped; not prep	1 pkg (10 oz)	83	tr
onion rings	9 oz pkg	658	36
onion rings	16 oz pkg	1170	64
onion rings; cooked	2 rings	81	5
whole; not prep	10 oz pkg	101	tr

ORANGE

CANDIED			
orange peel	1 oz	90	tr
CANNED			
Mandarin, Natural Style (S&W)	½ cup	60	0
Mandarin Oranges in Light Syrup (Dole)	½ cup	76	tr
Mandarin Selected Sections in Heavy Syrup (S&W)	½ cup	76	0
FRESH			
orange	1	62	tr
peel	1 Tbsp	tr	tr
peel, grated	1 tsp	0	0
JUICE			
Orange (Tree Top)	6 oz	90	0

FOOD	PORTION	CALORIES	FAT
Orange (Ocean Spray)	6 oz	90	1
Orange 100% Pure (Sippin Pak)	8.45 oz	110	0
Orange 100% Pure, Unsweetened (Kraft)	6 oz	90	0
Unsweetened 100% Juice (S&W)	6 oz	83	0
chilled	1 cup	110	2 g
fresh	1 cup	111	tr
frzn; as prep	1 cup	112	tr
frzn; not prep	6 oz container	339	tr

ORANGE EXTRACT

Virginia Dare	1 tsp	22	0

ORGAN MEAT

(*see* BRAINS, GIBLETS, GIZZARD, HEART, KIDNEY, LIVER)

ORIENTAL FOOD

(*see also* DINNER, RICE)

FOOD	PORTION	CALORIES	FAT
CANNED			
Chun King Divider Pak Beef Chow Mein	7 oz	100	2
Chun King Divider Pak Beef Chow Mein	8 oz	110	2
Chun King Divider Pak Beef Pepper Oriental	7 oz	110	4
Chun King Divider Pak Chicken Chow Mein	7 oz	110	4
Chun King Divider Pak Chicken Chow Mein	8 oz	120	4
Chun King Divider Pak Pork Chow Mein	7 oz	120	4

FOOD	PORTION	CALORIES	FAT
Chun King Divider Pak Shrimp Chow Mein	7 oz	100	2
Chun King Stir-Fry Entree, Chow Mein w/ Beef	6 oz	290	19
Chun King Stir-Fry Entree, Chow Mein w/ Chicken	6 oz	220	11
Chun King Stir-Fry Entree, Egg Foo Young	5 oz	140	8
Chun King Stir-Fry Entree, Pepper Steak	6 oz	250	17
Chun King Stir-Fry Entree, Sukiyaki	6 oz	290	19
La Choy Beef Pepper Oriental	¾ cup	90	2
La Choy Chow Mein, Beef	¾ cup	60	1
La Choy Chow Mein, Chicken	¾ cup	70	2
La Choy Chow Mein, Meatless	¾ cup	35	1
La Choy Chow Mein, Shrimp	¾ cup	45	1
La Choy Sweet & Sour Oriental w/ Chicken	¾ cup	240	2
La Choy Sweet & Sour Oriental w/ Pork	¾ cup	250	4
chop suey w/ meat	1 cup	144	7
chow mein noodle	½ cup	228	5
chow mein w/ chicken	1 cup	95	tr
FROZEN Benihana Oriental Lites, Chicken in Spicy Garlic Sauce	9 oz	270	4
Birds Eye Chinese Style International Recipe	½ cup	68	4
Birds Eye Chinese Style Stir-Fry Vegetable	½ cup	36	tr
Birds Eye Chow Mein Style International Recipe	½ cup	89	4
Birds Eye Japanese Style International Recipe	½ cup	88	4

FOOD	PORTION	CALORIES	FAT
Birds Eye Japanese Style Stir-Fry Vegetable	½ cup	29	tr
Birds Eye Mandarin Style International Recipe	½ cup	86	4
Budget Gourmet Slim Select Mandarin Chicken	10 oz	290	6
Budget Gourmet Slim Select Oriental Beef	10 oz	290	9
Budget Gourmet Teriyaki Chicken	12 oz	360	12
Chun King Beef Pepper Oriental	13 oz	309	3
Chun King Beef Terayaki	13 oz	379	2
Chun King Chicken Chow Mein	13 oz	361	5
Chun King Chicken Egg Rolls	7.25 oz	210	7
Chun King Crunchy Walnut Chicken	13 oz	305	5
Chun King Fried Rice w/ Chicken	8 oz	254	4
Chun King Fried Rice w/ Pork	8 oz	263	5
Chun King Hunan Pork	13 oz	324	6
Chun King Imperial Chicken	13 oz	294	1
Chun King Meat & Shrimp Egg Rolls	7.25 oz	214	8
Chun King Restaurant Style Egg Rolls	6 oz	202	7
Chun King Shrimp Egg Rolls	7.25 oz	189	6
Chun King Sweet & Sour Pork	13 oz	394	4
Chun King Szechuan Beef	13 oz	331	2
L'Orient Beef & Broccoli	11 oz	530	30
L'Orient Cantonese Chicken Chow Mein	11.5 oz	280	5
L'Orient Firecracker Chicken	10.5 oz	380	10
L'Orient Lemon Chicken	11 oz	400	15
L'Orient Orange Beef	10.75 oz	380	12
L'Orient Rock Sugar Glazed Pork	10.75 oz	360	15
La Choy Almond Chicken Egg Roll	2	450	21

FOOD	PORTION	CALORIES	FAT
La Choy Beef & Broccoli Egg Roll	2	380	13
La Choy Beef Pepper Oriental	⅔ cup	80	1
La Choy Chicken Egg Roll	3 sm	90	3
La Choy Chicken Chow Mein	⅔ cup	90	2
La Choy Lobster Egg Roll	1	180	5
La Choy Lobster Egg Roll	3 sm	80	2
La Choy Meat & Shrimp Egg Roll	3 sm	80	2
La Choy Shrimp Chow Mein	⅔ cup	70	1
La Choy Shrimp Egg Roll	3 sm	80	2
La Choy Shrimp Egg Roll	1	160	4
La Choy Spicy Oriental Chicken Egg Roll	2	300	10
La Choy Fresh & Lite Almond Chicken	9.75 oz	290	12
La Choy Fresh & Lite Beef Teriyaki	10 oz	280	7
La Choy Fresh & Lite Beef Broccoli	11 oz	290	7
La Choy Fresh & Lite Imperial Chicken Chow Mein	11 oz	270	7
La Choy Fresh & Lite Pepper Steak	10 oz	290	9
La Choy Fresh & Lite Shrimp w/ Lobster Sauce	10 oz	220	7
La Choy Fresh & Lite Spicy Chicken Oriental	9.75 oz	290	5
La Choy Fresh & Lite Sweet & Sour Chicken	10 oz	280	4
La Choy Sweet & Sour Pork Egg Roll	2	430	15
Lean Cuisine Chicken Chow Mein w/ Rice	11.25 oz	250	5
Lean Cuisine Shrimp & Chicken Cantonese w/ Noodles	10⅛ oz	260	9
Lean Cuisine Szechwan Beef w/ Noodles & Vegetables	9.25 oz	280	11

FOOD	PORTION	CALORIES	FAT
HOME RECIPE			
chicken teriyaki	¾ cup	399	27
chop suey w/ pork	1 cup	375	29
chow mein, chicken	1 cup	255	10
chow mein, pork	1 cup	425	24
chow mein, shrimp	1 cup	221	10
egg foo yong	1 (5.1 oz)	150	10
wonton, fried	½ cup	111	8
MIX			
Kikkoman Chow Mein Seasoning	1⅛ oz pkg	98	tr
Kikkoman Teriyaki Baste & Glaze	1 Tbsp	27	tr
La Choy Egg Foo Yung Dinner sauce; as prep	1 patty + ¼ cup sauce	125	7
La Choy Pepper Steak; as prep	¾ cup	210	9
La Choy Sukiyaki Dinner; as prep	¾ cup	210	9
La Choy Sweet & Sour; as prep as prep	¾ cup	410	21

OYSTER

FOOD	PORTION	CALORIES	FAT
CANNED			
Whole (Bumble Bee)	½ cup (3.5 oz)	100	4
eastern	1 cup	170	6
eastern	3 oz	58	2
FRESH			
eastern, raw	6 med	58	2
eastern, raw	1 cup	170	6
eastern; cooked	6 med	58	2
eastern; cooked	3 oz	117	4
pacific, raw	3 oz	69	2
pacific, raw	1 med	41	1

FOOD	PORTION	CALORIES	FAT
FROZEN			
Carnation Jumbo or Extra Select Breaded Oysters (King & Prince)	3.5 oz	130	2
HOME RECIPE			
eastern; breaded & fried	3 oz	167	11
eastern; breaded & fried	6 med	173	11
oysters rockefeller	3 oysters	66	2
stew	1 cup	278	18

PANCAKE

FOOD	PORTION	CALORIES	FAT
FROZEN, READY-TO-USE			
Batter; as prep (Aunt Jemima)	3 (4" diam)	210	3
Blueberry (Aunt Jemima)	3 (4" diam)	210	3
Blueberry Batter; as prep (Aunt Jemima)	3 (4" diam)	210	3
Buttermilk (Aunt Jemima)	3 (4" diam)	250	4
Buttermilk Batter; as prep (Aunt Jemima)	3 (4" diam)	210	2
Original (Aunt Jemima)	3 (4" diam)	260	4
Pancake (Morningstar Farms)	3.5 oz	232	5
Pancakes & Blueberry Sauce (Great Starts)	7 oz	410	10
Pancakes & Sausages (Great Starts)	6 oz	470	22
Pancakes w/ Strawberries (Great Starts)	7 oz	430	11
HOME RECIPE			
buckwheat	1 (6" diam)	137	3

FOOD	PORTION	CALORIES	FAT
buckwheat	1 (4" diam)	68	2
buttermilk	1 (6" diam)	164	5
buttermilk	1 (4" diam)	61	2
plain	1 (6" diam)	164	5
plain	1 (4" diam)	61	2
potato	1 (4" diam)	78	6
zucchini	1 (4" diam)	69	3
MIX			
Blueberry; as prep (Hungry Jack)	3 (4" diam)	320	15
Buttermilk; as prep (Hungry Jack)	3 (4" diam)	240	11
Buttermilk Complete; as prep (Hungry Jack)	3 (4" diam)	180	1
Buttermilk Complete Packets; as prep (Hungry Jack)	3 (4" diam)	180	3
Extra Lights; as prep (Hungry Jack)	3 (4" diam)	210	7
Extra Lights Complete; as prep (Hungry Jack)	3 (4" diam)	190	2
Pancake Mix; as prep (Estee)	3 (3" diam)	100	0
Pancake Mix; not prep (Health Valley)	1 oz	100	1
Panshakes (Hungry Jack)	3 (4" diam)	250	6

PANCAKE/WAFFLE SYRUP
(*see also* SYRUP)

FOOD	PORTION	CALORIES	FAT
Alaga Breakfast	2 Tbsp	108	0
Alaga Butter Lite	2 Tbsp	54	0
Alaga Honey Flavor	2 Tbsp	124	0
Alaga Lite	2 Tbsp	54	0

FOOD	PORTION	CALORIES	FAT
Estee	1 Tbsp	4	0
Golden Griddle (Best Foods)	1 Tbsp	55	0
Golden Griddle (Best Foods)	1 cup	885	0
Karo Pancake Syrup	1 Tbsp	60	0
Light Magic (Whitfield)	2 Tbsp	121	0
Log Cabin Syrup, Buttered	1 oz	106	tr
Log Cabin Syrup, Country Kitchen	1 oz	101	0
Log Cabin Syrup Lite	1 oz	61	tr
Log Cabin Syrup, Maple Honey	1 oz	106	0
Log Cabin Syrup, Regular	1 oz	99	tr
Tastee	2 Tbsp	121	0
Tastee Maple	2 Tbsp	113	0
Vermont Maid	1 Tbsp	50	0
Yellow Label (Whitfield)	2 Tbsp	125	0
Yellow Label, Butter Flavor (Whitfield)	2 Tbsp	117	0
Yellow Label, Maple Flavor (Whitfield)	2 Tbsp	117	0

PAPAYA

FOOD	PORTION	CALORIES	FAT
nectar	1 cup	142	tr
Papayas (Produce Marketing Assoc.)	½	80	0
papaya	1	117	tr

PARSNIP

FOOD	PORTION	CALORIES	FAT
cooked; sliced	½ cup	63	tr
raw; sliced	½ cup	50	tr

FOOD	PORTION	CALORIES	FAT
PASSION FRUIT			
passion fruit	1	18	tr
PASTA			
(see also NOODLES, PASTA DINNERS, PASTA SALAD)			
DRY			
Acini de Pepe (San Giorgio)	2 oz	210	1
All Shapes (Mueller's)	2 oz	210	1
Alphabets (P&R)	2 oz	210	1
Alphabets (San Giorgio)	2 oz	210	1
Alphabets (Skinner)	2 oz	210	1
Baby Pastina (San Giorgio)	2 oz	210	1
Bows, Medium & Small (P&R)	2 oz	220	3
Capellini (Delmonico)	2 oz	210	1
Capellini (P&R)	2 oz	210	1
Capellini (San Giorgio)	2 oz	210	1
Ditalini (San Giorgio)	2 oz	210	1
Elbow Macaroni (Delmonico)	2 oz	210	1
Elbow Macaroni (San Giorgio)	2 oz	210	1
Elbow Macaroni (Skinner)	2 oz	210	1
Elbow Macaroni, Regular & Large (P&R)	2 oz	210	1

FOOD	PORTION	CALORIES	FAT
Elbow Spaghetti (Delmonico)	2 oz	210	1
Elbows, Whole Wheat (Health Valley)	2 oz	170	1
Elbows w/ 4 Vegetables, Whole Wheat (Health Valley)	2 oz	170	1
Fettuccini (P&R)	2 oz	210	1
Fettucini (Skinner)	2 oz	210	1
Fetuccini, Egg (P&R)	2 oz	220	3
Fideo Enrollacio (Skinner)	2 oz	210	1
Flakes (San Giorgio)	2 oz	210	1
Fusilli Cut (San Giorgio)	2 oz	210	1
Fusilli Cut (P&R)	2 oz	210	1
Kluski (San Giorgio)	2 oz	220	3
Lasagna (Delmonico)	2 oz	210	1
Lasagna (Skinner)	2 oz	210	1
Lasagna Jumbo (P&R)	2 oz	210	1
Lasagna Spinach, Whole Wheat (Health Valley)	2 oz	170	1
Lasagna, Whole Wheat (Health Valley)	2 oz	170	1
Lasagne (Mueller's)	2 oz	210	1
Linguini (P&R)	2 oz	210	1

FOOD	PORTION	CALORIES	FAT
Linguini (San Giorgio)	2 oz	210	1
Linguini (Skinner)	2 oz	210	1
Linguini, Egg (Creamette)	2 oz	221	3
Macaroni (Ronzoni)	2 oz	209	tr
Manicotti (P&R)	2 oz	210	1
Manicotti (San Giorgio)	2 oz	210	1
Manicotti (Skinner)	2 oz	210	1
Mostaccioli (Delmonico)	2 oz	210	1
Mostaccioli (Skinner)	2 oz	210	1
Mostaccioli, Rigati (San Giorgio)	2 oz	210	1
Orzo (San Giorgio)	2 oz	210	1
Perciatelli (P&R)	2 oz	210	1
Perciatelli (San Giorgio)	2 oz	210	1
Pot Pie Bows (San Giorgio)	2 oz	220	3
Pot Pie Squares (San Giorgio)	2 oz	220	3
Racing Wheels (San Giorgio)	2 oz	210	1
Ribbon Pasta, Whole Wheat (Pritikin Foods)	2 oz	220	2
Rigatoni (Delmonico)	2 oz	210	1

FOOD	PORTION	CALORIES	FAT
Rigatoni (San Giorgio)	2 oz	210	1
Rigatoni (Skinner)	2 oz	210	1
Rings (P&R)	2 oz	210	1
Rippled Lasagne (San Giorgio)	2 oz	210	1
Ripplets (Skinner)	2 oz	210	1
Rotelle (Creamette)	2 oz	210	1
Rotini (Delmonico)	2 oz	210	1
Rotini (San Giorgio)	2 oz	210	1
Rotini, Rainbow (Creamette)	2 oz	210	1
Shell Macaroni (Skinner)	2 oz	210	1
Shells Jumbo (P&R)	2 oz	210	1
Shells, Large, Medium & Small (P&R)	2 oz	210	1
Shells, Large, Medium, Small & Jumbo (San Giorgio)	2 oz	210	1
Shells, Regular & Jumbo (Delmonico)	2 oz	210	1
Spaghetti (Delmonico)	2 oz	210	1
Spaghetti (San Giorgio)	2 oz	210	1
Spaghetti (Mueller's)	2 oz	210	1
Spaghetti (Skinner)	2 oz	210	1

FOOD	PORTION	CALORIES	FAT
Spaghetti, Egg (Creamette)	2 oz	221	3
Spaghetti, Regular & Thin (P&R)	2 oz	210	1
Spaghetti, Thin (Creamette)	2 oz	210	1
Spaghetti Wheels (Hanover)	½ cup	90	0
Spaghetti, Whole Wheat (Health Valley)	2 oz	170	1
Spaghetti, Whole Wheat (Pritikin Foods)	2 oz	220	2
Spaghetti w/ Amaranth, Whole Wheat (Health Valley)	2 oz	170	1
Spaghetti w/ Spinach, Whole Wheat (Health Valley)	2 oz	170	1
Spaghettini (Delmonico)	2 oz	210	1
Spaghettini (San Giorgio)	2 oz	210	1
Spinach Macaroni (Ronzoni)	2 oz	206	tr
Tubettini (San Giorgio)	2 oz	210	1
Twirls (Skinner)	2 oz	210	1
Twists, Tri Color (Mueller's)	2 oz	210	1
Vermicelli (Delmonico)	2 oz	210	1
Vermicelli (P&R)	2 oz	210	1
Vermicelli (San Girogio)	2 oz	210	1

FOOD	PORTION	CALORIES	FAT
Vermicelli (Skinner)	2 oz	210	1
Ziti (Creamette)	2 oz	210	1
Ziti Cut (Delmonico)	2 oz	210	1
Ziti Cut (San Giorgio)	2 oz	210	1

PASTA DINNERS
(see also DINNER, PASTA SALAD)

FOOD	PORTION	CALORIES	FAT
Chef Boy.ar.dee ABC's & 1,2,3's in Sauce	7.5 oz	160	1
Chef Boy.ar.dee ABC's & 1,2,3's w/ Mini Meatballs	7.5 oz	240	9
Chef Boy.ar.dee Beef Ravioli	7 oz	180	5
Chef Boy.ar.dee Beef Ravioli in Sauce	8.7 oz	240	6
Chef Boy.ar.dee Beef Ravioli in Tomato & Meat Sauce	7.5 oz	210	5
Chef Boy.ar.dee Beef-O-Getti	7.5 oz	220	9
Chef Boy.ar.dee Beefaroni	7.5 oz	220	8
Chef Boy.ar.dee Cheese Ravioli in Beef & Tomato Sauce	7.5 oz	200	3
Chef Boy.ar.dee Cheese Ravioli in Tomato Sauce	7.5 oz	200	5
Chef Boy.ar.dee Chicken Ravioli	7.5 oz	180	4
Chef Boy.ar.dee Dinosaurs in Spaghetti Sauce w/ Cheese Flavor	7.5 oz	155	1
Chef Boy.ar.dee Dinosaurs w/ Mini Meatballs	7.5 oz	235	8
Chef Boy.ar.dee Lasagna	7.5 oz	230	8
Chef Boy.ar.dee Macaroni Shells in Tomato Sauce	7.5 oz	150	1

FOOD	PORTION	CALORIES	FAT
Chef Boy.ar.dee Microwave Bowl ABC's & 1,2,3's w/ Mini Meatballs	7.5 oz	260	11
Chef Boy.ar.dee Microwave Bowl Beefaroni	7.5 oz	220	7
Chef Boy.ar.dee Microwave Bowl Lasagna	7.5 oz	230	9
Chef Boy.ar.dee Microwave Bowl Ravioli	7.5 oz	190	4
Chef Boy.ar.dee Microwave Bowl Spaghetti w/ Meatballs	7.5 oz	240	10
Chef Boy.ar.dee Microwave Bowl Tic Tac Toes w/ Meatballs	7.5 oz	260	11
Chef Boy.ar.dee Mini Bites	7.5 oz	260	12
Chef Boy.ar.dee Mini Cannelloni	7.5 oz	230	7
Chef Boy.ar.dee Mini Chicken Ravioli	7.5 oz	220	8
Chef Boy.ar.dee Mini Ravioli Beef	7.5 oz	210	5
Chef Boy.ar.dee Pac Man in Chicken Sauce	7.5 oz	170	7
Chef Boy.ar.dee Pac Man in Tomato Sauce	7.5 oz	150	1
Chef Boy.ar.dee Pac Man w/ Meatballs	7.5 oz	230	9
Chef Boy.ar.dee Roller Coasters	7.5 oz	230	9
Chef Boy.ar.dee Roller Coasters	7 oz	230	9
Chef Boy.ar.dee Smurf Beef in Spaghetti Sauce w/ Cheese Flavor	7.5 oz	150	1
Chef Boy.ar.dee Smurf Beef Ravioli & Pasta in Meat Sauce	7.5 oz	220	5
Chef Boy.ar.dee Smurf Pasta w/ Meatballs	7.5 oz	230	9
Chef Boy.ar.dee Spaghetti & Meatballs	7 oz	210	8
Chef Boy.ar.dee Spaghetti & Meatballs	8.5 oz	260	11

FOOD	PORTION	CALORIES	FAT
Chef Boy.ar.dee Spaghetti & Meatballs w/ Tomato Sauce	7.5 oz	230	8
Chef Boy.ar.dee Spaghetti & Meatballs w/ Tomato Sauce	7.8 oz	230	9
Chef Boy.ar.dee Spaghetti 'n Beef in Tomato Sauce	7 oz	220	8
Chef Boy.ar.dee Spaghetti 'n Beef in Tomato Sauce	7.5 oz	240	9
Chef Boy.ar.dee Tic Tac Toes in Spaghetti Sauce w/ Cheese Flavor	7.5 oz	160	1
Chef Boy.ar.dee Tic Tac Toes w/ Mini Meatballs	7.5 oz	240	9
Chef Boy.ar.dee Zooroni w/ Meatballs in Sauce	7.5 oz	240	8
Franco-American Beef Ravioli in Meat Sauce	7½ oz	230	5
Franco-American Beef RavioliO's in Meat Sauce	7½ oz	250	7
Franco-American Macaroni & Cheese	7⅜ oz	170	5
Franco-American PizzO's	7.5 oz	170	2
Franco-American Spaghetti in Tomato Sauce w/ Cheese	7⅜ oz	190	2
Franco-American Spaghetti w/ Meatballs in Tomato Sauce	7⅜ oz	220	8
Franco-American SpaghettiO's in Tomato & Cheese Sauce	7⅜ oz	170	2
Franco-American SpaghettiO's w/ Meatballs in Tomato Sauce	7⅜ oz	220	8
Franco-American SpaghettiO's w/ Sliced Beef Franks in Tomato Sauce	7⅜ oz	220	9
Estee Ravioli Beef	7.5 oz	210	8
Estee Spaghetti and Meatballs	7.5 oz	240	15
Lido Club Beef Ravioli	7.5 oz	190	4
Lido Club Spaghetti Rings & Little Meat Balls	7.5 oz	220	10

FOOD	PORTION	CALORIES	FAT
Mama Leone's Pasta Supreme Beef Ravioli	7.5 oz	240	7
Mama Leone's Pasta Supreme Cheese Ravioli	7.5 oz	200	2
Mama Leone's Pasta Supreme Mini Lasagna	7.5 oz	170	1
Mama Leone's Pasta Supreme Spaghetti in Tomato Sauce	7.5 oz	160	1
Mama Leone's Pasta Supreme Ziti in Meat Flavored Sauce	7.5 oz	170	4
spaghetti w/ meatballs & tomato sauce	1 cup	258	10
spaghetti w/ tomato sauce cheese	1 cup	190	2
DRY MIX Chef Boy.ar.dee Lasagna Dinner	1 serving (5.97 oz)	280	8
Chef Boy.ar.dee Spaghetti Dinner w/ Condensed Meat Sauce	1 serving (3.25 oz)	250	6
Chef Boy.ar.dee Spaghetti Dinner w/ Meat Sauce	1 serving (4.88 oz)	240	3
Chef Boy.ar.dee Spaghetti Dinner w/ Mushroom Sauce	1 serving (7.9 oz)	210	1
Kraft American Style Spaghetti Dinner; as prep	1 cup	310	8
Kraft Egg Noodle & Cheese Dinner; as prep	¾ cup	340	17
Kraft Macaroni & Cheese Dinner; as prep	¾ cup	290	13
Kraft Macaroni & Cheese Dinner Family Size; as prep	¾ cup	290	13
Kraft Macaroni & Deluxe Dinner; as prep	¾ cup	260	8
Kraft Spaghetti w/ Meat Sauce Dinner; as prep	1 cup	360	14
Kraft Spiral Macaroni & Cheese Dinner; as prep	¾ cup	330	17

FOOD	PORTION	CALORIES	FAT
Kraft Tangy Italian Style Spaghetti Dinner; as prep	1 cup	310	8
Lipton Pasta & Sauce, Cheddar Broccoli w/ Fusilli; as prep	½ cup	137	2
Lipton Pasta & Sauce, Creamy Garlic; as prep	½ cup	144	3
Lipton Pasta & Sauce, Creamy Mushroom; as prep	½ cup	143	3
Lipton Pasta & Sauce, Herb Tomato; as prep	½ cup	130	tr
Lipton Pasta & Sauce, Italiano; as prep	½ cup	135	2
Lipton Pasta & Sauce, Mushroom & Chicken Flavored; as prep	½ cup	134	tr
Lipton Pasta & Sauce, Oriental w/ Fusilli; as prep	½ cup	130	tr
Lipton Pasta & Sauce, Primavera; as prep	½ cup	143	2
Velveeta Shells and Cheese Dinner; as prep	¾ cup	260	10
FROZEN			
Armour Lite Tortellini w/ Meat	10 oz	250	10
Banquet Macaroni & Cheese	8 oz	344	17
Banquet Spaghetti w/ Meat Sauce	8 oz	270	8
Banquet Cookin' Bag, Chicken & Vegetables Primavera	4 oz	100	2
Birds Eye Pasta, Primavera Style International Recipe	½ cup	121	5
Budget Gourmet Cheese Manicotti w/ Meat Sauce	10 oz	450	26
Budget Gourmet Chicken w/ Fettucini	10 oz	400	21
Budget Gourmet Italian Sausage Lasagne	10 oz	420	20
Budget Gourmet Linguini w/ Shrimp	10 oz	330	15
Budget Gourmet Macaroni & Cheese	5.3 oz	210	8

FOOD	PORTION	CALORIES	FAT
Budget Gourmet Pasta Alfredo w/ Broccoli	5.5 oz	200	8
Budget Gourmet Pasta Shells & Beef	10 oz	340	14
Budget Gourmet Slim Select, Cheese Ravioli	10 oz	260	7
Budget Gourmet Slim Select, Fettucini w/ Meat Sauce	10 oz	290	10
Budget Gourmet Slim Select, Lasagne w/ Meat Sauce	10 oz	290	10
Budget Gourmet Slim Select, Linguini w/ Scallops & Clams	9.5 oz	280	11
Budget Gourmet Three Cheese Lasagna	10 oz	400	17
Budget Gourmet Tortellini Cheese	5.5 oz	180	6
Le Menu Light Style 3-Cheese Stuffed Shells	10 oz	280	8
Le Menu Light Style Chicken Cacciatore	10 oz	260	8
Le Menu Manicotti	8½ oz	300	12
Le Menu Vegetable Lasagna	11 oz	360	19
Lean Cuisine Linguine w/ Clam Sauce	9⅝ oz	260	7
Lean Cuisine Tuna Lasagna w/ Spinach Noodles & Vegetables	9¾ oz	280	10
Lean Cuisine Veal Lasagna	10¼ oz	280	8
Lean Cuisine Veal Primavera	9⅛ oz	250	9
Lean Cuisine Zucchini Lasagna	11 oz	260	7
Morton Lasagna w/ Garlic Bread	8.25 oz	320	10
Morton Spaghetti & Meatballs Dinner	10 oz	206	2
OH Boy! Lasagna w/ Meat & Sauce	6 oz	230	11
OH Boy! Spaghetti & Meatballs	7 oz	190	4
Sensible Chef Fettucini Alfredo w/ Chicken Casserole	9 oz	410	22

FOOD	PORTION	CALORIES	FAT
Sensible Chef Linguini w/ Shrimp & Clams Casserole	9 oz	190	3
Swanson Hungry Man Lasagna	18.75 oz	740	26
Swanson Lasagna w/ Meat	13.25 oz	470	19
Swanson Macaroni & Cheese	12 oz	390	16
Van De Kamp's Italian Classics Beef and Mushroom Lasagna	11 oz	430	25
Van De Kamp's Italian Classics, Sausage Lasagna	11 oz	440	25
Weight Watchers Baked Cheese Ravioli	9 oz	310	12
Weight Watchers Beef Salisbury Steak Romana	8.75 oz	320	13
Weight Watchers Cheese Manicotti	9.25 oz	300	13
Weight Watchers Chicken Fettucini	8.25 oz	300	10
Weight Watchers Italian Cheese Lasagna	12 oz	370	14
Weight Watchers Lasagna w/ Meat Sauce	11 oz	340	14
Weight Watchers Pasta Primavera	8.5 oz	290	13
Weight Watchers Pasta Rigati	11 oz	290	8
Weight Watchers Seafood Linguini	9 oz	220	8
Weight Watchers Spaghetti w/ Meat Sauce	10.5 oz	280	7
HOME RECIPE			
lasagna	2½" x 2½" (8.8 oz)	374	21
macaroni & cheese	¾ cup	323	17
manicotti	¾ cup	273	12
rigatoni w/ sausage sauce	¾ cup	260	12
spaghetti w/ meatballs & cheese	1 cup	407	19
spaghetti w/ meatballs & tomato sauce	1 cup	332	12

FOOD	PORTION	CALORIES	FAT

PASTA SALAD

FROZEN

FOOD	PORTION	CALORIES	FAT
Italian Pasta Salad (Hanover)	½ cup	60	0
Milano Pasta Salad (Hanover)	½ cup	60	0
Oriental Pasta Salad • (Hanover)	½ cup	80	0
Primavera Pasta Salad (Hanover)	½ cup	50	0

MIX

FOOD	PORTION	CALORIES	FAT
Country Buttermilk, Salad Bar Pasta; as prep (Best Foods)	½ cup	250	16
Creamy Buttermilk; as prep (Lipton)	½ cup	117	tr
Creamy Cucumber, Salad Bar Pasta; as prep (Best Foods)	½ cup	250	16
Creamy Italian; as prep (Lipton)	½ cup	122	1
Creamy Italian, Salad Bar Pasta; as prep (Best Foods)	½ cup	290	22
Garden Macaroni; as prep (Lipton)	½ cup	119	tr
Homestyle, Salad Bar Pasta; as prep (Best Foods)	½ cup	250	16
Lemon Dill; as prep (Lipton)	½ cup	115	tr
Robust Italian; as prep (Lipton)	½ cup	128	1
Sour Cream & Dill; as prep (Lipton)	½ cup	120	1
Zesty Italian Salad Bar Pasta; as prep (Best Foods)	½ cup	140	5

FOOD	PORTION	CALORIES	FAT
PATE			
CANNED			
chicken liver	1 Tbsp	109	2
chicken liver	1 oz	238	4
goose liver, smoked	1 oz	131	12
goose liver, smoked	1 Tbsp	60	6
liver	1 Tbsp	41	4
liver	1 oz	90	8
PEACH			
CANNED			
Clingstone Halves (S&W)	½ cup	100	0
Freestone Halves in Heavy Syrup (S&W)	½ cup	100	0
Freestone Sliced in Heavy Syrup (S&W)	½ cup	100	0
Yellow Cling Natural Lite (S&W)	½ cup	50	0
Yellow Cling Natural Style (S&W)	½ cup	90	0
Yellow Cling Sliced Premium in Heavy Syrup (S&W)	½ cup	100	0
Yellow Cling Whole, Spiced, in Heavy Syrup (S&W)	½ cup	90	0
halves in heavy syrup	1 cup	190	tr
halves, in juice	1 cup	109	tr
peaches, spiced, in heavy syrup	1 cup	180	tr
DRIED			
Peaches (Mariani)	¼ cup	140	0
halves	10	311	1

FOOD	PORTION	CALORIES	FAT
FRESH			
peach	1	37	tr
FROZEN			
peaches, sweetened, sliced	1 cup	235	tr
JUICE			
Peach	8 oz	120	0
(Smucker's)			
Pure & Light	6 oz	102	tr
(Dole)			
nectar	1 cup	134	tr

PEANUT BUTTER

FOOD	PORTION	CALORIES	FAT
BAMA Creamy Peanut Butter	2 Tbsp	200	17
BAMA Crunchy Peanut Butter	2 Tbsp	200	17
BAMA Jelly & Peanut Butter	2 Tbsp	150	7
Erewhon, Chunky Salted	2 Tbsp	190	14
Erewhon, Chunky, Unsalted	2 Tbsp	190	14
Erewhon, Creamy, Salted	2 Tbsp	190	14
Erewhon, Creamy, Unsalted	2 Tbsp	14	0
Estee	1 Tbsp	100	8
Health Valley Chunky	1 Tbsp	83	7
Health Valley Chunky, No Salt	1 Tbsp	83	7
Health Valley Creamy	1 Tbsp	83	7
Health Valley Creamy, No Salt	1 Tbsp	83	7
Home Brand Natural, Lightly Salted	2 Tbsp	210	17
Home Brand Natural, Unsalted	2 Tbsp	210	17
Home Brand, No-Sugar Added	2 Tbsp	180	16
Home Brand Real Peanut Butter	2 Tbsp	210	17
Jif Creamy	2 Tbsp	190	16
Jif Crunchy	2 Tbsp	190	16
Reese's Peanut Butter Flavored Chips	¼ cup	230	13

FOOD	PORTION	CALORIES	FAT
Sexton, Salt Free	1 Tbsp	98	8
Skippy Creamy	2 Tbsp	190	17
Skippy Creamy	1 cup	1540	135
Skippy Creamy; w/ 2 slices white bread	1 sandwich	340	19
Skippy Super Chunk	2 Tbsp	190	17
Skippy Super Chunk	1 cup	1540	137
Skippy Super Chunk; w/ 2 slices white bread	1 sandwich	340	19
Smucker's Goober Grape	2 Tbsp	180	10
Smucker's Goober Honey	2 Tbsp	180	10
Smucker's Natural	2 Tbsp	200	16
Smucker's Natural, No-Salt Added	2 Tbsp	200	16
Teddie Natural Peanut Butter w/ No Salt Added	2 Tbsp	200	17
chunk style	1 cup	1520	129
chunk style	2 Tbsp	188	16
smooth style	2 Tbsp	188	16
smooth style	1 cup	1517	129

PEANUTS

FOOD	PORTION	CALORIES	FAT
Cocktail, Oil Roasted (Planters)	1 oz	170	15
Cocktail, Oil Roasted, Unsalted (Planters)	1 oz	170	15
Dry Roasted (Guy's)	1 oz	170	14
Dry Roasted (Lance)	1⅛ oz	190	15
Dry Roasted (Planters)	1 oz	160	14
Dry Roasted, Honey Roasted (Planters)	1 oz	160	13

FOOD	PORTION	CALORIES	FAT
Dry Roasted, Unsalted (Planters)	1 oz	170	15
Honey Roasted (Planters)	1 oz	170	13
Honey Toasted P'nuts (Lance)	1⅜ oz	230	17
Honey Toasted P'nuts (Lance)	1¼ oz	210	16
Party Peanuts (Fisher)	1 oz	160	14
Peanuts (Beer Nuts)	1 oz	180	14
Redskin Oil Roasted (Planters)	1 oz	170	15
Redskin Salted (Lance)	1⅛ oz	190	15
Roasted w/ Shell (Lance)	1¾ oz	190	15
Roasted-in-shell, Salted (Planters)	1 oz	160	14
Roasted-in-shell, Unsalted (Planters)	1 oz	160	14
Salted (Lance)	1⅛ oz	190	15
Salted (Little Debbie)	1 pkg (1.25 oz)	230	18
Salted, Oil Roasted (Planters)	1 oz	170	15
Spanish Dry Roasted (Planters)	1 oz	160	14
Spanish Oil Roasted (Planters)	1 oz	170	15
Spanish Oil Roasted (Planters)	1 cup	851	72
Spanish, raw (Planters)	1 oz	150	12

FOOD	PORTION	CALORIES	FAT
Spanish, Salted (Guy's)	1 oz	170	14
Sweet 'n Crunchy (Planters)	1 oz	140	8
boiled	½ cup	102	7
dried	1 oz	161	14
dry-roasted	1 cup	855	73
dry-roasted	1 oz	164	14
oil roasted	1 oz	165	14
valencia, oil-roasted	1 cup	848	74
valencia, oil-roasted	1 oz	165	14
virginia, oil-roasted	1 oz	161	14
virginia, oil-roasted	1 cup	826	70

PEAR

FOOD	PORTION	CALORIES	FAT
CANNED			
Bartlett Halves in Heavy Syrup (S&W)	½ cup	100	0
Sliced Natural Style (S&W)	½ cup	80	0
halves in heavy syrup	1 cup	188	tr
halves in juice	1 cup	123	tr
halves in light syrup	1 cup	144	tr
halves in water pack	1 cup	71	tr
DRIED			
Pears (Mariani)	¼ cup	150	0
halves	10	459	1
FRESH			
pear	1	98	1
JUICE			
nectar	1 cup	149	tr

FOOD	PORTION	CALORIES	FAT

PEAS

CANNED
Crowder Peas Seasoned w/ Pork (Luck's)	7.5 oz	200	7
Early June or Sweet (Owatonna)	½ cup	70	0
Field Peas w/ Snaps Seasoned w/ Pork (Luck's)	7.5 oz	200	7
Peas (Libby)	½ cup	60	0
Peas (Seneca)	½ cup	60	0
Peas Natural Pack (Libby)	½ cup	60	1
Peas Natural Pack (Seneca)	½ cup	60	0
Petit Pois (S&W)	½ cup	70	0
Small Pea Baked Beans (B&M)	⅞ cup	300	7
Sweet Peas Perfections (S&W)	½ cup	70	0
Sweet Peas, Veri-Green (S&W)	½ cup	70	0
green	½ cup	61	tr

DRIED
Split Peas (Hurst Brand)	1 cup	277	tr
Whole Peas (Hurst Brand)	1 cup	272	1
split, raw	1 cup	671	2
split; cooked	1 cup	231	1
sprouts	½ cup	77	tr

FOOD	PORTION	CALORIES	FAT
FRESH			
edible-podded; cooked	½ cup	34	tr
green, raw	½ cup	63	tr
green; cooked	½ cup	67	tr
raw	½ cup	30	tr
FROZEN			
Chinese Pea Pods (Chun King)	6 oz	8	0
Chinese Pea Pods (LaChoy)	½ pkg	35	tr
Green (Birds Eye)	½ cup	77	tr
Green; cooked (Health Valley)	5.6 oz	126	tr
Peas w/ Cream Sauce (Birds Eye)	½ cup	117	6
Petite Peas (Hanover)	½ cup	70	0
Snow Peas (Hanover)	½ cup	35	0
Sweet Peas (Hanover)	½ cup	70	0
Tiny Tender (Birds Eye)	½ cup	62	tr
edible-podded; not prep	½ cup	30	tr
edible-podded; cooked	½ cup	42	tr
green; cooked	½ cup	63	tr
green; not prep	½ cup	55	tr
PECANS			
Chips, Halves or Pieces (Planters)	1 oz	190	20
dried	1 oz	190	19

FOOD	PORTION	CALORIES	FAT
dry roasted	1 oz	187	18
halves, dried	1 cup	721	73
oil roasted	1 oz	195	20

PECTIN

FOOD	PORTION	CALORIES	FAT
Certo Fruit Pectin	1 Tbsp	2	0
Sure-Jell Fruit Pectin	¼ pkg	38	0
Sure-Jell Light Fruit Pectin	¼ pkg	33	0

PEPPER

FOOD	PORTION	CALORIES	FAT
CANNED			
Hot Banana Pepper Rings (Vlasic)	1 oz	4	0
Mild Cherry Peppers (Vlasic)	1 oz	8	0
Mild Greek Pepperoncini (Vlasic)	1 oz	4	0
chili hot	1	18	tr
green & red, sweet	½ cup	13	tr
jalapeno; chopped	½ cup	17	tr
DRIED			
green; freeze dried	1 Tbsp	1	tr
red; freeze dried	1 Tbsp	1	tr
FRESH			
green, raw	1	18	tr
red, raw	1	18	tr
red; chopped, cooked	½ cup	12	tr
FROZEN			
Green, Diced (Southland)	2 oz	10	0
Sweet Red & Green, Cut (Southland)	2 oz	15	0

FOOD	PORTION	CALORIES	FAT
green & red, sweet; chopped, not prep	1 oz pkg	6	tr

PERCH

FRESH

cooked	1 fillet (1.6 oz)	54	1
cooked	3 oz	99	1
ocean perch, Atlantic, raw	3 oz	80	1
ocean perch, Atlantic, raw	1 fillet (2.2 oz)	60	1
ocean perch, Atlantic; cooked	1 fillet (1.8 oz)	60	1
ocean perch, Atlantic; cooked	3 oz	103	2
raw	3 oz	77	1
raw	1 fillet (2.1 oz)	55	1

FROZEN

Au Natural Perch Fillets (Mrs. Paul's)	4 oz	80	2
Batter-Dipped Ocean Perch (Van De Kamp's)	2 pieces	270	15
Breaded Ocean Perch (Van De Kamp's)	1 piece	170	12
Crispy Crunchy Perch Fillets (Mrs. Paul's)	2 fillets	320	19
Fishmarket Fresh Ocean Perch (Gorton's)	5 oz	140	3
Lightly Breaded Ocean Perch (Van De Kamp's)	5 oz	300	20
Microwave, Lightly Breaded Ocean Perch (Van De Kamp's)	5 oz	300	20
Today's Catch, Perch (Van De Kamp's)	5 oz	160	2

PERSIMMON

persimmon	1	32	tr

FOOD	PORTION	CALORIES	FAT
PHEASANT			
breast, meat, raw	½ breast (6.4 oz)	243	6
leg, meat, raw	3.6 oz	143	5
meat, raw	½ pheasant (12.4 oz)	470	13
meat & skin, raw	½ pheasant (14 oz)	723	37
PICKLE			
Bread & Butter Deli Chunks (Vlasic)	1 oz	25	0
Bread & Butter Old Fashioned Chunks (Vlasic)	1 oz	25	0
Bread & Butter Sweet Butter Chips (Vlasic)	1 oz	30	0
Bread & Butter Sweet Butter Stix (Vlasic)	1 oz	18	0
Bread 'N Butter Slices (Claussen)	1 slice	7	tr
Dill Spears (Claussen)	1 spear	4	tr
Half-The-Salt, Hamburger Dill Chips (Vlasic)	1 oz	2	0
Half-The-Salt, Kosher Crunch Dill (Vlasic)	1 oz	4	0
Half-The-Salt, Kosher Dill Spears (Vlasic)	1 oz	4	0
Half-The-Salt, Sweet Butter Chips (Vlasic)	1 oz	30	0
Hot & Spicy Garden Mix (Vlasic)	1 oz	4	0
Kosher Baby Dill (Vlasic)	1 oz	4	0

FOOD	PORTION	CALORIES	FAT
Kosher Crunchy Dill (Vlasic)	1 oz	4	0
Kosher Deli Dill (Vlasic)	1 oz	4	0
Kosher Dill Gherkins (Vlasic)	1 oz	4	0
Kosher Dill Spears (Vlasic)	1 oz	4	0
Kosher Halves (Claussen)	1 half	9	tr
Kosher Slices (Claussen)	1 slice	1	tr
Kosher Whole (Claussen)	1	9	tr
No Garlic Dill (Vlasic)	1 oz	4	0
No Garlic Dills (Claussen)	1	17	tr
Original Dill (Vlasic)	1 oz	2	0
Relish (Claussen)	1 Tbsp	14	tr
Zesty Crunchy Dill (Vlasic)	1 oz	4	0
Zesty Dill Spears (Vlasic)	1 oz	4	0

PIE
(see also PIE CRUST)

FOOD	PORTION	CALORIES	FAT
CANNED FILLING			
Mincemeat, Condensed (None Such)	¼ pkg	220	2
Mincemeat, Mellowed w/ Brandy Old Fashioned (S&W)	3 oz	177	2

FOOD	PORTION	CALORIES	FAT
Mincemeat, Ready-to-Use (None Such)	⅓ cup	200	1
Mincemeat, Ready-to-Use w/ Brandy & Rum (None Such)	⅓ cup	220	2
Pumpkin (Libby's)	1 cup	210	0
pumpkin pie mix	1 cup	282	tr
FROZEN			
Apple (Banquet)	3.33 oz	250	11
Apple (Mrs. Smith's)	⅛ of 9⅝" pie	390	17
Apple (Weight Watchers)	1	190	5
Apple Natural Juice (Mrs. Smith's)	½ of 9" pie	420	22
Apple Streusel Natural Juice (Mrs. Smith's)	½ of 9" pie	420	16
Banana (Banquet)	2.33 oz	180	10
Blackberry (Banquet)	3.33 oz	270	11
Blueberry (Banquet)	3.33 oz	270	11
Blueberry (Mrs. Smith's)	⅛ of 9⅝" pie	380	17
Boston Cream (Weight Watchers)	1	170	4
Cherry (Banquet)	3.33 oz	250	11
Cherry (Mrs. Smith's)	⅛ of 9⅝" pie	400	16
Cherry Natural Juice (Mrs. Smith's)	½ of 9" pie	410	18

FOOD	PORTION	CALORIES	FAT
Chocolate (Banquet)	2.33 oz	185	10
Coconut (Banquet)	2.33 oz	190	11
Coconut Custard (Mrs. Smith's)	⅛ of 9⅝″ pie	330	15
Lemon (Banquet)	2.33 oz	170	9
Mincemeat (Banquet)	3.33 oz	260	11
Peach (Banquet)	3.33 oz	245	11
Peach (Mrs. Smith's)	⅛ of 9⅝″ pie	365	16
Pecan Thaw 'n' Serve (Mrs. Smith's)	⅛ of 9⅝″ pie	510	23
Pumpkin (Banquet)	3.33 oz	200	8
Pumpkin Custard (Mrs. Smith's)	⅛ of 9⅝″ pie	310	11
Strawberry (Banquet)	2.33 oz	170	9
HOME RECIPE			
apple	⅐ of 9″ pie	402	19
banana cream	⅐ of 9″ pie	354	16
blackberry	⅐ of 9″ pie	372	15
blueberry	⅐ of 9″ pie	411	19
butterscotch	⅐ of 9″ pie	417	21
cherry	⅐ of 9″ pie	462	20
chess	⅐ of 9″ pie	682	42
chocolate	⅐ of 9″ pie	337	19
chocolate meringue	⅐ of 9″ pie	371	19
coconut custard	⅐ of 9″ pie	346	18

FOOD	PORTION	CALORIES	FAT
custard	1/7 of 9" pie	324	18
grasshopper	1/7 of 9" pie	396	20
key lime	1/7 of 9" pie	393	16
lemon chiffon	1/7 of 9" pie	381	21
lemon meringue	1/7 of 9" pie	399	16
mince	1/7 of 9" pie	441	26
peach	1/7 of 9" pie	409	20
pecan	1/7 of 9" pie	566	33
pineapple chiffon	1/7 of 9" pie	337	18
pumpkin	1/7 of 9" pie	287	15
pumpkin; as prep w/ Libby's Solid Pack Pumpkin	1/6 of 9" pie	330	17
raisin	1/7 of 9" pie	545	27
rhubarb	1/7 of 9" pie	414	19
squash	1/7 of 9" pie	311	17
strawberry	1/7 of 9" pie	282	12
MIX			
Banana Cream; as prep w/ whole milk (Jell-O)	1/6 of 8" pie	107	3
Banana Cream, No Bake Dessert; as prep (Jell-O)	1/8 pie	233	12
Chocolate Cream Pie, No Bake Dessert; as prep (Jell-O)	1/8 pie	260	17
Chocolate Mint, No Bake; as prep w/ whole milk (Royal)	1/8 pie	260	15
Chocolate Mousse No-Bake; as prep w/ whole milk (Royal)	1/8 pie	230	12
Chocolate Mousse Pie, No Bake Dessert; as prep (Jell-O)	1/8 pie	262	15

FOOD	PORTION	CALORIES	FAT
Coconut Cream; as prep w/ whole milk (Jell-O)	⅙ of 8" pie	115	5
Key Lime Pie Filling; as prep (Royal)	½ cup	160	3
Lemon; as prep (Jell-O)	⅙ of 8" pie	180	2
Lemon Meringue No-Bake; as prep (Royal)	⅛ pie	310	11
Lemon Pie Filling; as prep (Royal)	½ cup	160	3
Lite Cheese Cake No-Bake; as prep w/ 2% milk	⅛ pie	210	10
Real Cheese Cake No-Bake; as prep w/ whole milk	⅛ pie	280	9
SNACK Apple (Hostess)	1	403	20
Apple (Tastykake)	1	345	12
Berry (Hostess)	1	391	20
Blueberry (Hostess)	1	378	20
Blueberry (Tastykake)	1	359	12
Cherry (Hostess)	1	416	20
Cherry (Tastykake)	1	368	13
Chocolate Pudding (Tastykake)	1	443	16
Coconut Creme (Tastykake)	1	432	22
French Apple (Tastykake)	1	399	13

FOOD	PORTION	CALORIES	FAT
Lemon (Hostess)	1	416	21
Lemon (Tastykake)	1	361	13
Marshmallow Pies, Banana (Little Debbie)	1 pkg (1.4 oz)	170	6
Marshmallow Pies, Banana (Little Debbie)	1 pkg (3 oz)	360	12
Marshmallow Pies, Chocolate (Little Debbie)	1 pkg (1.38 oz)	170	6
Marshmallow Pies, Chocolate (Little Debbie)	1 pkg (3 oz)	370	13
Oatmeal Creme Pies (Little Debbie)	1 pkg (1.33 oz)	160	6
Peach (Hostess)	1	403	20
Peach (Tastykake)	1	343	12
Pecan Pie (Little Debbie)	1 pkg (1.83 oz)	170	2
Pecan Pie (Little Debbie)	1 pkg (3 oz)	280	3
Pineapple (Tastykake)	1	362	12
Pumpkin (Tastykake)	1	356	14
Raisin Creme Pie (Little Debbie)	1 pkg (1.17 oz)	140	6
Raisin Creme Pie (Little Debbie)	1 pkg (2.5 oz)	290	10
Strawberry (Tastykake)	1	373	12
Tasty Klair (Tastykake)	1	436	19
Vanilla Pudding (Tastykake)	1	437	19

FOOD	PORTION	CALORIES	FAT

PIE CRUST
(*see also* PIE)

FROZEN

Patty Shells (Pepperidge Farm)	1	210	15
Pie Shell (Mrs. Smith's)	⅛ of 9⅝" shell	130	8
Puff Pastry Sheets (Pepperidge Farm)	¼ sheet	260	17

HOME RECIPE

piecrust	1 for 9" pie	900	60

MIX

Pie Crust Sticks (Pillsbury)	⅙ of a 2 crust pie	270	17

REFRIGERATED

Pillsbury All Ready	⅛ of a 2 crust pie	240	15

PIEROGI

FROZEN

Potato Cheese (Mrs. T's)	1	70	1
Potato Onion (Mrs. T's)	1	50	tr
Sauerkraut (Mrs. T's)	1	60	0

HOME RECIPE

pierogi	¾ cup	307	19

PIGEON PEAS

cooked	½ cup	86	1
cooked	1 cup	204	1
raw	1 cup	704	3

FOOD	PORTION	CALORIES	FAT
PIGNOLIA (*see* PINE NUTS)			
PIGS' EARS & FEET			
ears, frzn, raw	1 ear (4 oz)	263	17
ears, frzn; simmered	1 ear (3.7 oz)	183	12
feet, pickled	1 oz	58	5
feet, pickled	1 lb	923	73
feet, raw	3.3 oz	251	18
feet; simmered	2.5 oz	138	9
PIKE			
northern, raw	3 oz	75	1
northern, raw	½ fillet (6.9 oz)	175	1
northern; cooked	½ fillet (5.4 oz)	176	1
northern; cooked	3 oz	96	1
roe, raw	3.5 oz	130	2
walleye, red, raw	3 oz	79	1
walleye, raw	1 fillet (5.6 oz)	147	2
PIMENTO			
All Types (Dromedary)	1 oz	10	0
PINE NUTS			
pignolia, dried	1 oz	146	14
pignolia, dried	1 Tbsp	51	5
pinyon, dried	1 oz	161	17
PINEAPPLE			
DRIED Pineapple Nuggets (Del Monte)	.9 oz	90	0

FOOD	PORTION	CALORIES	FAT
CANDIED			
slices	1 oz	179	tr
CANNED			
All Cuts in Juice (Dole)	½ cup	70	tr
All Cuts in Syrup (Dole)	½ cup	95	tr
Hawaiian 100% Sliced (S&W)	2 slices	90	0
Hawaiian 100% Sliced (S&W)	½ cup	70	0
chunks in heavy syrup	1 cup	199	tr
chunks in juice	1 cup	150	tr
crushed	1 cup	199	tr
sliced in water pack	1 slice	19	tr
tidbits	1 cup	199	tr
tidbits in juice	1 cup	150	tr
tidbits in water pack	1 cup	79	tr
FRESH			
Chiquita	1 cup	90	1
diced	1 cup	77	tr
FROZEN			
chunks, sweetened	½ cup	104	tr
JUICE			
Pineapple (Mott's)	9.5 oz	169	0
Pineapple (Tree Top)	6 oz	100	0
Unsweetened (S&W)	6 oz	100	0
frzn; as prep	1 cup	129	tr
frzn; not prep	6 oz container	387	tr
juice	1 cup	139	tr

FOOD	PORTION	CALORIES	FAT
PINK BEANS			
cooked	1 cup	252	1
raw	1 cup	721	2
PINTO BEANS			
CANNED			
Pinto Beans Seasoned w/ Pork (Luck's)	7.25 oz	220	6
Pinto Beans w/ Onions, Seasoned w/ Pork (Luck's)	7.5 oz	220	6
Pintos w/ Jalapeno (Ranch Style)	7.5 oz	180	2
Premium Pintos (Ranch Style)	7.5 oz	160	1
pinto	1 cup	186	1
DRIED			
Pinto (Hurst Brand)	1 cup	265	tr
cooked	1 cup	235	1
raw	1 cup	656	2
FROZEN			
cooked	3 oz	152	tr
raw	10 oz pkg	484	1
SPROUTS			
cooked	3½ oz	22	tr
raw	3½ oz	62	1
PINYON (see PINE NUTS)			
PISTACHIO			
Dry Roasted (Planters)	1 oz	170	15

FOOD	PORTION	CALORIES	FAT
Natural (Planters)	1 oz	170	5
Pistachios (Lance)	1⅛ oz	180	14
Red Pistachios (Planters)	1 oz	170	15
Roasted Shelled Pistachios (Dole)	1 oz	163	14
dried	1 oz	164	14
dried	1 cup	739	62
dry roasted	1 oz	172	15

PIZZA

FROZEN

FOOD	PORTION	CALORIES	FAT
Canadian Style Bacon (Celeste)	1 (9.25 oz)	550	26
Cheese (Celeste)	1 (6.5 oz)	500	24
Cheese French Bread (Weight Watchers)	5.12 oz	320	11
Cheese (Weight Watchers)	5.75 oz	320	8
Croissant Pastry, Cheese (Pepperidge Farm)	1	490	27
Croissant Pastry Deluxe (Pepperidge Farm)	1	520	27
Croissant Pastry, Hamburger (Pepperidge Farm)	1	510	27
Croissant Pastry, Pepperoni (Pepperidge Farm)	1	490	25
Deluxe (Celeste)	1 (8.25 oz)	600	32
Deluxe Combination (Weight Watchers)	6.75 oz	300	8

FOOD	PORTION	CALORIES	FAT
Deluxe French Bread (Weight Watchers)	6.12 oz	330	12
Pepperoni (Celeste)	1 (6.75 oz)	540	29
Pepperoni (Weight Watchers)	5.87 oz	320	9
Pepperoni French Bread (Weight Watchers)	5.25 oz	330	13
Pizza Round (Lamb-Weston)	4.8 oz	370	18
Sausage (Celeste)	1 (7.5 oz)	580	32
Sausage & Mushroom (Celeste)	1 (9.25 oz)	600	32
Sausage (Weight Watchers)	6.25 oz	310	8
Supreme (Celeste)	1 (9 oz)	690	39
cheese	½ of 10″ pie	140	4
HOME RECIPE cheese & sausage	⅛ of 14″ pie	266	16
MIX Chef Boy.ar.dee 2 Complete Cheese Pizzas	1 serving (3.16 oz)	210	5
Chef Boy.ar.dee 2 Complete Pepperoni Pizzas	1 serving (3.75 oz)	210	7
Chef Boy.ar.dee Complete Cheese Pizza	1 serving (3.84 oz)	230	6
Chef Boy.ar.dee Complete Pepperoni Pizza	1 serving (4.16 oz)	250	9
Chef Boy.ar.dee Complete Sausage Pizza	1 serving (4.22 oz)	270	10
Chef Boy.ar.dee Plain Pizza	1 serving (3.5 oz)	180	3

FOOD	PORTION	CALORIES	FAT
Chef Boy.ar.dee Quick & Easy Crust Mix	1 serving (1.5 oz)	150	2
Ragu Mix for Homemade Pizza Crust	¼ crust	170	2
Ragu Mix for Homemade Pizza Crust, pizza recipe; as prep	¼ pizza	300	11
SAUCE Chef Boy.ar.dee Pizza Sauce w/ Cheese	3.88 oz	90	6
Contadina Original Quick & Easy	¼ cup	30	1
Contadina Pizza Sauce w/ Italian Cheese	¼ cup	30	1
Contadina Pizza Sauce w/ Pepperoni	¼ cup	40	2
Ragu Pizza Quick Sauce, Chunky Style	3 Tbsp	45	2
Ragu Pizza Quick Sauce Chunky Style; as prep, muffin recipe	2 muffins	220	7
Ragu Pizza Quick Sauce Pepperoni	3 Tbsp	50	3
Ragu Pizza Quick Sauce Pepperoni; as prep, muffin recipe	2 muffins	230	8
Ragu Pizza Quick Sauce Sausage	3 Tbsp	40	2
Ragu Pizza Quick Sauce Sausage; as prep, muffin recipe	2 muffins	220	7
Ragu Pizza Quick Sauce Traditional	3 Tbsp	40	2
Ragu Pizza Quick Sauce Traditional; as prep, muffin recipe	2 muffin halves	220	7
Ragu Pizza Quick Sauce w/ Mushrooms	3 Tbsp	40	2
Ragu Pizza Quick Sauce w/ Mushrooms; as prep, muffin recipe	2 muffins	220	7
Ragu Pizza Sauce Extra Tomatoes	3 Tbsp	25	1
Ragu Pizza Sauce Extra Tomatoes; as prep, pizza recipe	¼ pizza	280	10

FOOD	PORTION	CALORIES	FAT

PLANTAINS

raw	1 (6.3 oz)	218	tr
sliced; cooked	½ cup	89	tr

PLUM

CANNED

Purple Plums, Halves, Fancy, Unpeeled in Extra Heavy Syrup (S&W)	½ cup	135	0
Purple Plums, Whole, Fancy, Unpeeled in Extra Heavy Syrup (S&W)	½ cup	135	0
purple, in heavy syrup	3	119	tr
purple, in juice	3	55	tr

FRESH

plum	1	36	tr

POI

cooked	½ cup	134	tr

POKEBERRY SHOOTS

cooked	½ cup	16	tr
raw	½ cup	18	tr

POLLOCK

Atlantic, raw	½ fillet (6.8 oz)	177	2
Atlantic, raw	3 oz	78	1
walleye, raw	3 oz	68	1
walleye, raw	1 fillet (2.7 oz)	62	1
walleye; cooked	3 oz	96	1
walleye; cooked	1 fillet (2.1 oz)	68	1

FOOD	PORTION	CALORIES	FAT
POMEGRANATE			
pomegranate	1	104	tr
POMPANO			
Florida, raw	3 oz	140	8
Florida, raw	1 fillet (3.9 oz)	184	11
Florida; cooked	3 oz	179	10
Florida; cooked	1 fillet (3.1 oz)	185	11
POPCORN			
(see also CHIPS, PRETZELS, SNACKS)			
Bachman Popcorn	1 oz	160	11
Cracker Jack	1 oz	120	3
Jiffy Pop, Microwave Butter Flavor; as prep	4 cups	140	7
Jiffy Pop, Microwave Regular; as prep	4 cups	140	7
Jiffy Pop, Pan Butter Flavor; as prep	4 cups	130	6
Jiffy Pop, Pan Regular; as prep	4 cups	130	6
Lance Cheese Popcorn	1 pkg (⅞ oz)	130	8
Lance Cheese Popcorn	1 oz	150	9
Lance Plain	1 pkg (1 oz)	140	8
Planters Microwave Butter; as prep	3 cups	140	10
Planters Microwave Natural; as prep	3 cups	140	9
Planters; as prep	3 cups	20	0
Wise Tender Eating Baby Popcorn	½ oz	70	6
Wise w/ Real Premium White Cheddar Cheese	½ oz	70	5
air-popped	1 cup	30	tr
popped w/ vegetable oil	1 cup	55	3
sugar syrup coated	1 cup	135	1

FOOD	PORTION	CALORIES	FAT

POPOVER

popover (home recipe)	1 (1.4 oz)	98	4

PORK

(*see also* BACON, CANADIAN BACON, HAM, LUNCHEON MEATS/COLD CUTS, SAUSAGE)

The values for cooked pork may differ slightly from values for raw pork. When meat is cooked some moisture and fat is lost, changing the nutritive value slightly. As a rule of thumb, it can be assumed that a 4 oz raw portion will equal a 3 oz cooked portion of meat.

FRESH

center loin chop, lean & fat; braised	1 chop (2.6 oz)	266	19
center loin chop, lean & fat; broiled	1 chop (3.1 oz)	275	19
center loin chop, lean & fat; pan-fried	1 chop (3.1 oz)	333	27
center loin chop, lean & fat, raw	1 chop (4.4 oz)	341	27
center loin chop, lean & fat; roasted	1 chop (3.1 oz)	268	19
center loin chop, lean only; braised	1 chop (2.1 oz)	166	8
center loin chop, lean only; broiled	1 chop (2.5 oz)	166	8
center loin chop, lean only; pan-fried	1 chop (2.4 oz)	178	11
center loin chop, lean only, raw	1 chop (3.4 oz)	155	7
center loin chop, lean only; roasted	1 chop (2.4 oz)	180	10
center loin, lean & fat; braised	3 oz	301	22
center loin, lean & fat; broiled	3 oz	269	19
center loin, lean & fat; pan-fried	3 oz	318	26
center loin, lean & fat; roasted	3 oz	259	18
center loin, lean only; broiled	3 oz	196	9
center loin, lean only; pan-fried	3 oz	226	14
center loin, lean only; roasted	3 oz	204	11
ham, fresh, shank half, lean & fat; roasted	3 oz	258	19
ham, fresh, shank half, lean only; roasted	3 oz	183	9

FOOD	PORTION	CALORIES	FAT
ham, fresh, whole, lean & fat; roasted	3 oz	250	18
ham, fresh, whole, lean only; roasted	3 oz	187	9
ham, fresh, rump half, lean & fat; roasted	3 oz	233	23
ham, fresh, rump half, lean only; roasted	3 oz	187	9
leg, rump half, lean & fat, raw	3 oz	198	15
leg, rump half, lean only, raw	3 oz	87	5
leg, shank half, lean & fat, raw	3 oz	240	14
leg, shank half, lean only, raw	3 oz	117	5
leg, whole, lean & fat, raw	3 oz	222	18
leg, whole, lean only, raw	3 oz	117	5
loin, blade, lean & fat; braised	3 oz	348	29
loin, blade, lean & fat; broiled	3 oz	334	29
loin, blade, lean & fat; pan-fried	3 oz	352	31
loin, blade, lean & fat; roasted	3 oz	310	26
loin, blade, lean only; braised	3 oz	266	18
loin, blade, lean only; broiled	3 oz	255	18
loin, blade, lean only; pan-fried	3 oz	240	17
loin, blade, lean only; roasted	3 oz	238	16
loin blade chop, lean & fat; braised	1 chop (2.4 oz)	275	23
loin blade chop, lean & fat; broiled	1 chop (3.1 oz)	321	27
loin blade chop, lean & fat; pan-fried	1 chop (3.1 oz)	368	33
loin blade chop, lean only; braised	1 chop (1.8 oz)	156	10
loin blade chop, lean only; broiled	1 chop (2.1 oz)	177	13
loin blade chop, lean only; pan-fried	1 chop (2.2 oz)	175	12
loin blade chop, lean only; roasted	1 chop (2.5 oz)	198	14
loin center rib chop, lean & fat, raw	1 chop (3.9 oz)	322	26
loin center rib chop, lean only, raw	1 chop (3 oz)	138	6

FOOD	PORTION	CALORIES	FAT
loin chop, lean & fat, raw	1 chop (4 oz)	345	29
loin chop, lean & fat; braised	1 chop (2.5 oz)	261	20
loin chop; lean & fat; broiled	1 chop (2.7 oz)	295	23
loin chop, lean & fat; pan-fried	1 chop (2.9 oz)	337	29
loin chop, lean & fat; roasted	1 chop (2.9 oz)	262	20
loin chop, lean only, raw	1 chop (3 oz)	142	7
loin chop; lean only; braised	1 chop (1.8 oz)	147	8
loin chop, lean only; broiled	1 chop (2.1 oz)	165	10
loin chop, lean only; pan-fried	1 chop (2 oz)	157	9
loin chop, lean only; roasted	1 chop (2.3 oz)	167	9
loin, lean & fat; braised	3 oz	312	24
loin, lean & fat; broiled	3 oz	294	23
loin, lean & fat; roasted	3 oz	271	21
loin, lean only; braised	3 oz	232	12
loin, lean only; broiled	3 oz	218	13
loin, lean only; roasted	3 oz	204	12
lungs, raw	3.5 oz	83	3
lungs; braised	3 oz	84	3
pancreas, raw	4 oz	225	15
pancreas; braised	3 oz	186	9
rib chop, lean & fat; braised	1 chop (2.2 oz)	246	18
rib chop, lean & fat; broiled	1 chop (2.6 oz)	264	20
rib chop, lean & fat; pan-fried	1 chop (2.9 oz)	343	29
rib chop, lean & fat; roasted	1 chop (2.6 oz)	252	19
rib chop, lean only; braised	1 chop (1.8 oz)	147	8
rib chop, lean only; broiled	1 chop (2.1 oz)	162	9
rib chop, lean only; pan-fried	1 chop (2 oz)	160	9
rib chop, lean only; roasted	1 chop (2.2 oz)	162	9
salt pork	1 oz	212	23

FOOD	PORTION	CALORIES	FAT
shoulder, arm picnic, cured, lean & fat; roasted	3 oz	238	18
shoulder, arm picnic, cured, lean only; roasted	3 oz	145	6
shoulder, arm picnic, lean & fat; braised	3 oz	293	22
shoulder, arm picnic, lean & fat, raw	3 oz	231	19
shoulder, arm picnic, lean & fat; roasted	3 oz	281	22
shoulder, arm picnic, lean only; braised	3 oz	211	10
shoulder, arm picnic, lean only, raw	3 oz	120	5
shoulder, arm picnic, lean only; roasted	3 oz	194	11
shoulder blade Boston steak, lean & fat; braised	1 steak (5.6 oz)	594	46
shoulder blade Boston steak, lean & fat; broiled	1 steak (6.5 oz)	647	53
shoulder blade Boston steak, lean & fat, raw	1 steak (9.6 oz)	737	62
shoulder blade Boston steak, lean & fat; roasted	1 steak (6.5 oz)	594	47
shoulder blade Boston steak, lean only; braised	1 steak (4.6 oz)	382	23
shoulder blade Boston steak, lean only; broiled	1 steak (5.3 oz)	413	28
shoulder blade Boston steak, lean only, raw	1 steak (7.4 oz)	346	19
shoulder blade Boston steak, lean only; roasted	1 steak (5.5 oz)	404	27
shoulder, whole, lean & fat, raw	3 oz	234	19
shoulder, whole, lean only, raw	3 oz	132	7
shoulder, blade roll, cured, lean & fat; roasted	3 oz	244	20

FOOD	PORTION	CALORIES	FAT
shoulder, Boston blade, lean only; braised	3 oz	250	15
shoulder, Boston blade, lean only; broiled	3 oz	233	16
shoulder, Boston blade, lean only; roasted	3 oz	218	14
shoulder, Boston blade, lean & fat; braised	3 oz	316	24
shoulder, Boston blade, lean & fat; broiled	3 oz	297	24
shoulder, Boston blade, lean & fat; roasted	3 oz	273	21
shoulder, whole, lean & fat; roasted	3 oz	277	22
shoulder, whole, lean only; roasted	3 oz	207	13
sirloin chop, lean & fat; braised	1 chop (2.4 oz)	250	18
sirloin chop, lean & fat; broiled	1 chop (2.8 oz)	278	21
sirloin chop, lean & fat; raw	1 chop (4.2 oz)	328	27
sirloin chop, lean & fat; roasted	1 chop (2.8 oz)	244	17
sirloin chop, lean only; braised	1 chop (1.9 oz)	149	7
sirloin chop, lean only; broiled	1 chop (2.3 oz)	165	9
sirloin chop, lean only; raw	1 chop (3.2 oz)	139	6
sirloin chop, lean only; roasted	1 chop (2.5 oz)	175	10
spareribs, lean & fat; braised	3 oz	338	26
spareribs, lean & fat, raw	3 oz	243	20
spleen; braised	3 oz	127	3
spleen, raw	4 oz	113	3
tail; simmered	3 oz	336	30
tail, raw	4 oz	427	38
tenderloin, lean only, raw	3 oz	96	2
tenderloin; lean only; roasted	3 oz	141	4
top loin chop, lean & fat, raw	1 chop (4 oz)	360	30
top loin chop, lean only, raw	1 chop (3.1 oz)	142	7

FOOD	PORTION	CALORIES	FAT
POT PIE			
Beef (Banquet)	7 oz	439	29
Beef (Morton)	7 oz	430	31
Beef (Swanson)	8 oz	410	21
Chicken (Banquet)	7 oz	429	27
Chicken (Morton)	7 oz	415	27
Chicken (Swanson)	8 oz	420	26
Chunky Beef (Swanson)	10 oz	550	29
Chunky Chicken (Swanson)	10 oz	580	33
Chunky Turkey (Swanson)	10 oz	540	31
Hungry-Man Beef (Swanson)	16 oz	680	33
Hungry-Man Chicken (Swanson)	16 oz	730	41
Hungry-Man Turkey (Swanson)	16 oz	690	38
Macaroni & Cheese (Swanson)	7 oz	220	9
Turkey (Banquet)	7 oz	423	26
Turkey (Morton)	7 oz	420	27
Turkey (Swanson)	8 oz	410	24
HOME RECIPE beef; baked	4¼" diam	558	33

FOOD	PORTION	CALORIES	FAT
chicken	1 (11 oz)	706	46
turkey	1 (10.6 oz)	710	47

POTATOES
(*see also* CHIPS)

FOOD	PORTION	CALORIES	FAT
CANNED			
New Potatoes, Extra Small (S&W)	½ cup	45	0
Potatoes (Libby)	½ cup	45	0
Potatoes (Seneca)	½ cup	45	0
Scalloped Potatoes Flavored w/ Ham (Lunch Bucket)	8.25 oz	250	12
potatoes	½ cup	54	tr
FRESH			
Yukon Gold	1 (5.3 oz)	110	0
baked, flesh & skin	1 (6.5 oz)	220	tr
baked, flesh only	1 (5 oz)	145	tr
baked, skin only	skin from 1 potato	115	tr
boiled	½ cup	68	tr
boiled	1 (4.7 oz)	119	tr
flesh & skin; microwaved	1 (7 oz)	212	tr
flesh only; microwaved	1 (5.5 oz)	156	tr
flesh only, raw	1 (3.9 oz)	88	tr
skin only, raw	1 (1.3 oz)	22	tr
FROZEN			
Bacon & Cheddar Baked Potato Entree (Idaho Original)	11 oz	982	74
Broccoli and Cheese Baked Potato (Weight Watchers)	1	280	7

FOOD	PORTION	CALORIES	FAT
Cheddar Browns (Ore Ida)	3 oz	90	2
Cheddared Potatoes (Budget Gourmet)	5.5 oz	230	13
Cheddared Potatoes & Broccoli (Budget Gourmet)	5 oz	130	4
Chicken & Almond Baked Potato Entree (Idaho Original)	11 oz	433	18
Chicken Divan Baked Potato (Weight Watchers)	1	300	6
Cottage Fries (Ore Ida)	3 oz	120	5
Crinkle Cuts French Fries (Lamb-Weston)	3 oz	130	4
Crinkle Cuts, Lites (Ore Ida)	3 oz	90	2
Crinkle Cuts, Microwave (Ore Ida)	3.5 oz	180	8
Crispers! (Ore Ida)	3 oz	230	15
Crispy Crowns (Ore Ida)	3 oz	160	9
Crispy Crowns w/ Onion (Ore Ida)	3 oz	170	9
Deep Fries, Crinkle Cuts (Heinz)	3 oz	150	6
Deep Fries, Shoestrings (Heinz)	3 oz	200	10
French Fries (Heinz)	3 oz	160	6
French Fries, Golden Crinkles (Ore Ida)	3 oz	120	4
French Fries, Golden Fries (Ore Ida)	3 oz	120	4

FOOD	PORTION	CALORIES	FAT
French Fries, Lites (Ore Ida)	3 oz	90	2
French Fries, Pixie Crinkles (Ore Ida)	3 oz	140	6
French Fries, Shoestrings (Ore Ida)	3 oz	140	6
Fries Country Style Dinner (Ore Ida)	3 oz	110	3
Golden Patties (Ore Ida)	2.5 oz	140	8
Hash Browns, Microwave (Ore Ida)	2 oz	180	8
Hash Browns, Shredded (Ore Ida)	3 oz	70	tr
Hash Browns, Southern Style (Ore Ida)	3 oz	70	tr
Hash Browns, Southern Style w/ Butter & Onions (Heinz)	3 oz	110	7
Home Browns, Hash Browns (Lamb-Weston)	1 piece (2.25 oz)	150	9
Italian Baked Potato Entree (Idaho Original)	11 oz	443	21
MunchSkins (Lamb-Weston)	3 oz	120	4
Nacho Potatoes (Budget Gourmet)	5 oz	180	10
Natural Cuts, Skin-On (Lamb-Weston)	3 oz	120	4
Natural Slices, Skin-On (Lamb-Weston)	3 oz	120	3
Natural Trim Fries, Skin-On (Lamb-Weston)	3 oz	140	5
New Potatoes in Sour Cream Sauce (Budget Gourmet)	5 oz	120	6

FOOD	PORTION	CALORIES	FAT
O'Brien Potatoes (Ore Ida)	3 oz	60	tr
Primavera Baked Potato Entree (Idaho Original)	11 oz	499	26
Regular Cut French Fries (Lamb-Weston)	3 oz	130	4
Shoestring French Fries (Lamb-Weston)	3 oz	140	5
Shoestrings, Lites (Ore Ida)	3 oz	90	4
Steak House Fries (Lamb-Weston)	3 oz	120	4
Stuffed Potatoes w/ Cheddar Cheese (OH Boy!)	6 oz	142	4
Stuffed Potatoes w/ Real Bacon (OH Boy!)	6 oz	116	3
Stuffed Potatoes w/ Sour Cream & Chives (OH Boy!)	6 oz	129	5
Tater Puffs (Lamb-Weston)	3 oz	150	7
Tater Tots (Ore Ida)	3 oz	140	7
Tater Tots, Microwave (Ore Ida)	2 oz	200	9
Tater Tots w/ Bacon Flavored Vegetable Protein (Ore Ida)	3 oz	140	6
Tater Tots w/ Onion (Ore Ida)	3 oz	140	6
Tater Wedges (Lamb-Weston)	2 pieces (4 oz)	200	10
Three Cheese Potatoes (Budget Gourmet)	5.75 oz	230	11
Wedges, Home Style (Ore Ida)	3 oz	100	3

FOOD	PORTION	CALORIES	FAT
Western Style Baked Potato Entree (Idaho Original)	11 oz	567	25
Whole Small (Ore Ida)	3 oz	70	tr
french fried; not prep	10 strips	107	4
french-fried, cottage cut; cooked	10 strips	109	4
french-fried; cooked	10 strips	111	4
hashed brown; cooked	½ cup	170	9
hashed brown; not prep	12 oz pkg	280	2
hashed brown w/ butter sauce; not prep	6 oz pkg	229	11
potato puffs; as prep	½ cup	138	7
whole; not prep	½ cup	71	tr
HOME RECIPE au gratin	½ cup	160	9
au gratin w/ cheese	½ cup	178	10
hash brown	½ cup	163	11
mashed	½ cup	111	4
O'Brien	1 cup	157	3
potato pancakes	1	495	13
scalloped	½ cup	105	5
MIX Creamy Italian-Style Potatoes w/ Parmesan Cheese; as prep (French's)	½ cup	130	4
Creamy Stroganoff Potatoes; as prep (French's)	½ cup	130	4
Crispy Top Scalloped Potatoes w/ Savory Onion; as prep (French's)	½ cup	140	5
Mashed; not prep (Country Store)	⅓ cup	70	0

FOOD	PORTION	CALORIES	FAT
Potato Salad, Classic Idaho; as prep (Lipton)	½ cup	94	tr
Potato Salad, German; as prep (Lipton)	½ cup	99	tr
Potatoes & Sauce Au Gratin; as prep (Lipton)	½ cup	108	tr
Potatoes & Sauce, Beef & Mushroom; as prep (Lipton)	½ cup	95	tr
Potatoes & Sauce, Cheddar Bacon; as prep (Lipton)	½ cup	106	1
Potatoes & Sauce, Cheddar Broccoli; as prep (Lipton)	½ cup	104	1
Potatoes & Sauce, Chicken Flavored Mushroom; as prep (Lipton)	½ cup	90	tr
Potatoes & Sauce, Italiano; as prep (Lipton)	½ cup	107	2
Potatoes & Sauce, Nacho; as prep (Lipton)	½ cup	103	1
Potatoes & Sauce, Scalloped; as prep (Lipton)	½ cup	102	2
Potatoes & Sauce, Sour Cream & Chives; as prep (Lipton)	½ cup	113	2
Real Cheese Scalloped Potatoes; as prep (French's)	½ cup	140	5
Real Sour Cream & Chives Potatoes; as prep (French's)	½ cup	150	6
Spuds Mashed; as prep (French's)	½ cup	140	7

FOOD	PORTION	CALORIES	FAT
Tangy Au Gratin; as prep (French's)	½ cup	140	6
au gratin; as prep	4.5 oz	127	6
au gratin; not prep	1 pkg (5.5 oz)	490	6
mashed, dehydrated, flakes; as prep	½ cup	361	1
mashed, dehydrated, flakes; not prep	½ cup	118	6
mashed, granules; as prep w/ whole milk	½ cup	137	7
mashed, granules; not prep	½ cup	80	tr
scalloped; as prep	4½ oz	127	6
scalloped; not prep	1 pkg (5.5 oz)	558	7
READY-TO-USE salad	½ cup	179	10

POTATO STARCH

Potato Starch (Manischewitz)	1 cup	570	0

POUT

ocean, raw	3 oz	67	1
ocean, raw	½ fillet (6.2 oz)	140	2

PRESERVES
(see JAM/JELLY/PRESERVES)

PRETZELS
(see also CHIPS, POPCORN, SNACKS)

Bachman Pretzel Rolls	1 rod (1 oz)	110	2
Estee Unsalted	5	25	tr
J&J Soft Pretzels	1 oz	76	tr
Lance Pretzel Twist	1.5 oz	150	1

FOOD	PORTION	CALORIES	FAT
Lance Pretzels	1 oz	100	1
Mister Salty Butter Flavored Rings	23	110	2
Mister Salty Butter Flavored Sticks	90	110	1
Mister Salty Dutch	2	110	1
Mister Salty Junior	29	110	2
Mister Salty Mini	16	110	1
Mister Salty Mini Mix	23	110	1
Mister Salty Rings	22	110	2
Mister Salty Sticks	90	110	1
Mister Salty Twists	5	110	2
Mister Salty Veri-Thin Sticks	45	110	1
Planters	1 oz	110	1
Quinlan Artificial Butter Tiny Thins	1 oz	108	1
Quinlan Beers	1 oz	110	1
Quinlan Cheese Tiny Thins	1 oz	109	2
Quinlan Logs	1 oz	103	tr
Quinlan Party Thins	1 oz	109	tr
Quinlan Philly Style	1 oz	107	tr
Quinlan Rods	1 oz	100	tr
Quinlan Sour Cheese Tiny Thins	1 oz	100	0
Quinlan Sour Thins Dough Hard	1 oz	100	0
Quinlan Sticks	1 oz	105	tr
Quinlan Thins	1 oz	104	tr
Quinlan Tiny Thins	1 oz	109	2
Quinlan Tiny Thins, No-Salt	1 oz	115	2
Quinlan Ultra Thins	1 oz	106	tr
Seyfert's Butter Pretzel Rods	1 oz	110	1
thin slim sticks	47 pieces	110	1
twist, tiny	14 pieces	109	1

FOOD	PORTION	CALORIES	FAT

PRUNES

FOOD	PORTION	CALORIES	FAT
CANNED			
in heavy syrup	5	90	tr
DRIED			
Prunes, Pitted (Mariani)	¼ cup	140	1
Prunes, Whole (Mariani)	¼ cup	140	1
cooked w/o sugar	½ cup	113	tr
prunes	10	201	tr
JUICE			
Country Style (Mott's)	6 oz	130	0
Prune (Mott's)	6 oz	130	0
Unsweetened (S&W)	6 oz	120	0
juice	1 cup	181	tr

PUDDING
(*see also* CUSTARD, PUDDING POPS)

FOOD	PORTION	CALORIES	FAT
HOME RECIPE			
bread w/ raisins	½ cup	180	5
corn	½ cup	97	1
corn	⅔ cup	181	9
pumpkin	½ cup	170	5
rice w/ raisins	½ cup	246	6
tapioca	½ cup	169	6
MIX			
Banana Creme, Instant (Jello-O)	1 pkg (3.5 oz)	360	tr
Butter Pecan, Instant (Jell-O)	1 pkg (3.5 oz)	383	3

FOOD	PORTION	CALORIES	FAT
Butterscotch (Jell-O)	1 pkg (3.6 oz)	364	tr
Butterscotch; as prep (Estee)	½ cup	70	tr
Butterscotch, Instant (Jell-O)	1 pkg (3.5 oz)	358	tr
Chocolate (Jell-O)	1 pkg (3.5 oz)	346	1
Chocolate; as prep (Estee)	½ cup	70	tr
Chocolate Fudge (Jell-O)	1 pkg (3.5 oz)	345	1
Chocolate Tapioca Americana (Jell-O)	1 pkg (3.5 oz)	378	2
Coconut Cream, Instant (Jell-O)	1 pkg (3.5 oz)	416	9
French Vanilla (Jell-O)	1 pkg	365	tr
French Vanilla, Instant (Jell-O)	1 pkg (3.5 oz)	360	tr
Lemon; as prep (Estee)	½ cup	70	tr
Lemon, Instant (Jell-O)	1 pkg (3.5 oz)	376	tr
Milk Chocolate (Jell-O)	1 pkg (3.5 oz)	362	2
Pineapple Cream, Instant (Jell-O)	1 pkg (3.5 oz)	363	tr
Pistachio, Instant (Jell-O)	1 pkg (3.5 oz)	383	3
Vanilla; as prep (Estee)	½ cup	70	tr
Vanilla, Instant (Jell-O)	1 pkg (3.5 oz)	374	tr

FOOD	PORTION	CALORIES	FAT
MIX WITH 2% MILK			
Butterscotch, Instant, Sugar Free; as prep (Jell-O)	½ cup	88	2
Butterscotch, Sugar Free Instant; as prep (Royal)	½ cup	100	2
Chocolate Fudge, Instant, Sugar Free; as prep (Jell-O)	½ cup	100	3
Chocolate, Instant, Sugar Free; as prep (Jell-O)	½ cup	96	3
Chocolate Sugar Free; as prep (Jell-O)	½ cup	91	3
Chocolate, Sugar Free Instant; as prep (Royal)	½ cup	110	3
Pistachio, Instant, Sugar Free; as prep (Jell-O)	½ cup	94	3
Vanilla, Instant, Sugar Free; as prep (Jell-O)	½ cup	90	2
Vanilla Sugar Free; as prep (Jell-O)	½ cup	82	2
Vanilla, Sugar Free Instant; as prep (Royal)	½ cup	100	2
MIX WITH SKIM MILK			
Butterscotch (D-Zerta)	½ cup	69	tr
Butterscotch w/ Nutrasweet; as prep (D-Zerta)	½ cup	69	tr
Chocolate w/ Nutrasweet; as prep (D-Zerta)	½ cup	65	tr
Vanilla (D-Zerta)	½ cup	69	tr

FOOD	PORTION	CALORIES	FAT
Vanilla w/ Nutrasweet; as prep (D-Zerta)	½ cup	69	tr
MIX WITH WHOLE MILK			
Banana Cream; as prep (Royal)	½ cup	160	4
Banana Cream, Instant; as prep (Royal)	½ cup	180	5
Banana Creme Instant; as prep (Jell-O)	½ cup	168	5
Butter Pecan Instant; as prep (Jell-O)	½ cup	174	5
Butterscotch; as prep (Jell-O)	½ cup	171	4
Butterscotch; as prep (Royal)	½ cup	160	4
Butterscotch Instant; as prep (Jell-O)	½ cup	168	5
Butterscotch Instant; as prep (Royal)	½ cup	180	5
Chocolate; as prep (Jell-O)	½ cup	165	5
Chocolate; as prep (Royal)	½ cup	180	4
Chocolate Chocolate Chip Instant; as prep (Royal)	½ cup	190	4
Chocolate Fudge; as prep (Jell-O)	½ cup	164	5
Chocolate Fudge Instant; as prep (Jell-O)	½ cup	174	5
Chocolate Instant; as prep (Jell-O)	½ cup	176	5
Chocolate Instant; as prep (Royal)	½ cup	190	5
Chocolate Mint Instant; as prep (Royal)	½ cup	190	4

FOOD	PORTION	CALORIES	FAT
Chocolate Tapioca Americana; as prep (Jell-O)	½ cup	173	5
Coconut Cream Instant; as prep (Jell-O)	½ cup	182	6
Custard; as prep (Royal)	½ cup	150	5
Dark 'n Sweet; as prep (Royal)	½ cup	180	4
Dark 'n Sweet Instant; as prep (Royal)	½ cup	190	4
Flan w/ Caramel Sauce; as prep (Royal)	½ cup	150	5
French Vanilla; as prep (Jell-O)	½ cup	171	4
French Vanilla Instant; as prep (Jell-O)	½ cup	168	5
Golden Egg Custard Americana; as prep (Jell-O)	½ cup	167	6
Lemon Instant; as prep (Jell-O)	½ cup	172	5
Lemon Instant; as prep (Royal)	½ cup	180	5
Milk Chocolate; as prep (Jell-O)	½ cup	168	5
Milk Chocolate Instant; as prep (Jell-O)	½ cup	178	5
Pineapple Cream Instant; as prep (Jell-O)	½ cup	168	5
Pistachio Instant; as prep (Jell-O)	½ cup	172	5
Pistachio Nut Instant; as prep (Royal)	½ cup	170	4
Rice Americana; as prep (Jell-O)	½ cup	177	4

FOOD	PORTION	CALORIES	FAT
Toasted Butter Almond Instant; as prep (Royal)	½ cup	170	4
Toasted Coconut Instant; as prep (Royal)	½ cup	170	4
Vanilla; as prep (Jell-O)	½ cup	162	4
Vanilla; as prep (Royal)	½ cup	160	4
Vanilla Instant; as prep (Jell-O)	½ cup	171	5
Vanilla Instant; as prep (Royal)	½ cup	180	5
Vanilla Tapioca Americana; as prep (Jell-O)	½ cup	166	4
READY-TO-USE			
Banana Snack Pack (Hunt's)	4.25 oz	180	9
Butterscotch Snack Pack (Hunt's)	4.25 oz	180	7
Butterscotch Sugar Free (Diamond Crystal)	½ cup	80	tr
Chocolate Fudge Snack Pack (Hunt's)	4.25 oz	170	9
Chocolate Marshmallow Snack Pack (Hunt's)	4.25 oz	170	7
Chocolate Snack Pack (Hunt's)	4.25 oz	180	7
Chocolate Sugar Free (Diamond Crystal)	½ cup	70	tr
German Chocolate Snack Pack (Hunt's)	4.25 oz	190	8
Lemon Snack Pack (Hunt's)	4.25 oz	150	3
Rice Snack Pack (Hunt's)	4.25 oz	190	10

FOOD	PORTION	CALORIES	FAT
Tapioca Snack Pack (Hunt's)	4.25 oz	120	5
Vanilla Snack Pack (Hunt's)	4.25	180	7
Vanilla Sugar Free (Diamond Crystal)	½ cup	80	tr

PUDDING POPS
(*see also* ICE CREAM AND FROZEN DESSERTS, PUDDING)

FOOD	PORTION	CALORIES	FAT
Chocolate Covered Chocolate Pudding Pop (Jell-O)	1 pop	130	8
Chocolate Covered Vanilla Pudding Pops (Jell-O)	1 pop	130	8
Chocolate Fudge Pudding Pops (Jell-O)	1 pop	73	2
Chocolate Pudding Pops (Jell-O)	1 pop	80	2
Chocolate w/ Chocolate Chips Pudding Pops (Jell-O)	1 pop	82	3
Chocolate/Caramel Swirl Pudding Pops (Jell-O)	1 pop	78	2
Chocolate/Vanilla Swirl Pudding Pops (Jell-O)	1 pop	77	2
Double Chocolate Swirl Pudding Pops (Jell-O)	1 pop	74	2
Milk Chocolate Pudding Pops (Jell-O)	1 pop	75	2
Vanilla Pudding Pops (Jell-O)	1 pop	75	2
Vanilla w/ Chocolate Chips (Jell-O)	1 pop	82	3

FOOD	PORTION	CALORIES	FAT
PUMPKIN			
CANNED			
Pumpkin (Owatonna)	½ cup	40	1
Solid Pack (Libby's)	1 cup	80	1
pumpkin	½ cup	41	tr
FRESH			
mashed; cooked	½ cup	24	tr
flowers, raw	1	0	0
flowers; cooked	½ cup	10	tr
raw; cubed	½ cup	15	tr
SEEDS			
seeds, dried	1 oz	154	13
seeds, whole; roasted	1 oz	127	6
PURSLANE			
cooked	½ cup	10	tr
raw	1 cup	7	tr
QUAHOG (*see* CLAM)			
QUAIL			
breast, meat only, raw	2 oz	69	2
meat & skin, raw	3.8 oz	210	13
meat, raw	3.2 oz	123	4
QUICHE			
lorraine (home recipe)	⅙ of 9″ pie	379	27

FOOD	PORTION	CALORIES	FAT
RABBIT			
stewed	3.5 oz	216	10
RADISH			
DRIED			
oriental	½ cup	157	tr
seeds, sprouted, raw	½ cup	8	tr
FRESH			
Chinese; cooked	½ cup	13	tr
daikon; cooked	½ cup	13	tr
oriental, sliced, raw	½ cup	8	tr
raw	10	7	tr
white icicle, sliced, raw	½ cup	7	tr
RAISINS			
California Seedless (Cinderella)	½ cup	250	0
Golden Raisins (Dole)	½ cup	260	0
Raisins (Dole)	½ cup	260	0
raisins	1 cup	434	1
raisins, golden	1 cup	437	1
DRIED			
Yogurt Raisins (Del Monte)	.9 oz	120	5
Yogurt Raisins Strawberry (Del Monte)	.9 oz	120	5
HOME RECIPE			
raisin sauce	2 Tbsp	51	tr

FOOD	PORTION	CALORIES	FAT

RASPBERRIES

FOOD	PORTION	CALORIES	FAT
CANNED			
whole in heavy syrup	½ cup	117	tr
FRESH			
raspberries	1 cup	61	1
FROZEN			
Red Raspberries Whole in Lite Syrup (Birds Eye)	½ cup	99	tr
sweetened	1 cup	256	tr
JUICE			
Pure & Light (Dole)	6 oz	87	tr
Red Raspberry (Smucker's)	8 oz	120	0

RELISH

FOOD	PORTION	CALORIES	FAT
Dill (Vlasic)	1 oz	2	0
Hamburger (Vlasic)	1 oz	40	0
Hot Dog (Vlasic)	1 oz	40	1
Sandwich Spred (Hellman's)	1 Tbsp	55	5
Sweet (Vlasic)	1 oz	40	0
chow chow	1 Tbsp	8	0
chutney, apple cranberry	1 Tbsp	16	0
cranberry orange	½ cup	246	tr

RHUBARB

FOOD	PORTION	CALORIES	FAT
rhubarb	1 cup	26	tr

FOOD	PORTION	CALORIES	FAT

RICE
   (see also RICE CAKE*)*

BROWN

FOOD	PORTION	CALORIES	FAT
Pritikin Pilaf Brown Rice	½ cup	90	tr
Pritikin Spanish Brown Rice	½ cup	100	tr
S&W Quick Natural Long Grain; cooked	2 oz	63	0
bran	1 oz	80	tr

CANNED

FOOD	PORTION	CALORIES	FAT
Ranch Style Spanish Rice	7.5 oz	160	3

FROZEN

FOOD	PORTION	CALORIES	FAT
Birds Eye French Style International Rice	½ cup	106	tr
Birds Eye Italian Style International Rice	½ cup	119	tr
Birds Eye Rice & Peas w/ Mushrooms	⅔ cup	108	tr
Birds Eye Spanish Style International Rice	½ cup	111	tr
Budget Gourmet Oriental Rice & Vegetables	5.75 oz	210	10
Budget Gourmet Rice Pilaf w/ Green Beans	5.5 oz	240	9

HOME RECIPE

FOOD	PORTION	CALORIES	FAT
pilaf	½ cup	84	3
spanish	¾ cup	363	27

MIX, DRY

FOOD	PORTION	CALORIES	FAT
Cajun Rice; as prep (Lipton)	½ cup	121	tr
Fried Rice Seasoning Mix (Kikkoman)	1 oz pkg	91	tr
Rice & Sauce & Peas; as prep (Lipton)	½ cup	128	tr

FOOD	PORTION	CALORIES	FAT
Rice & Sauce Almondine; as prep (Lipton)	½ cup	140	2
Rice & Sauce Beef Flavored; as prep (Lipton)	½ cup	124	tr
Rice & Sauce Chicken Flavored; as prep (Lipton)	½ cup	126	1
Rice & Sauce Florentine; as prep (Lipton)	½ cup	134	1
Rice & Sauce, Herbs & Butter; as prep (Lipton)	½ cup	127	2
Rice & Sauce, Long Grain & Wild Mushroom & Herb; as prep (Lipton)	½ cup	42	2
Rice & Sauce, Long Grain & Wild Oriental Recipe; as prep (Lipton)	½ cup	121	tr
Rice & Sauce Mushroom; as prep (Lipton)	½ cup	123	tr
Rice & Sauce Oriental; as prep (Lipton)	½ cup	131	1
Rice & Sauce, Rice Medley; as prep (Lipton)	½ cup	124	tr
Rice & Sauce, Spanish; as prep (Lipton)	½ cup	120	tr
Rice & Sauce w/ Vegetables, Broccoli & Cheddar; as prep (Lipton)	½ cup	128	2
Rice Asparagus w/ Hollandaise Sauce; as prep (Lipton)	½ cup	123	tr
Rice Pilaf; as prep (Lipton)	½ cup	117	tr
Rice Salad, Herbal Vinaigrette; as prep (Lipton)	½ cup	111	tr

FOOD	PORTION	CALORIES	FAT
Stir-Fry Entree (Chun King)	.25 oz	20	0
WHITE			
Long Grain; cooked (S&W)	2 oz	61	0
Minute Rice; as prep (General Foods)	⅔ cup	142	2
Minute Rice, Drumstick; as prep (General Foods)	½ cup	143	4
Minute Rice, Fried; as prep (General Foods)	½ cup	164	5
Minute Rice, Long Grain & Wild; as prep (General Foods)	½ cup	149	5
Minute Rice, Rib Roast; as prep (General Foods)	½ cup	152	4

RICE CAKE

FOOD	PORTION	CALORIES	FAT
7 Grain Rice Cakes (Pritikin Foods)	1	35	0
Crispy Rice Cakes, Sodium Free (Chico-San)	1	35	0
Crispy Rice Cakes, Very Low Sodium (Chico-San)	1	35	0
Plain Rice Cakes (Pritikin Foods)	1	35	0
Sesame Rice Cakes (Pritikin Foods)	1	35	0

ROCKFISH

FOOD	PORTION	CALORIES	FAT
Pacific, raw	1 fillet (6.7 oz)	180	3
Pacific, raw	3 oz	80	1
Pacific; cooked	3 oz	103	2
Pacific; cooked	1 fillet (5.2 oz)	180	3

FOOD	PORTION	CALORIES	FAT

ROE
(*see* INDIVIDUAL FISH NAMES)

FOOD	PORTION	CALORIES	FAT
raw	1 oz	39	2
raw	3 oz	119	5

ROLL
(*see also* BISCUIT, CROISSANT, ENGLISH MUFFIN, MUFFIN, POPOVER, SCONE)

FROZEN

FOOD	PORTION	CALORIES	FAT
All Butter Cinnamon Roll w/ Icing (Sara Lee)	1	290	10
All Butter Cinnamon Roll w/o Icing (Sara Lee)	1	230	10
Apple Sweet Roll (Weight Watchers)	1	190	5

HOME RECIPE

FOOD	PORTION	CALORIES	FAT
sweet roll	1 (1.8 oz)	143	4

MIX

FOOD	PORTION	CALORIES	FAT
Hot Roll Mix; as prep (Pillsbury)	2	240	4

READY-TO-EAT

FOOD	PORTION	CALORIES	FAT
Butter Crescent (Pepperidge Farm)	1	110	6
Club Brown 'n Serve (Pepperidge Farm)	1	100	1
Dark Bread (Hollywood)	1	40	tr
Dinner (Roman Meal)	1	45	tr
Frankfurt Rolls (Country Kitchen)	1	120	2
French Twist (Pepperidge Farm)	1	110	1
Golden Twist (Pepperidge Farm)	1	110	6

FOOD	PORTION	CALORIES	FAT
Hamburger (Pepperidge Farm)	1	130	2
Hamburger (Shop 'n Save)	1	120	2
Hamburger Bun (Roman Meal)	1	113	2
Hotdog Bun (Roman Meal)	1	104	2
Light Pan Dinner Rolls Special Formula (Hollywood)	1	60	tr
Light Sliced Rolls Special Formula (Hollywood)	1	80	tr
Onion Sandwich Buns w/Poppy Seeds (Pepperidge Farm)	1	150	3
Parker House (Pepperidge Farm)	1	60	1
Potato Rolls (Martin's)	1	130	2
Sandwich w/ Sesame Seeds (Pepperidge Farm)	1	160	3
Sourdough Style French (Pepperidge Farm)	1	100	1
REFRIGERATED Hungry Jack Butter Tastin' Cinnamon w/ Icing	2	290	14
Pillsbury Best Quick Cinnamon Rolls w/ Icing	1	210	9
Pillsbury Butterflake	1	110	4
Pillsbury Cinnamon w/ Icing	2	230	9
Pillsbury Crescent	1	200	11

ROUGHY
orange, raw | 3 oz | 107 | 6 |

FOOD	PORTION	CALORIES	FAT
RUTABAGA			
cubed, raw	½ cup	25	tr
mashed; cooked	½ cup	41	tr
SABLEFISH			
FRESH			
raw	3 oz	166	13
raw	½ fillet (6.8 oz)	377	30
SMOKED			
sablefish	1 oz	72	6
sablefish	3 oz	218	17
SALAD			
(*see also* PASTA SALAD)			
Holiday Coleslaw (Fresh Chef Salads)	4 oz	200	15
HOME RECIPE			
chef	1.5 cups	386	28
popeye	½ cup	204	21
taco salad	1 cup	292	20
tossed	1 cup	32	tr
waldorf	½ cup	79	6
SALAD DRESSING			
HOME RECIPE			
french	1 Tbsp	88	10
french	2 Tbsp	177	20
vinegar & oil	1 Tbsp	72	8
vinegar & oil	2 Tbsp	140	16
MIXES			
Bleu Cheese & Herbs (Good Seasons)	1 pkg	4	tr

FOOD	PORTION	CALORIES	FAT
Bleu Cheese & Herbs; as prep (Good Seasons)	1 Tbsp	72	8
Buttermilk Farm Style; as prep (Good Seasons)	1 Tbsp	58	6
Cheese Garlic; as prep (Good Seasons)	1 Tbsp	72	8
Cheese Italian; as prep (Good Seasons)	1 Tbsp	72	8
Classic Herb; as prep (Good Seasons)	1 Tbsp	83	9
Garlic & Herbs; as prep (Good Seasons)	1 Tbsp	84	9
Italian; as prep (Good Seasons)	1 Tbsp	71	8
Italian Lite; as prep (Good Seasons)	1 Tbsp	27	3
Italian Mild; as prep (Good Seasons)	1 Tbsp	73	8
Italian No Oil; as prep (Good Seasons)	1 Tbsp	7	tr
Lemon & Herbs; as prep (Good Seasons)	1 Tbsp	83	9
Zesty Italian; as prep (Good Seasons)	1 Tbsp	71	8
Zesty Italian Lite; as prep (Good Seasons)	1 Tbsp	31	3
READY-TO-USE Bacon & Buttermilk (Kraft)	1 Tbsp	80	8
Bacon & Tomato (Kraft)	1 Tbsp	70	7
Blue Cheese (Diamond Crystal)	1 Tbsp	20	1
Blue Cheese (Roka Brand)	1 Tbsp	60	6

FOOD	PORTION	CALORIES	FAT
Blue Cheese Chunky (Kraft)	1 Tbsp	70	6
Blue Cheese, Lite (Wish-Bone)	1 Tbsp	38	4
Buttermilk & Chives Creamy (Kraft)	1 Tbsp	80	8
Buttermilk Creamy (Kraft)	1 Tbsp	80	8
Buttermilk, Lite (Wish-Bone)	1 Tbsp	53	5
Ceasar (Wish-Bone)	1 Tbsp	78	8
Caesar Golden (Kraft)	1 Tbsp	70	7
Coleslaw (Kraft)	1 Tbsp	70	6
Creamy Italian (Pritikin Foods)	1 Tbsp	12	0
Cucumber Creamy (Kraft)	1 Tbsp	70	8
Dijon Classic Creamy (Wish-Bone)	1 Tbsp	62	6
Dijon Classic Vinaigrette (Wish-Bone)	1 Tbsp	61	6
Famous Chef Style (Ott's)	1 Tbsp	40	3
French (Catalina)	1 Tbsp	70	6
French (Kraft)	1 Tbsp	60	6
French (Pritikin Foods)	1 Tbsp	10	0
French, Deluxe (Wish-Bone)	1 Tbsp	59	6
French, Lite (Wish-Bone)	1 Tbsp	31	3

FOOD	PORTION	CALORIES	FAT
Garlic Creamy (Kraft)	1 Tbsp	50	5
Garlic Creamy (Wish-Bone)	1 Tbsp	74	8
Garlic French (Wish-Bone)	1 Tbsp	56	5
Home Style (Diamond Crystal)	1 Tbsp	20	1
Italian (Presto)	1 Tbsp	70	7
Italian (Pritikin Foods)	1 Tbsp	6	0
Italian Chef Style (Ott's)	1 Tbsp	80	9
Italian Creamy (Wish-Bone)	1 Tbsp	56	5
Italian Creamy w/ Real Sour Cream (Kraft)	1 Tbsp	60	6
Italian Herbal Classics (Wish-Bone)	1 Tbsp	70	7
Italian Oil-Free (Kraft)	1 Tbsp	4	0
Italian Robusto (Wish-Bone)	1 Tbsp	70	7
Oil & Vinegar (Kraft)	1 Tbsp	70	7
Onion & Chive (Wish-Bone)	1 Tbsp	37	3
Onion & Chives, Creamy (Kraft)	1 Tbsp	70	7
Ranch (Pritikin Foods)	1 Tbsp	18	0
Ranch, Lite (Wish-Bone)	1 Tbsp	42	4
Rancher's Choice Creamy (Kraft)	1 Tbsp	80	8

FOOD	PORTION	CALORIES	FAT
Red Wine Vinaigrette (Wish-Bone)	1 Tbsp	50	4
Red Wine Vinegar & Oil (Kraft)	1 Tbsp	50	4
Romano & Parmesan, Creamy (Wish-Bone)	1 Tbsp	89	9
Russian (Kraft)	1 Tbsp	60	5
Russian (Pritikin Foods)	1 Tbsp	12	0
Russian (Wish-Bone)	1 Tbsp	47	3
Russian, Lite (Wish-Bone)	1 Tbsp	22	tr
Thousand Island (Diamond Crystal)	1 Tbsp	20	1
Thousand Island (Kraft)	1 Tbsp	60	5
Thousand Island (Wish-Bone)	1 Tbsp	69	5
Thousand Island & Bacon (Kraft)	1 Tbsp	60	6
Thousand Island Lite (Wish-Bone)	1 Tbsp	40	3
Vinaigrette (Pritikin Foods)	1 Tbsp	10	0
Zesty Italian (Kraft)	1 Tbsp	70	8
Zesty Tomato (Pritikin Foods)	1 Tbsp	18	0
blue cheese	1 Tbsp	77	8
french	1 Tbsp	67	6
italian	1 Tbsp	69	7
russian	1 Tbsp	76	8

FOOD	PORTION	CALORIES	FAT
sesame seed	1 Tbsp	68	7
thousand island	1 Tbsp	59	6
READY-TO-USE, REDUCED CALORIE			
Bacon & Tomato Reduced Calorie (Kraft)	1 Tbsp	30	2
Bacon and Tomato (Estee)	1 Tbsp	8	tr
Bacon Creamy Reduced Calorie (Kraft)	1 Tbsp	30	2
Bleu Cheese (Walden Farms)	1 Tbsp	27	2
Bleu Cheese Natural (Magic Mountain)	1 Tbsp	5	tr
Blue Cheese (Estee)	1 Tbsp	8	tr
Blue Cheese Chunky Reduced Calorie (Kraft)	1 Tbsp	30	2
Blue Cheese Reduced Calorie (Roka Brand)	1 Tbsp	14	1
Buttermilk Creamy (Estee)	1 Tbsp	6	0
Buttermilk Creamy Reduced Calorie (Kraft)	1 Tbsp	30	3
Creamy Cucumber Reduced Calorie (Herb Magic)	1 Tbsp	8	0
Creamy Italian w/ Parmesan (Walden Farms)	1 Tbsp	35	3
Cucumber Creamy Reduced Calorie (Kraft)	1 Tbsp	30	3
Dijon Creamy (Estee)	1 Tbsp	8	tr
French (Walden Farms)	1 Tbsp	33	2
French Reduced Calorie (Kraft)	1 Tbsp	25	2

FOOD	PORTION	CALORIES	FAT
French Style Natural (Magic Mountain)	1 Tbsp	4	tr
Garlic Creamy w/ Red Wine Vinegar (Estee)	1 Tbsp	2	0
Herb & Spice No Oil (Magic Mountain)	1 Tbsp	2	tr
Herb Basket Reduced Calorie (Herb Magic)	1 Tbsp	6	0
Italian (Walden Farms)	1 Tbsp	9	tr
Italian Creamy (Estee)	1 Tbsp	4	0
Italian Creamy Reduced Calorie (Kraft)	1 Tbsp	25	2
Italian French (Estee)	1 Tbsp	4	0
Italian No Sugar Added (Walden Farms)	1 Tbsp	6	tr
Italian Reduced Calorie (Herb Magic)	1 Tbsp	4	0
Italian Reduced Calorie (Kraft)	1 Tbsp	6	0
Italian Sodium Free (Walden Farms)	1 Tbsp	9	tr
Northern Italian Natural (Magic Mountain)	1 Tbsp	2	tr
Ranch (Walden Farms)	1 Tbsp	35	2
Rancher's Choice Creamy Reduced Calorie (Kraft)	1 Tbsp	30	3
Reduced Calorie (Catalina)	1 Tbsp	16	0
Russian Reduced Calorie (Kraft)	1 Tbsp	30	1
Sweet & Sour Reduced Calorie (Herb Magic)	1 Tbsp	18	0

FOOD	PORTION	CALORIES	FAT
Thousand Island (Estee)	1 Tbsp	6	0
Thousand Island (Walden Farms)	1 Tbsp	24	2
Thousand Island Reduced Calorie (Herb Magic)	1 Tbsp	8	0
Thousand Island Reduced Calorie (Kraft)	1 Tbsp	30	2
Vinaigrette Reduced Calorie (Herb Magic)	1 Tbsp	6	0
Zesty Tomato Reduced Calorie (Herb Magic)	1 Tbsp	14	0
french	1 Tbsp	22	1
italian	1 Tbsp	16	2
russian	1 Tbsp	23	1
thousand island	1 Tbsp	24	2

SALMON

FOOD	PORTION	CALORIES	FAT
CANNED			
Keta (Libby's)	½ can (3.8 oz)	140	6
Pink (Bumble Bee)	3 oz	137	7
Pink (Libby's)	½ can (3.8 oz)	150	7
Pink Skinless (Bumble Bee)	3.25 oz	120	5
Red (Bumble Bee)	3 oz	154	9
chum w/ bone	3 oz	120	5
chum w/ bone	1 can (13.9 oz)	521	20
pink w/ bone	3 oz	118	5

FOOD	PORTION	CALORIES	FAT
pink w/ bone	1 can (15.9 oz)	631	27
sockeye w/ bone	3 oz	130	6
sockeye w/ bone	1 can (12.9 oz)	566	27
FRESH Salmon Steak (Health Valley)	3.5 oz	220	15
Atlantic, raw	3 oz	121	5
Atlantic, raw	½ fillet (6.9 oz)	281	13
chinook, raw	½ fillet (6.9 oz)	356	21
chinook, raw	3 oz	153	9
chum, raw	3 oz	102	3
chum, raw	½ fillet (6.9 oz)	237	7
coho, raw	½ fillet (6.9 oz)	289	12
coho, raw	3 oz	124	5
coho; cooked	3 oz	157	6
coho; cooked	½ fillet (5.4 oz)	286	12
pink, raw	½ fillet (5.6 oz)	185	5
pink, raw	3 oz	99	3
sockeye, raw	½ fillet (6.9 oz)	333	17
sockeye, raw	3 oz	143	7
sockeye; cooked	3 oz	183	9
sockeye; cooked	½ fillet (5.4 oz)	334	17
HOME RECIPE salmon cake	3.4 oz	241	15
salmon casserole	¾ cup	416	26
salmon rice loaf	½" slice (6.2 oz)	299	16
SMOKED chinook	1 oz	33	1
chinook	3 oz	99	4

FOOD	PORTION	CALORIES	FAT
SALSIFY			
sliced; cooked	½ cup	46	tr
sliced, raw	½ cup	55	tr
SALT SUBSTITUTE			
Nu-Salt	1 pkg (1g)	0	0
Salt-It Salt Substitute (Estee)	½ tsp	0	0
Salt Substitute (Morton)	1 tsp	tr	0
Seasoned Salt Substitute (Morton)	1 tsp	2	tr
SALT/SEASONED SALT (see also SALT SUBSTITUTE)			
Garlic Salt (Morton)	1 tsp	3	tr
Kosher Salt (Morton)	1 tsp	0	0
Lite Salt Mixture (Morton)	1 tsp	tr	0
Nature's Seasons Seasoning Blend (Morton)	1 tsp	3	tr
Salt Iodized (Morton)	1 tsp	tr	0
Salt Non-Iodized (Morton)	1 tsp	0	0
Seasoned Salt (Morton)	1 tsp	4	tr
SAPODILLA			
sapodilla	1	140	2

FOOD	PORTION	CALORIES	FAT

SARDINE

CANNED

Food	Portion	Calories	Fat
Sardines in Mustard Sauce (Port Clyde Foods)	1 can (3.75 oz)	175	11
Sardines in Soybean Oil (Port Clyde Foods)	1 can (3.75 oz)	225	18
Sardines in Tomato Sauce (Port Clyde Foods)	1 can (3.75 oz)	170	11
Atlantic in oil w/ bone	1 can (3.2 oz)	192	11
Atlantic in oil w/ bone	2 oz	50	3
Pacific in brine & mustard	1 lg (.7 oz)	39	2
Pacific w/ tomato sauce w/ bone	1 can (13 oz)	658	44
Pacific w/ tomato sauce w/ bone	1 oz	68	5

SAUCE

(*see also* GRAVY, PIZZA, SPAGHETTI SAUCE, TOMATO)

DRY

Food	Portion	Calories	Fat
Bar-B-Q Sauce Mix (Diamond Crystal)	2 oz	35	1
Brown Sauce Mix (Diamond Crystal)	2 oz	15	tr
Cheese Sauce Mix (Diamond Crystal)	2 oz	50	2
Cream Sauce Mix (Diamond Crystal)	2 oz	40	1
Italian Sauce Mix (Diamond Crystal)	3 oz	50	tr
Marinade For Meat (Kikkoman)	1 oz pkg	64	tr
Sweet & Sour Sauce Mix (Kikkoman)	2⅛ oz pkg	228	tr
Sweet 'n Sour Entree Mix Chun King	3.8 oz	370	0

FOOD	PORTION	CALORIES	FAT
Teriyaki Sauce Mix (Kikkoman)	1½ oz pkg	125	tr
bearnaise; as prep w/ milk & butter	1 cup	701	68
bearnaise; not prep	1 pkg (.9 oz)	90	2
cheese; as prep w/ milk	1 cup	307	17
cheese; not prep	1 pkg (1.2 oz)	158	9
curry; as prep w/ milk	1 cup	270	15
curry; not prep	1 pkg (1.2 oz)	151	8
hollandaise w/ butterfat; as prep w/ water	1 cup	237	20
hollandaise w/ butterfat; not prep	1 pkg (1.2 oz)	187	16
hollandaise w/ oil; as prep w/ water	1 cup	703	68
hollandaise w/ oil; not prep	1 pkg (.9 oz)	93	2
mushroom; as prep w/ milk	1 cup	228	10
mushroom; not prep	1 pkg (1 oz)	99	3
sourcream; as prep w/ milk	1 cup	509	30
sourcream; not prep	1 pkg (1.2 oz)	180	11
stroganoff; as prep w/ milk & water	1 cup	271	11
stroganoff; not prep	1 pkg (1.6 oz)	161	4
sweet & sour; as prep w/ water & vinegar	1 cup	294	tr
sweet & sour; not prep	1 pkg (2 oz)	220	tr
teriyaki; as prep w/ water	1 cup	131	1
teriyaki; not prep	1 pkg (1.6 oz)	130	1
white; as prep w/ milk	1 cup	241	13
white; not prep	1 pkg (1.7 oz)	230	13
HOME RECIPE hollandaise	2 Tbsp	130	14
BOTTLED A-1 Steak Sauce (Heublein)	1 Tbsp	14	tr

FOOD	PORTION	CALORIES	FAT
Barbecue (Mauil's)	3.5 oz	123	2
Barbecue Beer Flavor, Non-Alcoholic (Mauil's)	3.5 oz	128	2
Barbecue Sauce (Estee)	1 Tbsp	18	tr
Barbecue Sauce (Kraft)	2 Tbsp	40	1
Barbecue Sauce (Ott's)	1 Tbsp	14	tr
Barbecue Sauce, Garlic Flavored (Kraft)	2 Tbsp	40	0
Barbecue Sauce, Hickory Smoke (Open Pit)	1 Tbsp	25	0
Barbecue Sauce, Hickory Smoke Flavor (Kraft)	2 Tbsp	40	1
Barbecue Sauce, Hickory Smoke, Flavored w/ Flavored Onion Bits (Kraft)	2 Tbsp	50	1
Barbecue Sauce, Hot (Kraft)	2 Tbsp	40	1
Barbecue Sauce, Hot, Hickory Smoke Flavored (Kraft)	2 Tbsp	40	1
Barbecue Sauce, Italian Seasoning (Kraft)	2 Tbsp	45	1
Barbecue Sauce, Kansas City Style (Kraft)	2 Tbsp	45	1
Barbecue Sauce, Mesquite Smoke (Kraft)	2 Tbsp	45	1
Barbecue Sauce, Onion Bits (Kraft)	2 Tbsp	50	1
Barbecue Sauce, Original (Bull's Eye)	2 Tbsp	50	0
Barbecue Sauce, Smoky (Ott's)	1 Tbsp	14	tr

FOOD	PORTION	CALORIES	FAT
Barbecue Sauce, Thick 'n Tangy Hickory (Open Pit)	1 Tbsp	25	0
Barbecue Sauce, Thick 'n Spicy, Chunky (Kraft)	2 Tbsp	50	1
Barbecue Sauce, Thick 'n Spicy, Hickory Smoked (Kraft)	2 Tbsp	50	1
Barbecue Sauce, Thick 'n Spicy, Kansas City Style (Kraft)	2 Tbsp	60	1
Barbecue Sauce, Thick 'n Spicy, Original (Kraft)	2 Tbsp	50	1
Barbecue Sauce, Thick 'n Spicy w/ Honey (Kraft)	2 Tbsp	60	1
Barbecue, Smoky (Maull's)	3.5 oz	124	tr
Barbecue, Sweet-n-Mild (Maull's)	3.5 oz	167	2
Barbecue, Sweet-n-Smoky (Maull's)	3.5 oz	160	tr
Barbecue w/ Onion Bits (Maull's)	3.5 oz	126	2
Bolognese (Fresh Chef)	4 oz	130	7
Cocktail (Sauceworks)	1 Tbsp	12	0
Cocktail Sauce (Estee)	1 Tbsp	10	tr
Diable Sauce (Escoffier)	1 Tbsp	20	0
Newburg Sauce w/ Sherry (Snow's)	⅓ cup	120	8

FOOD	PORTION	CALORIES	FAT
Pesto (Fresh Chef)	4 oz	630	60
Rib Sauce (Gold's)	1 oz	60	0
Robert Sauce (Escoffier)	1 Tbsp	20	0
Steak Sauce (Estee)	½ oz	15	tr
Steak Sauce (Steak Supreme)	1 Tbsp	20	0
Stir-Fry Sauce (Kikkoman)	1 tsp	6	tr
Sweet & Sour (La Choy)	1 Tbsp	30	tr
Sweet & Sour Sauce (Kikkoman)	1 Tbsp	18	tr
Sweet 'n Sour (Sauceworks)	1 Tbsp	20	0
Sweet 'n Sour (Contadina)	½ cup	150	3
Tartar Sauce (Best Foods)	1 Tbsp	70	8
Tartar Sauce (Bright Day)	1 Tbsp	50	5
Tartar Sauce (Hellman's)	1 Tbsp	70	8
Tartar Sauce (Kraft)	1 Tbsp	70	8
Tartar Sauce (Sauceworks)	1 Tbsp	70	8
Tartar Sauce, Natural Lemon & Herb Flavor (Sauceworks)	1 Tbsp	70	8
Teriyaki Marinade & Sauce (La Choy)	1 oz	30	0

FOOD	PORTION	CALORIES	FAT
Teriyaki Sauce (Kikkoman)	1 Tbsp	15	tr
Tabasco (McIlhenny)	¼ tsp	tr	tr
Welsh Rarebit Cheese Sauce (Snow's)	½ cup	170	11
Worchestershire (Lea & Perrins)	1 Tbsp	59	tr
barbecue	1 cup	188	5
teriyaki	1 Tbsp	15	0
teriyaki	1 oz	30	0

SAUERKRAUT

FOOD	PORTION	CALORIES	FAT
CANNED			
Old Fashioned Sauerkraut (Vlasic)	1 oz	4	0
Sauerkraut (Claussen)	½ cup	17	tr
Sauerkraut (Libby)	½ cup	20	0
Sauerkraut (Seneca)	½ cup	20	0
canned	½ cup	22	tr
JUICE			
Sauerkraut Juice (S&W)	5 oz	14	0

SAUSAGE
(*see also* HOT DOGS, SAUSAGE SUBSTITUTE)

FOOD	PORTION	CALORIES	FAT
Biscuit & Sausage (Great Starts)	4.75 oz	410	23
Bratwurts, Smoked (Oscar Mayer)	1 (2.7 oz)	237	21
Breakfast Sausage, Turkey (Bil Mar Foods)	1 oz	58	4

FOOD	PORTION	CALORIES	FAT
Churro (J&J Snack Foods)	1.4 oz	141	9
Country Sausage, Lower Salt (Armour)	1 oz	110	11
Country Sausage, Lower Salt Links (Armour)	1 oz	110	11
Country Sausage, Lower Salt Patties (Armour)	1.5 oz	160	16
Italian Smoked, Cooked, Cured (Oscar Mayer)	1 (2.6 oz)	264	24
Kielbasa	1 oz	83	8
Knockwurst (Health Valley)	3.5 oz	280	15
Knockwurst (Hebrew National)	1 (3 oz)	260	25
Little Friers, Prok; cooked (Oscar Mayer)	1 (.7 oz)	82	8
Polish (Oscar Mayer)	1 (2.7 oz)	229	20
Polish Kielbasa (Mr. Turkey)	3 oz	177	13
Pork Breakfast Patties (Jones)	1 (2 oz)	136	11
Pork Brown & Serve Links (Jones)	1 (.8 oz)	55	5
Pork Brown & Serve Patties (Jones)	1 (2 oz)	136	11
Pork Sausage (Armour)	1 oz	110	11
Pork Sausage Links (Armour)	1 oz	110	11
Pork Sausage Patties (Armour)	1.5 oz	160	16
Pork, Light Breakfast Links (Jones)	1 (.8 oz)	55	5

FOOD	PORTION	CALORIES	FAT
Pork, Light Breakfast Links (Jones)	1 (2 oz)	136	11
Sausage Biscuits, Microwave (Jimmy Dean)	1	210	14
Smoked (Oscar Mayer)	1 oz	83	8
Smoked Sausage (Bil Mar Foods)	3 oz	142	10
Smokies, Beef (Oscar Mayer)	1 (1.5 oz)	123	11
Smokies, Cheese (Oscar Mayer)	1 (1.5 oz)	127	11
Smokies, Links (Oscar Mayer)	1 (1.5 oz)	124	11
Smokies, Little (Oscar Mayer)	1 (.3 oz)	28	3
bockwurst, pork	1 link (65 g)	200	18
bockwurst, pork	1 oz	87	8
bratwurst, pork; cooked	1 link (85 g)	256	22
bratwurst, pork; cooked	1 oz	85	7
bratwurst, pork & beef	1 link (70 g)	226	19
bratwurst, pork & beef	1 oz	92	8
country-style, pork; cooked	1 patty (1 oz)	100	8
country-style, pork; cooked	1 link (½ oz)	48	4
italian, pork, raw	1 link (2.3 oz)	315	13
italian, pork, raw	1 link (4 oz)	391	16
italian, pork; cooked	1 link (67 g)	216	17
italian, pork; cooked	1 link (83 g)	268	21
kielbasa	1 oz	88	8
kielbasa, pork	1 slice (26 g)	81	7
knockwurst, pork & beef	1 link (68 g)	209	19
knockwurst, pork & beef	1 oz	87	8
polish, pork	1 link (8 oz)	739	65

FOOD	PORTION	CALORIES	FAT
polish, pork	1 oz	92	8
pork & beef; cooked	1 patty (1 oz)	107	10
pork & beef; cooked	1 link (½ oz)	52	5
pork, country-style, raw	1 patty (2 oz)	238	23
pork, country-style, raw	1 link (1 oz)	118	11
pork, raw	1 patty (2 oz)	238	23
pork, raw	1 link (1 oz)	118	11
pork; cooked	1 patty (1 oz)	100	8
pork; cooked	1 link (½ oz)	48	4
smoked, beef; cooked	1 sausage (1.4 oz)	134	12
smoked, pork	1 link (2⅓ oz)	256	22
smoked, pork	1 sm link (½ oz)	62	5
smoked, pork & beef	1 link (2⅓ oz)	229	21
smoked, pork & beef	1 sm link (½ oz)	54	5
vienna, canned, beef & pork	1 sausage (½ oz)	45	4

SAUSAGE SUBSTITUTE

FOOD	PORTION	CALORIES	FAT
Grillers; frzn (Morningstar Farms)	3.5 oz	290	19
Linketts (Loma Linda)	2 (2.6 oz)	150	8
Links; frzn (Morningstar Farms)	3.5 oz	237	18
Little Links (Loma Linda)	2 (1.6 oz)	80	5

SCALLOP

FRESH

FOOD	PORTION	CALORIES	FAT
raw	3 oz	75	1

FOOD	PORTION	CALORIES	FAT
raw	2 lg	26	tr
raw	5 sm	26	tr
FROZEN			
French Fried Scallops (Mrs. Paul's)	3.5 oz	230	9
Lightly Breaded Scallops (King & Prince)	3.5 oz	120	tr
HOME RECIPE			
breaded & fried	2 lg	67	3

SCONE

FOOD	PORTION	CALORIES	FAT
apricot scone (home recipe)	1	232	7
scone (home recipe)	1 (1.4 oz)	130	6

SCROD

FOOD	PORTION	CALORIES	FAT
FROZEN			
Ready-To-Bake Scrod (King & Prince)	5 oz	252	16
Ready-To-Bake Scrod (King & Prince)	8 oz	403	26
Seafood Lover's Baked Scrod (Gorton's)	1 pkg	320	18

SCUP

FOOD	PORTION	CALORIES	FAT
raw	3 oz	89	2
raw	1 fillet (2.2 oz)	67	2

SEA BASS
(see BASS)

SEASONING

FOOD	PORTION	CALORIES	FAT
Herb Seasoning (American Heart Association)	¼ tsp	tr	tr

FOOD	PORTION	CALORIES	FAT
Instead of Salt, All Purpose (Health Valley)	¾ tsp	11	tr
Instead of Salt, Chicken (Health Valley)	¾ tsp	8	tr
Instead of Salt, Fish (Health Valley)	¾ tsp	11	tr
Instead of Salt, Steak & Hamburger (Health Valley)	½ tsp	6	tr
Instead of Salt, Vegetable (Health Valley)	1 tsp	13	tr
Lemon Herb Seasoning (American Heart Association)	¼ tsp	tr	tr
Original Herb Seasoning (American Heart Association)	¼ tsp	tr	tr
Savorex (Loma Linda)	1 tsp	16	tr

SEA TROUT
(*see* TROUT)

SESAME

FOOD	PORTION	CALORIES	FAT
Sesame Nut Mix, Dry Roasted (Planters)	1 oz	160	12
Sesame Nut Mix, Oil Roasted (Planters)	1 oz	160	13
seeds	1 tsp	16	2
seeds, dried	1 Tbsp	52	5
seeds, dried	1 cup	825	72
seeds; roasted & toasted	1 oz	161	14
sesame butter	1 Tbsp	95	8
tahini, from roasted & toasted kernels	1 Tbsp	89	8
tahini, from unroasted kernels	1 Tbsp	85	8

FOOD	PORTION	CALORIES	FAT
SHAD			
American, raw	3 oz	167	12
American, raw	1 fillet (6.5 oz)	362	25
roe, raw	3.5 oz	130	2
SHALLOT			
freeze-dried	1 Tbsp	3	0
fresh, chopped	1 Tbsp	7	tr
SHARK			
raw	3 oz	111	4
batter-dipped & fried (home recipe)	3 oz	194	12
SHEEPSHEAD FISH			
cooked	1 fillet (6.5 oz)	234	3
cooked	3 oz	107	1
raw	3 oz	92	2
raw	1 fillet (8.4 oz)	257	6

SHELLFISH
(*see* INDIVIDUAL NAMES, SHELLFISH SUBSTITUTE)

SHELLFISH SUBSTITUTE

Kibun Sea Pasta w/ dressing	½ pkg	220	7
Kibun Sea Pasta w/o dressing	½ pkg	110	1
Kibun Sea Pasta w/ Shrimp, w/ dressing	½ pkg	210	9
Kibun Sea Pasta w/ Shrimp, w/o dressing	½ pkg	140	1
Kibun Sea Stix, Salad Style	4 oz	110	tr
Kibun Sea Stix, Whole Leg	4 oz	110	tr
Kibun Sea Tails	4 oz	110	tr

FOOD	PORTION	CALORIES	FAT
Louis Kemp Crab Delights	2 oz	60	tr
SeaLegs, Imitation Lobster Meat	3 oz	80	1
crab, imitation	3 oz	87	1
scallop, imitation	3 oz	84	tr
shrimp, imitation	3 oz	86	1
surimi	1 oz	28	tr
surimi	3 oz	84	1

SHELLIE BEANS

shellie beans, canned	½ cup	37	tr

SHRIMP

CANNED

Canned Shrimp (Robinson)	2 oz	58	1
canned	1 cup	154	3
canned	3 oz	102	2

FRESH

cooked	4 large	22	tr
cooked	3 oz	84	1
raw	3 oz	90	1
raw	4 large	30	tr

FROZEN

Cooked in the Shell (King & Prince)	4 oz	70	tr
Cooked in the Shell (King & Prince)	3.5 oz	65	tr
Fried Shrimp (Mrs. Paul's)	3 oz	200	11
Gourmet Hand Breaded Shrimp Butterfly (King & Prince)	3.5 oz	150	tr

FOOD	PORTION	CALORIES	FAT
Gourmet Hand Breaded Shrimp Round (King & Prince)	3.5 oz	150	tr
Shrimp a la Monterey (King & Prince)	3.5 oz	190	7
Shrimp a la Monterey (King & Prince)	2 oz	107	4
Shrimp & Clams w/ Linguini (Mrs. Paul's)	10 oz	280	6
Shrimp Cajun Style (Mrs. Paul's)	10.5 oz	200	4
Shrimp Del Ray (King & Prince)	3 oz	85	6
Shrimp Del Ray (King & Prince)	1.5 oz	43	3
Shrimp Oriental (Mrs. Paul's)	11 oz	280	5
Shrimp Primavera (Mrs. Paul's)	11 oz	240	4
Shrimp Scampi (Gorton's)	1 pkg	350	24
Supreme Hand Breaded Shrimp Butterfly (King & Prince)	3.5 oz	130	tr
Supreme Hand Breaded Shrimp Round (King & Prince)	3.5 oz	140	tr
Western Style Breaded Shrimp (King & Prince)	3.5 oz	115	tr
HOME RECIPE			
jambalaya	¾ cup	188	5
breaded & fried	3 oz	206	10
breaded & fried	4 lg	73	4
stew	1 cup	207	14

FOOD	PORTION	CALORIES	FAT
READY-TO-USE Fried Shrimp (American Original Foods)	4 oz	253	12

SMELT

rainbow, raw	3 oz	83	2
rainbow, cooked	3 oz	106	3

SNACKS
    (*see also* CHIPS; FRUIT SNACKS; NUTS, MIXED; POPCORN; PRETZELS)

FOOD	PORTION	CALORIES	FAT
Cheddar Lites (Health Valley)	.2 oz	40	2
Cheddar Lites w/ Green Onion (Health Valley)	.2 oz	40	1
Cheese Balls (Lance)	1 pkg (1⅛ oz)	190	13
Cheese Balls (Lance)	1 oz	160	11
Cheetos Crunchy Cheese Flavored	1 oz	160	10
Cheetos Puffed Balls, Cheese Flavored	1 oz	160	10
Cheetos Puffs Cheese Flavored	1 oz	160	10
Cheez Balls (Planters)	1 oz	160	11
Cheez Curls (Planters)	1 oz	160	11
Cheez Doodles, Crunchy	1 oz	160	10
Cheez Doodles, Puffed	1 oz	150	9
Cheez Waffies	1 oz	140	8
Combos, Cracker Cheddar	1.8 oz	240	10
Combos, Cracker Peanut Butter	1.8 oz	240	10
Combos, Pretzel Cheddar	1.8 oz	240	9
Combos, Pretzel Nacho	1.8 oz	240	9

FOOD	PORTION	CALORIES	FAT
Combos, Pretzel Pizza	1.8 oz	240	9
Cornnuts, Barbecue	1 oz	110	4
Cornnuts, Nacho Cheese	1 oz	110	4
Cornnuts, Original	1 oz	120	4
Cornnuts, Unsalted	1 oz	120	4
Crunchy Cheese Twists (Lance)	1 pkg (1.5 oz)	230	13
Crunchy Cheese Twists (Lance)	1 oz	150	9
Doo Dads, Cheddar 'n Herb (Nabisco)	½ cup	140	6
Doo Dads, Original (Nabisco)	½ cup	140	6
Doo Dads, Zesty Cheese (Nabisco)	½ cup	140	6
Funyuns (Frito-Lay)	1 oz	140	6
Gold-N-Chee (Lance)	1⅜ oz	180	8
Gold-N-Chee (Lance)	1 oz	130	6
Munchos	1 oz	150	9
Pork Skins (Lance)	½ oz	80	5
Pork Skins, Regular (Lance)	½ oz	80	5
Sour Cream & Onion Puffs (Planters)	1 oz	160	10
Tostada, Nacho (Lance)	1 oz	140	7
Tostada, Regular (Lance)	1 oz	150	8
Wheat Snax (Estee)	1 oz	110	1

FOOD	PORTION	CALORIES	FAT

SNAIL
(*see* WHELK)

SNAP BEANS

CANNED

seasoned	½ cup	18	tr
snap beans	½ cup	18	tr

FRESH

cooked	½ cup	22	tr
raw	½ cup	17	tr

FROZEN

snap beans	½ cup	18	tr

SNAPPER

cooked	1 fillet (6 oz)	217	3
cooked	3 oz	109	1
raw	3 oz	85	1
raw	1 fillet (7.6 oz)	217	3

SODA
(*see also* DRINK MIXER)

Apple (Crush)	6 oz	90	0
Apple Sparkling (Welch's)	12 oz	180	0
Birch Beer Diet (Shasta)	12 oz	4	0
Black Cherry (Shasta)	12 oz	162	0
Cherry (Crush)	6 oz	100	0

FOOD	PORTION	CALORIES	FAT
Cherry Cola (Shasta)	12 oz	140	0
Citrus Mist (Shasta)	12 oz	170	0
Club (Schweppes)	6 oz	0	0
Club Soda (Shasta)	12 oz	0	0
Coca-Cola	6 oz	77	0
Coca-Cola, Caffeine-Free	6 oz	77	0
Coca-Cola, Cherry	6 oz	76	0
Coca-Cola, Classic	6 oz	72	0
Cola (Shasta)	8 oz	98	0
Cola (Shasta)	12 oz	147	0
Cola, Diet (Shasta)	8 oz	0	0
Collins (Shasta)	12 oz	118	0
Creme (Shasta)	12 oz	154	0
Diet Apple (Crush)	6 oz	10	0
Diet Cherry Coca Cola	6 oz	tr	0
Diet Coke	6 oz	tr	0
Diet Coke, Caffeine-Free	6 oz	tr	0
Diet Minute Maid Lemon Lime	6 oz	10	0
Diet Minute Maid Orange	6 oz	4	0
Diet Orange (Crush)	6 oz	12	0
Diet Sprite	6 oz	2	0
Diet Sun-Drop	6 oz	4	0

FOOD	PORTION	CALORIES	FAT
Dr Pepper	1 oz	13	0
Dr Pepper Diet	1 oz	tr	0
Dr. Diablo (Shasta)	12 oz	140	0
Fanta Ginger Ale	6 oz	63	0
Fanta Grape	6 oz	86	0
Fanta Orange	6 oz	88	0
Fanta Root Beer	6 oz	78	0
Fresca	6 oz	2	0
Fruit Punch (Shasta)	12 oz	173	0
Ginger Ale (Health Valley)	13 oz	153	1
Ginger Ale (Schweppes)	6 oz	63	0
Ginger Ale (Shasta)	8 oz	80	0
Ginger Ale (Shasta)	12 oz	120	0
Ginger Ale Diet (Schweppes)	6 oz	tr	0
Ginger Ale Diet (Shasta)	8 oz	0	0
Ginger Beer (Schweppes)	6 oz	68	0
Grape (Crush)	6 oz	100	0
Grape (Schweppes)	6 oz	92	0
Grape (Shasta)	12 oz	177	0
Grape, Sparkling (Welch's)	12 oz	180	0
Grapefruit (Schweppes)	6 oz	77	0

FOOD	PORTION	CALORIES	FAT
Lemon Lime (Schweppes)	6 oz	71	0
Lemon Lime (Shasta)	8 oz	97	0
Lemon Lime (Shasta)	12 oz	146	0
Lemon Lime Diet (Shasta)	8 oz	0	0
Like Cola	1 oz	13	0
Like Cola Sugar Free	1 oz	tr	0
Mello Yellow	6 oz	87	0
Minute Maid Lemon Lime	6 oz	71	0
Minute Maid Orange	6 oz	87	0
Mr. PIBB	6 oz	71	0
Orange (Crush)	6 oz	100	0
Orange (Shasta)	12 oz	177	0
Orange, Sparkling (Welch's)	12 oz	180	0
Orange, Sparkling (Schweppes)	6 oz	86	0
Pepper Free	1 oz	12	0
Pepper Free Diet	1 oz	tr	0
Pineapple (Crush)	6 oz	100	0
Ramblin' Root Beer	6 oz	88	0
Red Berry (Shasta)	12 oz	158	0
Red Pop (Shasta)	12 oz	158	0
Root Beer (Health Valley)	13 oz	120	1

FOOD	PORTION	CALORIES	FAT
Root Beer (Hires)	6 oz	90	0
Root Beer (Schweppes)	6 oz	75	0
Root Beer (Shasta)	12 oz	154	0
Root Beer, Sugar Free (Hires)	6 oz	2	0
Sarsaparilla (Health Valley)	13 oz	153	1
Seltzer (Schweppes)	6 oz	0	0
Seltzer, Flavored (Schweppes)	6 oz	0	0
Seltzer, Light Black Cherry Cider (Crystal Geyser)	6 oz	60	0
Seltzer, Light Cranberry-Raspberry (Crystal Geyser)	6 oz	60	0
Seltzer, Light Kiwi Lemonade (Crystal Geyser)	6 oz	60	0
Seltzer, Light Natural Peach (Crystal Geyser)	6 oz	60	0
Seltzer, Light Vanilla Creme (Crystal Geyser)	6 oz	60	0
Seltzer, No Salt Added, No Calories (Manischewitz)	8 oz	0	0
7 Up	1 oz	12	0
7 Up Cherry	1 oz	13	0
7 Up Cherry Diet	1 oz	tr	0
7 Up Diet	1 oz	tr	0
7 Up Gold	1 oz	13	0
7 Up Gold Diet	1 oz	tr	0
Shasta Free Cola	12 oz	151	0
Sprite	6 oz	71	0

FOOD	PORTION	CALORIES	FAT
Strawberry (Crush)	6 oz	90	0
Strawberry (Shasta)	12 oz	147	0
Strawberry, Sparkling (Welch's)	12 oz	180	0
Sun-Drop	6 oz	90	0
TAB	6 oz	tr	0
TAB Caffeine-Free	6 oz	tr	0
Tonic Water (Shasta)	12 oz	0	0
Wild Berry (Health Valley)	13 oz	142	1
club	12 oz	0	0
cola	12 oz	151	tr
cream	12 oz	191	0
ginger ale	12 oz	124	0
grape	12 oz	161	0
lemon lime	12 oz	149	0
orange	12 oz	177	0
pepper type	12 oz	151	tr
root beer	12 oz	152	0
tonic water	12 oz	125	0

SOLE

FOOD	PORTION	CALORIES	FAT
FROZEN			
Au Natural Sole Fillets (Mrs. Paul's)	4 oz	90	2
Fillet of Sole w/ Lemon Butter Sauce (Gorton's)	1 pkg	250	14
Fishmarket Fresh Sole (Gorton's)	5 oz	110	1

FOOD	PORTION	CALORIES	FAT
Light Breaded Sole Fillets (Mrs. Paul's)	1 fillet	280	13
Lightly Breaded Sole (Van De Kamp's)	5 oz	293	18
Microwave, Lightly Breaded Sole (Van De Kamp's)	5 oz	290	18
Sole a la Monterey (King & Prince)	6 oz	221	13
Sole a la Monterey (King & Prince)	8 oz	295	18
Sole in Wine Sauce (Gorton's)	1 pkg	140	4
Today's Catch, Baby Sole (Van De Kamp's)	5 oz	100	1

SOUFFLE

HOME RECIPE

cheese	1 cup	308	25
grand marnier	1 cup	109	4
lemon, chilled	1 cup	176	tr
raspberry, chilled	1 cup	173	tr
spinach	1 cup	218	18

SOUP

CANNED

5 Bean Chunky (Health Valley)	7.5 oz	80	2
Barley w/ Beef; as prep w/ water (Campbell)	1 cup	86	1
Bean (Health Valley)	4 oz	115	3
Bean w/ Bacon, Special Request (Campbell's)	8 oz	120	4

FOOD	PORTION	CALORIES	FAT
Bean w/ Bacon, Special Request (Campbell's)	8 oz	120	4
Beef Broth (College Inn)	1 cup	18	0
Beef Broth (Health Valley)	4 oz	10	0
Beef Broth (Pritikin Foods)	6⅞ oz	20	tr
Beef Broth (Swanson)	7.25 oz	20	1
Beefy Noodle Soup w/ Vegetables, Hearty (Lipton)	8 oz	85	tr
Borscht (Gold's)	8 oz	100	0
Borscht Lo-Cal (Gold's)	8 oz	20	1
Borscht, Low Calorie (Manischewitz)	8 oz	20	0
Borscht w/ Beets (Manischewitz)	8 oz	80	0
Chicken Broth (College Inn)	1 cup	35	3
Chicken Broth (Health Valley)	4 oz	15	1
Chicken Broth (Pritikin Foods)	6⅞ oz	14	0
Chicken Broth (Swanson)	7.25 oz	30	2
Chicken Gumbo (Pritikin Foods)	7⅜ oz	60	1
Chicken Noodle Soup, Hearty (Lipton)	8 oz	79	1
Chicken Soup w/ Ribbon Pasta (Pritikin Foods)	7.25 oz	60	tr

FOOD	PORTION	CALORIES	FAT
Chicken Vegetable (Pritikin Foods)	7.25 oz	70	tr
Chicken Vegetable, Chunky (Estee)	7.5 oz	120	6
Chicken w/ Rice, Special Request (Campbell's)	8 oz	60	2
Clam Chowder (Health Valley)	4 oz	80	3
Country Vegetable (Lunch Bucket)	1 container (8.25 oz)	90	1
Cream Of Broccoli, Calif. International Soup Classics (Lipton)	9 oz	86	3
Lentil (Health Valley)	4 oz	90	3
Lentil Soup (Pritikin Foods)	7⅜ oz	100	0
Manhattan Clam Chowder (Pritikin Foods)	7⅜ oz	70	tr
Manhattan Clam Chowder; as prep w/ water (Snow's)	7.5 oz	70	2
Minestrone (Health Valley)	7.5 oz	90	3
Minestrone, Chunky (Estee)	7.5 oz	160	5
Minestrone, Chunky (Health Valley)	4 oz	70	1
Minestrone Soup (Pritikin Foods)	7⅜ oz	110	tr
Mushroom (Health Valley)	4 oz	70	3
Mushroom (Pritikin Foods)	7⅜ oz	60	tr
Navy Bean (Pritikin Foods)	7⅜ oz	130	tr

FOOD	PORTION	CALORIES	FAT
New England Chowder (American Original Foods)	4 oz	64	1
New England Chowder; as prep w/ milk (American Original Foods)	4 oz	145	6
New England Clam Chowder; as prep w/ milk (Snow's)	7.5 oz	140	6
New England Corn Chowder; as prep w/ milk (Snow's)	7.5 oz	150	6
New England Fish Chowder; as prep w/ milk (Snow's)	7.5 oz	130	6
New England Seafood Chowder; as prep w/ milk (Snow's)	7.5 oz	130	6
New England Clam Chowder (Pritikin Foods)	7⅜ oz	118	tr
New England Clam Chowder; as prep w/ whole milk (Gorton's)	¼ can	140	5
Potato (Health Valley)	4 oz	70	2
Schav (Gold's)	8 oz	25	0
Seafood Soup, Spicy (Port Clyde Foods)	7.5 oz	68	1
Split Pea, Green (Health Valley)	4 oz	70	0
Split Pea Soup (Pritikin Foods)	7.5 oz	130	tr
Tomato (Health Valley)	4 oz	60	2
Tomato Soup w/ Tomato Pieces (Pritikin Foods)	7.5 oz	70	0

FOOD	PORTION	CALORIES	FAT
Turkey Vegetable Soup w/ Ribbon Pasta (Pritikin Foods)	7⅜ oz	50	tr
Vegetable (Health Valley)	7.5 oz	80	1
Vegetable Beef (Lunch Bucket)	1 container (8.25 oz)	140	5
Vegetable Beef, Chunky (Estee)	7.5 oz	140	7
Vegetable Chicken, Chunky (Health Valley)	4 oz	120	7
Vegetable Soup (Pritikin Foods)	7⅜ oz	70	0
asparagus, cream of; as prep w/ milk	1 cup	161	8
asparagus, cream of; as prep w/ water	1 cup	87	4
bean w/ frankfurters; as prep w/ water	1 cup	187	7
bean w/ frankfurters; not prep	1 can (11.25 oz)	454	17
bean black; as prep w/ water	1 cup	116	2
bean black; not prep	1 can (11 oz)	285	4
bean w/ bacon; as prep w/ water	1 cup	173	6
bean w/ bacon; not prep	1 can (11.5 oz)	420	14
bean w/ ham, chunky, ready-to-serve	1 can (19.25 oz)	519	19
bean w/ ham, chunky, ready-to-serve	1 cup	231	9
beef broth, ready-to-serve	1 can (14 oz)	27	1
beef broth, ready-to-serve	1 cup	16	1
beef chunky, ready-to-serve	1 cup	171	5
beef chunky, ready-to-serve	1 can (19 oz)	383	12

FOOD	PORTION	CALORIES	FAT
beef noodle; as prep w/ water	1 cup	84	3
beef noodle; not prep	1 can (10.75 oz)	204	7
black bean turtle soup	1 cup	218	tr
celery, cream of; as prep w/ milk	1 can (10.75 oz)	400	24
celery, cream of; as prep w/ milk	1 cup	165	10
celery, cream of; as prep w/ water	1 cup	90	6
celery, cream of; not prep	1 can (10.75 oz)	219	14
cheese; as prep w/ milk	1 cup	230	15
cheese; as prep w/ milk	1 can (11 oz)	558	35
cheese; as prep w/ water	1 can (11 oz)	377	25
cheese; as prep w/ water	1 cup	155	10
cheese; not prep	1 can (11 oz)	377	25
chicken, vegetable, chunky, ready-to-serve	1 can (19 oz)	374	11
chicken vegetable, chunky, ready-to-serve	1 cup	167	5
chicken vegetable; as prep w/ water	1 cup	74	3
chicken vegetable; not prep	1 can (10.5 oz)	181	7
chicken & dumplings; as prep w/ water	1 cup	406	6
chicken & dumplings; not prep	1 can (10.5 oz)	236	13
chicken broth; as prep w/ water	1 can (10.75 oz)	95	3
chicken broth; as prep w/ water	1 cup	39	1
chicken broth; not prep	1 can (10.75 oz)	94	3
chicken, chunky, ready-to-serve	1 cup	178	7
chicken, chunky, ready-to-serve	1 can (10.75 oz)	216	8
chicken, cream of; as prep w/ milk	1 cup	191	11

FOOD	PORTION	CALORIES	FAT
chicken, cream of; as prep w/ water	1 can (10.75 oz)	464	28
chicken, cream of; as prep w/ water	1 cup	116	7
chicken, cream of; not prep	1 can (10.75 oz)	283	18
chicken gumbo; as prep w/ water	1 cup	56	1
chicken gumbo; not prep	1 can (10.75 oz)	137	3
chicken noodle w/ meatballs, ready-to-serve	1 cup	99	4
chicken noodle w/ meatballs, ready-to-serve	1 can (20 oz)	227	8
chicken noodle; as prep w/ water	1 cup	75	2
chicken noodle; not prep	1 can (10.5 oz)	182	6
chicken rice, chunky, ready-to-serve	1 can (19 oz)	286	7
chicken rice, chunky, ready-to-serve	1 cup	127	3
chicken rice; as prep w/ water	1 cup	251	2
chicken rice; not prep	1 can (10.5 oz)	146	5
chicken rice; not prep	1 can (10.5 oz)	146	5
chili beef; as prep w/ water	1 cup	169	7
chili beef; not prep	1 can (11.25 oz)	411	16
clam chowder, Manhattan, chunky, ready-to-serve	1 cup	133	3
clam chowder, Manhattan, chunky, ready-to-serve	1 can (19 oz)	299	8
clam chowder, Manhattan; as prep w/ water	1 cup	78	2
clam chowder, Manhattan; not prep	1 can (10.75 oz)	187	5
clam chowder, New England; as prep w/ milk	1 cup	163	7
clam chowder, New England; as prep w/ water	1 cup	95	3

FOOD	PORTION	CALORIES	FAT
clam chowder, New England; not prep	1 can (10.75 oz)	214	8
consomme w/ gelatin; as prep w/ water	1 cup	29	0
consomme w/ gelatin; not prep	1 can (10.5 oz)	71	0
crab, ready-to-serve	1 cup	76	2
crab, ready-to-serve	1 can (13 oz)	114	2
escarole, ready-to-serve	1 can (19.5 oz)	61	4
escarole, ready-to-serve	1 cup	27	2
gazpacho, ready-to-serve	1 cup	57	2
gazpacho, ready-to-serve	1 can (13 oz)	87	3
lentil w/ ham, ready-to-serve	1 can (13 oz)	320	6
lentil w/ ham, ready-to-serve	1 cup	140	3
minestrone, chunky, ready-to-serve	1 cup	127	3
minestrone, chunky, ready-to-serve	1 can (19 oz)	285	6
minestrone; as prep w/ water	1 cup	83	3
minestrone; not prep	1 can (10.5 oz)	202	6
mushroom w/ beef stock; as prep w/ water	1 can (10.75 oz)	208	10
mushroom w/ beef stock; as prep w/ water	1 cup	85	4
mushroom w/ beef stock; not prep	1 can (10.75 oz)	208	10
mushroom, cream of; as prep w/ milk	1 can (10.75 oz)	494	33
mushroom, cream of; as prep w/ milk	1 cup	203	14
mushroom, cream of; as prep w/ water	1 cup	129	9
mushroom, cream of; not prep	1 can (10.75 oz)	313	23
onion; as prep w/ water	1 cup	57	2
onion; not prep	1 can (10.5 oz)	138	4

FOOD	PORTION	CALORIES	FAT
oyster stew; as prep w/ milk	1 cup	134	8
oyster stew; as prep w/ milk	1 can (10.5 oz)	325	19
oyster stew; as prep w/ water	1 cup	59	4
oyster stew; not prep	1 can (10.5 oz)	144	9
pea, green; as prep w/ milk	1 can (11.25 oz)	579	17
pea, green; as prep w/ milk	1 cup	239	7
pea, green; as prep w/ water	1 cup	164	3
pea, green; not prep	1 can (11.25 oz)	398	7
pepperpot; as prep w/ water	1 cup	103	5
pepperpot; not prep	1 can (10.5 oz)	251	11
potato, cream of; as prep w/ milk	1 can (10.75 oz)	360	16
potato, cream of; as prep w/ milk	1 cup	148	6
potato, cream of; as prep w/ water	1 cup	73	2
potato, cream of; not prep	1 can (10.75 oz)	178	6
scotch broth; as prep w/ water	1 cup	80	3
scotch broth; not prep	1 can (10.5 oz)	195	6
shrimp, cream of; as prep w/ milk	1 can (10.75 oz)	400	23
shrimp, cream of; as prep w/ milk	1 cup	165	9
shrimp, cream of; as prep w/ water	1 cup	90	5
shrimp, cream of; not prep	1 can (10.75 oz)	219	13
split pea w/ ham, chunky, ready-to-serve	1 cup	184	4
split pea w/ ham, chunky, ready-to-serve	1 can (19 oz)	413	9
split pea w/ ham; as prep w/ water	1 cup	189	4
split pea w/ ham; not prep	1 can (11.5 oz)	459	11

FOOD	PORTION	CALORIES	FAT
stockpot; as prep w/ water	1 cup	100	4
stockpot; not prep	1 can (11 oz)	242	9
tomato beef w/ noodle; as prep w/ water	1 cup	140	4
tomato beef w/ noodle; not prep	1 can (10.75 oz)	341	10
tomato bisque; as prep w/ milk	1 can (11 oz)	481	16
tomato bisque; as prep w/ milk	1 cup	198	7
tomato bisque; as prep w/ water	1 cup	123	3
tomato bisque; not prep	1 can (11 oz)	300	6
tomato rice; as prep w/ water	1 cup	120	3
tomato rice; not prep	1 can (11 oz)	291	7
tomato; as prep w/ milk	1 can (10.75 oz)	389	15
tomato; as prep w/ milk	1 cup	160	6
tomato; as prep w/ water	1 cup	86	2
tomato; not prep	1 can (10.75 oz)	208	5
turkey, chunky, ready-to-serve	1 can (18.75 oz)	306	10
turkey, chunky, ready-to-serve	1 cup	136	4
turkey noodle; as prep w/ water	1 cup	69	2
turkey noodle; not prep	1 can (10.75 oz)	168	5
turkey vegetable as prep w/ water	1 cup	74	3
turkey vegetable; not prep	1 can (10.5 oz)	179	7
vegetable, chunky, ready-to-serve	1 cup	122	4
vegetable, chunky, ready-to-serve	1 can (19 oz)	274	8
vegetable w/ beef; as prep w/ water	1 cup	79	2
vegetable w/ beef; not prep	1 can (10.75 oz)	192	5

FOOD	PORTION	CALORIES	FAT
vegetable w/ beef broth; as prep w/ water	1 cup	81	2
vegetable w/ beef broth; not prep	1 can (10.5 oz)	197	5
vegetarian vegetable; as prep w/ water	1 cup	72	2
vegetarian vegetable; not prep	1 can (10.5 oz)	176	5
vichyssoise	1 cup	148	6
vichyssoise	1 can (10.75 oz)	360	16
DRY Beef; as prep (Diamond Crystal)	6 oz	30	1
Beef Bouillon, Instant (Wylers)	1 tsp	6	tr
Beef Bouillon, Instant, Cube (Wylers)	1	6	tr
Beef Bouillon, Instant, Low Sodium (Lite Line)	1 tsp	12	tr
Beef Flavor Bouillon; as prep (Diamond Crystal)	6 oz	17	tr
Beef Noodle; as prep (Estee)	6 oz	20	tr
Broth & Brown Seasoning (George Washington)	1 serving	6	0
Broth & Golden Seasoning (George Washington)	1 serving	6	0
Broth & Onion Seasoning (George Washington)	1 serving	12	0
Broth & Vegetable Seasoning (George Washington)	1 serving	12	0
Chicken; as prep (Diamond Crystal)	6 oz	30	1
Chicken Bouillon, Instant (Wylers)	1 tsp	8	tr

FOOD	PORTION	CALORIES	FAT
Chicken Bouillon, Instant, Cube (Wylers)	1	8	tr
Chicken Bouillon, Instant, Low Sodium (Lite Line)	1 tsp	12	tr
Chicken Flavor Bouillon; as prep (Diamond Crystal)	6 oz	20	1
Chicken Noodle Instant; as prep (Estee)	6 oz	25	tr
Cream; as prep (Diamond Crystal)	6 oz	90	3
Minestrone Soup Mix; as prep (Manischewitz)	6 oz	50	tr
Mushroom, Instant; as prep (Estee)	6 oz	40	2
Onion Bouillon, Instant (Wylers)	1 tsp	10	tr
Onion Instant; as prep (Estee)	6 oz	25	tr
Split Pea Soup Mix; as prep (Manischewitz)	6 oz	45	tr
Tomato; as prep (Diamond Crystal)	6 oz	70	2
Tomato, Instant; as prep (Estee)	6 oz	40	tr
Vegetable Bouillon, Instant (Wylers)	1 tsp	6	tr
Vegetable Soup Mix; as prep (Manischewitz)	6 oz	50	tr
asparagus, cream of; as prep w/ water	1 cup	59	2
asparagus, cream of; not prep	1 pkg (2.2 oz)	234	7
bean w/ bacon; as prep w/ water	1 cup	105	2
bean w/ bacon; not prep	1 pkg (1 oz)	105	2
beef broth; as prep w/ water	1 cup	19	1

FOOD	PORTION	CALORIES	FAT
beef broth; as prep w/ water	1 cube	6	tr
beef broth; not prep	1 pkg (.2 oz)	14	1
beef broth, cube; as prep w/ water	1 cup	8	tr
beef noodle; as prep w/ water	6 oz	30	1
beef noodle; as prep w/ water	1 cup	41	1
beef noodle; not prep	1 pkg (.3 oz)	30	1
cauliflower; as prep w/ water	1 cup	68	2
cauliflower; not prep	1 pkg (.7 oz)	68	2
celery, cream of; as prep w/ water	1 cup	63	2
celery, cream of; not prep	1 pkg (.6 oz)	62	2
chicken vegetable; as prep w/ water	1 cup	49	1
chicken vegetable; not prep	1 pkg (.4 oz)	37	1
chicken broth; as prep w/ water	1 cup	21	1
chicken broth; not prep	1 pkg (.2 oz)	16	1
chicken broth, cube; as prep w/ water	1 cup	13	tr
chicken broth, cube; not prep	1 cube	9	tr
chicken, cream of; as prep w/ water	1 cup	107	5
chicken, cream of; not prep	1 pkg (.6 oz)	80	4
chicken noodle; as prep w/ water	1 cup	53	1
chicken noodle; not prep	1 pkg (2.6 oz)	257	6
chicken rice; as prep w/ water	1 cup	60	1
chicken rice; not prep	1 pkg (.6 oz)	60	1
clam chowder, Manhattan; not prep	1 pkg (.7 oz)	65	2
clam chowder, New England; not prep	1 pkg (.8 oz)	95	4
consomme, w/ gelatin; as prep w/ water	1 cup	17	tr
consomme, w/ gelatin; not prep	1 pkg (2 oz)	77	tr
leek; as prep w/ water	1 cup	71	2

FOOD	PORTION	CALORIES	FAT
leek; not prep	1 pkg (2.7 oz)	294	9
minestrone; as prep w/ water	1 cup	79	2
minestrone; not prep	1 pkg (2.7 oz)	279	6
mushroom; as prep w/ water	1 cup	96	5
mushroom; not prep	1 pkg (2.6 oz)	328	17
mushroom, instant; not prep	1 pkg (.6 oz)	74	4
onion; as prep w/ water	1 cup	28	1
onion; not prep	1 pkg (1.4 oz)	115	2
onion french; not prep	1 pkg (1.4 oz)	115	2
oxtail; as prep w/ water	1 cup	71	3
oxtail; not prep	1 pkg (2.6 oz)	280	10
pea, green; as prep w/ water	1 cup	133	2
pea, green; not prep	1 pkg (4 oz)	402	5
pea, split; as prep w/ water	1 cup	133	2
pea, split; not prep	1 pkg (4 oz)	402	5
tomato vegetable; as prep w/ water	1 cup	55	1
tomato vegetable; not prep	1 pkg (1.4 oz)	125	2
tomato; as prep w/ water	1 cup	102	2
tomato; not prep	1 pkg (.7 oz)	77	2
vegetable beef; as prep w/ water	1 cup	53	1
vegetable beef; not prep	1 pkg (2.6 oz)	256	5
vegetable, cream of; as prep w/ water	1 cup	105	6
vegetable, cream of; not prep	1 pkg (.62 oz)	79	4
FROZEN Boston Clam Chowder (Kettle Ready)	8 oz	199	11
Split Pea w/ Ham (Kettle Ready)	8 oz	189	5
Won Ton (La Choy)	½ pkg	50	1

FOOD	PORTION	CALORIES	FAT
HOME RECIPE			
black bean turtle soup	1 cup	241	1
corn & cheese chowder	¾ cup	215	12
corn chowder	1 cup	233	11
gazpacho	1 cup	46	tr
greek	¾ cup	63	2
hot & sour	1 cup	74	2
lentil	1 cup	175	2
mock turtle	1 cup	256	14
potato	1 cup	201	12
seafood chowder	1 cup	170	6
vegetable	1 cup	70	tr
vegetable beef	1 cup	320	25
wonton	1 cup	205	3

SOUR CREAM
(*see also* SOUR CREAM SUBSTITUTE)

FOOD	PORTION	CALORIES	FAT
LOW FAT			
Lean Cream (Land O'Lakes)	1 Tbsp	20	1
Lean Cream w/ Chives (Land O'Lakes)	1 Tbsp	20	1
Lite Delite (Friendship)	2 Tbsp	35	2
REGULAR			
Friendship	2 Tbsp	55	5
Land O'Lakes	1 Tbsp	32	2
Land O'Lakes	1 Tbsp	25	3
half & half	1 Tbsp	20	2
sour cream	1 Tbsp	26	3
sour cream	1 cup	493	48

FOOD	PORTION	CALORIES	FAT
SOUR CREAM SUBSTITUTE			
Formagg Sour, Sour Cream Style	1 oz	40	3
imitation, nondairy	1 oz	59	6
imitation, nondairy	1 cup	479	45
sour cream, nonbutterfat	1 Tbsp	21	2
sour cream, nonbutterfat	1 cup	417	39

SOY
(*see also* ICE CREAM NON-DAIRY, TEXTURED VEGETABLE PROTEIN, TOFU)

FOOD	PORTION	CALORIES	FAT
Soy Moo Soybean Milk (Health Valley)	8.5 oz	120	6
Soy Sauce (Kikkoman)	1 Tbsp	10	tr
Soy Sauce Lite (Kikkoman)	1 Tbsp	11	tr
Soy Sauce Mix (Diamond Crystal)	1 tsp	5	tr
lecithin	1 Tbsp	120	14
soy milk	1 cup	79	5
soy sauce	1 Tbsp	7	tr
soy sauce, shoyu	1 Tbsp	9	tr
soy sauce, tamari	1 Tbsp	11	tr
soybean sprouts	½ cup	45	2
soybeans; cooked	1 cup	298	15
soybeans, dry roasted	½ cup	387	19
soybeans, raw	1 cup	774	37
soybeans, roasted	½ cup	405	22
soybeans, roasted & toasted	1 oz	129	7

SPAGHETTI
(*see* PASTA, SPAGHETTI SAUCE)

FOOD	PORTION	CALORIES	FAT

SPAGHETTI SAUCE
(*see also* PIZZA, TOMATO)

BOTTLED

FOOD	PORTION	CALORIES	FAT
Chef Boy.ar.dee, Meatless	4 oz	60	1
Chef Boy.ar.dee w/ Ground Beef	4 oz	90	3
Chef Boy.ar.dee w/ Mushrooms	4 oz	70	2
Estee Spaghetti Sauce	4 oz	70	0
Prego Al Fresco Garden Tomato Sauce	4 oz	100	5
Prego Al Fresco Garden Tomato Sauce w/ Mushrooms	4 oz	100	5
Prego Al Fresco Garden Tomato Sauce w/ Peppers	4 oz	100	6
Prego Spaghetti Sauce	4 oz	140	6
Prego Spaghetti Sauce, Meat Flavored	4 oz	150	6
Prego Spaghetti Sauce, No-Salt-Added	4 oz	100	6
Prego Spaghetti Sauce w/ Mushrooms	4 oz	140	5
Prego Plus w/ Beef Sirloin & Onion	4 oz	160	7
Prego Plus w/ Mushrooms & Chunk	4 oz	130	5
Prego Plus w/ Sausage & Green Peppers	4 oz	170	9
Prego Plus w/ Veal & Sliced Mushrooms	4 oz	150	5
Pritikin Foods Spaghetti Sauce	4 oz	60	0
Pritikin Foods Spaghetti Sauce w/ Mushrooms	4 oz	60	0
Ragu Chunky Gardenstyle, Extra Tomatoes, Garlic & Onions	4 oz	80	2
Ragu Chunky Gardenstyle, Extra Tomatoes, Garlic & Onions w/ pasta	4 oz + 5 oz pasta	290	3

FOOD	PORTION	CALORIES	FAT
Ragu Chunky Gardenstyle, Green Peppers & Mushrooms	4 oz	80	2
Ragu Chunky Gardenstyle, Green Peppers & Mushrooms w/ pasta	4 oz + 5 oz pasta	290	3
Ragu Chunky Gardenstyle, Italian Garden Combination	4 oz	80	2
Ragu Chunky Gardenstyle, Italian Garden Combination w/ pasta	4 oz + 5 oz pasta	290	3
Ragu Chunky Gardenstyle, Mushrooms & Onions	4 oz	80	2
Ragu Chunky Gardenstyle, Mushrooms & Onions w/ pasta	4 oz + 5 oz pasta	290	3
Ragu Chunky Gardenstyle, Sweet Green & Red Peppers	4 oz	80	2
Ragu Chunky Gardenstyle, Sweet Green & Red Peppers w/ pasta	4 oz + 5 oz pasta	290	3
Ragu Extra Thick & Zesty, Flavored w/ Meat	4 oz	100	4
Ragu Extra Thick & Zesty, Flavored w/ Meat w/ pasta	4 oz + 5 oz pasta	310	5
Ragu Extra Thick & Zesty, Plain	4 oz	100	4
Ragu Extra Thick & Zesty, Plain, w/ pasta	4 oz + 5 oz pasta	310	5
Ragu Extra Thick & Zesty, w/ Mushrooms	4 oz	110	5
Ragu Extra Thick & Zesty, w/ Mushrooms w/ pasta	4 oz + 5 oz pasta	320	6
Ragu Homestyle, Flavored w/ Meat	4 oz	70	2
Ragu Homestyle, Flavored w/ Meat w/ pasta	4 oz + 5 oz pasta	280	3
Ragu Homestyle, Plain	4 oz	70	2
Ragu Homestyle, Plain w/ pasta	4 oz + 5 oz pasta	280	3
Ragu Homestyle w/ Mushrooms	4 oz	70	2

FOOD	PORTION	CALORIES	FAT
Ragu Homestyle w/ Mushrooms w/ pasta	4 oz + 5 oz pasta	280	3
Ragu Old World Style, Flavored w/ Meat	4 oz	80	2
Ragu Old World Style, Flavored w/ Meat w/ pasta	4 oz + 5 oz pasta	290	3
Ragu Old World Style, Marinara Sauce	4 oz	90	4
Ragu Old World Style, Marinara Sauce w/ pasta	4 oz + 5 oz pasta	300	5
Ragu Old World Style, Plain	4 oz	80	3
Ragu Old World Style, Plain w/ pasta	4 oz + 5 oz pasta	290	4
Ragu Old World Style w/ Extra Cheese	4 oz	80	3
Ragu Old World Style w/ Extra Cheese w/ pasta	4 oz + 5 oz pasta	290	4
Ragu Old World Style w/ Extra Garlic	4 oz	80	3
Ragu Old World Style w/ Extra Garlic w/ pasta	4 oz + 5 oz pasta	290	4
Ragu Old World Style w/ Mushrooms	4 oz	80	4
Ragu Old World Style w/ Mushrooms w/ pasta	4 oz + 5 oz pasta	290	5
Ragu Thick & Hearty, Flavored w/ Leaner Ground Beef	4 oz	120	4
Ragu Thick & Hearty, Flavored w/ Leaner Ground Beef w/ pasta	4 oz + 5 oz pasta	330	5
Ragu Thick & Hearty, Marinara	4 oz	110	4
Ragu Thick & Hearty, Marinara w/ pasta	4 oz + 5 oz pasta	320	5
Ragu Thick & Hearty, Plain	4 oz	110	4
Ragu Thick & Hearty, Plain w/ pasta	4 oz + 5 oz pasta	320	5

FOOD	PORTION	CALORIES	FAT
Ragu Thick & Hearty w/ Mushrooms	4 oz	110	4
Ragu Thick & Hearty w/ Mushrooms w/ pasta	4 oz + 5 oz pasta	320	5
marinara sauce	1 cup	171	8
spaghetti sauce	15½ oz	479	21
MIX spaghetti sauce; not prep	1 pkg (1.5 oz)	118	tr
sauce w/ mushrooms; not prep	1 pkg (1.4 oz)	118	4

SPARE RIBS
(*see* PORK)

SPICES
(*see* HERBS/SPICES)

SPINACH

FOOD	PORTION	CALORIES	FAT
CANNED Northwest Premium (S&W)	½ cup	25	0
Spinach (Libby)	½ cup	25	0
Spinach (Seneca)	½ cup	25	0
spinach	½ cup	25	1
FRESH cooked	½ cup	21	tr
chopped; raw	½ cup	6	tr
FROZEN Chopped (Birds Eye)	⅓ cup	22	tr
Chopped; cooked (Health Valley)	7.2 oz	57	tr

FOOD	PORTION	CALORIES	FAT
Creamed (Birds Eye)	⅓ cup	59	4
Leaf (Birds Eye)	⅓ cup	22	tr
Leaf; cooked (Health Valley)	6.7 oz	53	tr
Spinach Au Gratin (Budget Gourmet)	6 oz	120	5
frzn; cooked	½ cup	27	tr
frzn; not prep	10 oz pkg	68	tr

SPORTS DRINKS

thirst quencher	1 cup	60	tr

SPOT

raw	3 oz	105	4
raw	1 fillet (2.2 oz)	79	3

SQUAB

breast, raw	3.5 oz	135	5
meat & skin, raw	6.9 oz	584	47
meat, raw	5.9 oz	239	13

SQUASH
(*see also* ZUCCHINI)

CANNED			
crookneck, sliced	½ cup	14	tr
FRESH			
acorn; cooked, mashed	½ cup	41	tr
acorn; cubed, baked	½ cup	57	tr
butternut; baked	½ cup	41	tr
crookneck; cooked, sliced	½ cup	18	tr

FOOD	PORTION	CALORIES	FAT
hubbard; baked	½ cup	51	tr
hubbard; cooked, mashed	½ cup	35	tr
scallop; cooked	½ cup	14	tr
spaghetti; cooked	½ cup	23	tr
summer, all varieties, raw; sliced	½ cup	13	tr
summer; cooked, sliced	½ cup	18	tr
winter, all varieties, raw; cubed	½ cup	21	tr
winter; cooked, cubed	½ cup	39	1
FROZEN Butternut (Southland)	4 oz	45	0
Prepared Squash (Southland)	3.6 oz	80	2
Winter Cooked (Birds Eye)	⅓ cup	45	tr
butternut; cooked, mashed	½ cup	47	tr
crookneck; cooked, sliced	½ cup	24	tr
SEEDS seeds, dried	1 oz	154	13
seeds, whole; roasted	1 oz	127	6

SQUID

fried	3 oz	149	6
raw	3 oz	78	1

STRAWBERRY

FRESH strawberries	1 cup	45	1
FROZEN Strawberries, Halved, in Lite Syrup (Birds Eye)	½ cup	87	tr

FOOD	PORTION	CALORIES	FAT
Strawberries, Halved, Quick Thaw (Birds Eye)	½ cup	119	tr
Strawberries, Whole, in Lite Syrup (Birds Eye)	½ cup	81	tr
sweetened	1 cup	200	tr
unsweetened	1 cup	52	tr
JUICE Smucker's	8 oz	130	0

STUFFING/DRESSING

HOME RECIPE bread; as prep w/ water & fat	½ cup	251	15
bread; as prep w/ water, egg & fat	½ cup	107	7
sausage	½ cup	292	11
MIX Beef (Stove Top)	½ cup	165	8
Chicken (Stove Top)	½ cup	181	9
Chicken, Flexible Serve (Stove Top)	½ cup	180	9
Chicken w/ Rice (Stove Top)	½ cup	184	9
Corn Bread (Pepperidge Farm)	1 oz	110	1
Cornbread (Stove Top)	½ cup	163	8
Cornbread, Flexible Serve (Stove Top)	½ cup	180	9
Cube (Pepperidge Farm)	1 oz	110	1
Herb Homestyle, Flexible Serve (Stove Top)	½ cup	180	9

FOOD	PORTION	CALORIES	FAT
Herb Seasoned (Pepperidge Farm)	1 oz	110	1
Long Grain & Wild Rice (Stove Top)	½ cup	184	9
Pork (Stove Top)	½ cup	179	9
San Francisco Style Americana (Stove Top)	½ cup	162	8
Savory Herbs (Stove Top)	½ cup	180	9
Select Chicken Florentine (Stove Top)	½ cup	203	12
Select Garden Herb (Stove Top)	½ cup	219	13
Select Vegetable & Almond (Stove Top)	½ cup	227	15
Select Wild Rice & Mushroom (Stove Top)	½ cup	172	9
Turkey (Stove Top)	½ cup	179	9

STURGEON

FOOD	PORTION	CALORIES	FAT
FRESH			
cooked	3 oz	115	4
raw	3 oz	90	3
SMOKED			
sturgeon	3 oz	147	4
sturgeon	1 oz	48	1

SUCKER

FOOD	PORTION	CALORIES	FAT
white, raw	3 oz	79	2
white, raw	1 fillet (5.6 oz)	147	4

FOOD	PORTION	CALORIES	FAT

SUGAR
(*see also* FRUCTOSE, SUGAR SUBSTITUTE, SYRUP)

FOOD	PORTION	CALORIES	FAT
brown	1 cup	836	0
cube	1 cube	27	0
powdered	1 cup	493	0
white	1 cup	770	0

SUGAR SUBSTITUTE
(*see also* FRUCTOSE)

FOOD	PORTION	CALORIES	FAT
Adolph's	1 tsp	0	0
Diamond	1 tsp	tr	0
Spoon For Spoon	1 tsp	2	0
Sucaryl	1 tsp	0	0
Sugar Twin	1 tsp	tr	0
Sweet 'n Low	1 tsp	12	0
Sweet 'N Low, Brown Sugar Substitute	1/10 tsp	2	0
Sweet 'N Low, Granulated	1 pkg (1 g)	4	0
Sweet 'N Low, Liquid	10 drops	0	0
Sweet Top	1/8 tsp	0	0
Sweet'n It (Estee)	6 drops	0	0
Sprinkle Sweet	1 tsp	2	0

SUNDAE TOPPING
(*see* ICE CREAM TOPPING)

SUNFISH

FOOD	PORTION	CALORIES	FAT
pumpkinseed, raw	3 oz	76	1

SUNFLOWER SEEDS

FOOD	PORTION	CALORIES	FAT
Sunflower (Planters)	1 oz	160	14

FOOD	PORTION	CALORIES	FAT
Sunflower Nuts, Dry Roasted (Planters)	1 oz	160	14
Sunflower Nuts, Dry Roasted, Unsalted (Planters)	1 oz	170	15
Sunflower Nuts, Oil Roasted (Planters)	1 oz	170	15
dried	1 oz	162	14
dry roasted	1 oz	165	14
oil roasted	1 oz	175	16
sunflower butter	1 Tbsp	93	8
toasted	1 oz	176	16

SURF

CANNED surf (American Original Foods)	4 oz	100	tr
FRESH surf (American Original Foods)	4 oz	90	tr

SWEET POTATO
  (see also YAM)

CANNED in syrup pack	½ cup	106	tr
mashed	½ cup	233	tr
pieces	1 cup	183	tr
FRESH baked in skin	1 (3½ oz)	118	tr
mashed	½ cup	172	tr
raw	1 (4.6 oz)	136	tr
FROZEN frzn; baked	½ cup	88	tr

FOOD	PORTION	CALORIES	FAT
SWISS CHARD			
cooked	½ cup	18	tr
chopped, raw	½ cup	3	tr
SWORDFISH			
cooked	1 piece (3.7 oz)	164	5
cooked	3 oz	132	4
raw	3 oz	103	3
raw	1 piece (4.8 oz)	164	5

SYRUP
(*see also* ICE CREAM TOPPING, PANCAKE/WAFFLE SYRUP)

FOOD	PORTION	CALORIES	FAT
All Flavors Fruit Syrup (Smucker's)	2 Tbsp	100	0
Blueberry (Estee)	1 Tbsp	4	0
Corn Syrup, Dark (Karo)	1 Tbsp	60	0
Corn Syrup, Dark (Karo)	1 cup	975	0
Corn Syrup, Light (Karo)	1 Tbsp	60	0
Corn Syrup, Light (Karo)	1 cup	960	0
Fruit Flavored, all varieties (Smucker's)	1 Tbsp	50	tr
Maple Rich (Home Brands)	1 oz	110	0

TAHINI
(*see* SESAME)

TAMARIND

FOOD	PORTION	CALORIES	FAT
tamarind	1	5	tr

FOOD	PORTION	CALORIES	FAT

TANGERINE

FRESH
| tangerine | 1 | 37 | tr |

JUICE
Mandarin Tangerine (Dole)	6 oz	97	tr
frzn, sweetened; as prep	1 cup	110	tr
frzn; not prep	6 oz container	344	tr
sweetened	1 cup	125	tr

TAPIOCA

| Minute Tapioca (General Foods) | 1 Tbsp | 35 | tr |

TEA/HERBAL TEA

Almond Orange (Bigelow)	5 oz	tr	tr
Almond Sunset (Celestial Seasonings)	1 cup	3	tr
Apple Orchard (Bigelow)	1 cup	5	tr
Apple Spice (Bigelow)	5 oz	tr	tr
Chamomile (Bigelow)	5 oz	tr	tr
Chamomile (Celestial Seasonings)	1 cup	2	tr
Chamomile Mint (Bigelow)	5 oz	tr	tr
Cinnamon Apple Spice (Celestial Seasonings)	1 cup	3	tr
Cinnamon Orange (Bigelow)	5 oz	tr	tr

FOOD	PORTION	CALORIES	FAT
Cinnamon Rose (Celestial Seasonings)	1 cup	2	tr
Country Peach Spice (Celestial Seasonings)	1 cup	3	tr
Cranberry Cove (Celestial Seasonings)	1 cup	3	tr
Early Riser (Bigelow)	1 cup	3	tr
Emperor's Choice (Celestial Seasonings)	1 cup	4	tr
Feeling Free (Bigelow)	1 cup	1	tr
Fruit & Almond (Bigelow)	1 cup	1	tr
Ginseng Plus (Celestial Seasonings)	1 cup	3	tr
Grandma's Tummy Mints (Celestial Seasonings)	1 cup	2	tr
Hibiscus & Rose Hips (Bigelow)	5 oz	1	tr
I Love Lemon (Bigelow)	1 cup	1	tr
Lemon & C (Bigelow)	5 oz	tr	tr
Lemon Mist (Celestial Seasonings)	1 cup	2	tr
Lemon Zinger (Celestial Seasonings)	1 cup	4	tr
Looking Good (Bigelow)	1 cup	1	tr
Mandarin Orange Spice (Celestial Seasonings)	1 cup	5	tr
Mellow Mint (Celestial Seasonings)	1 cup	2	tr
Mint Blend (Bigelow)	5 oz	tr	tr

FOOD	PORTION	CALORIES	FAT
Mint Magic (Celestial Seasonings)	1 cup	1	tr
Mint Medley (Bigelow)	1 cup	1	tr
Mo's 24 (Celestial Seasonings)	1 cup	2	tr
Nice Over Ice (Bigelow)	1 cup	1	tr
Orange & C (Bigelow)	5 oz	tr	tr
Orange & Spice (Bigelow)	1 cup	1	tr
Orange Zinger (Celestial Seasonings)	1 cup	5	tr
Peppermint (Bigelow)	5 oz	tr	tr
Peppermint (Celestial Seasonings)	1 cup	2	tr
Raspberry Patch (Celestial Seasonings)	1 cup	4	tr
Red Zinger (Celestial Seasonings)	1 cup	4	tr
Roastaroma (Celestial Seasonings)	1 cup	11	tr
Roasted Grain & Carob (Bigelow)	5 oz	3	tr
Sleepytime (Celestial Seasonings)	1 cup	5	tr
Spearmint (Bigelow)	5 oz	tr	tr
Spearmint (Celestial Seasonings)	1 cup	5	tr
Strawberry Fields (Celestial Seasonings)	1 cup	4	tr
Sunburst C (Celestial Seasonings)	1 cup	3	tr

FOOD	PORTION	CALORIES	FAT
Sweet Dreams (Bigelow)	1 cup	1	tr
Take-A-Break (Bigelow)	1 cup	3	tr
Wild Forest Blueberry (Celestial Seasonings)	1 cup	2	tr
REGULAR			
Amaretto Nights (Celestial Seasonings)	1 cup	3	tr
Apple Spice and Tea (Celestial Seasonings)	1 cup	tr	tr
Bavarian Chocolate Orange (Celestial Seasonings)	1 cup	7	tr
Caffeine-Free (Celestial Seasonings)	1 cup	4	tr
Chinese Fortune (Bigelow)	1 cup	1	tr
Cinnamon Stick (Bigelow)	1 cup	1	tr
Cinnamon Vienna (Celestial Seasonings)	1 cup	2	tr
Classic English Breakfast (Celestial Seasonings)	1 cup	3	tr
Constant Comment (Bigelow)	1 cup	1	tr
Darjeeling Blend (Bigelow)	1 cup	1	tr
Darjeeling Gardens (Celestial Seasonings)	1 cup	3	tr
Earl Gray (Bigelow)	1 cup	1	tr
English Teatime (Bigelow)	1 cup	1	tr
Extraordinary Earl Grey (Celestial Seasonings)	1 cup	3	tr

FOOD	PORTION	CALORIES	FAT
Fruit Tea Fruit Cooler; as prep (Lipton)	8 oz	87	0
Iced Berry Tea; as prep (Crystal Light)	8 oz	3	0
Iced Tea (SIPPS)	8.45 oz	100	0
Iced Tea (Shasta)	12 oz	124	0
Irish Cream Mist (Celestial Seasonings)	1 cup	3	tr
Lemon Lift (Bigelow)	1 cup	1	tr
Lemons and Tea (Celestial Seasonings)	1 cup	tr	tr
Morning Thunder (Celestial Seasonings)	1 cup	3	tr
Orange Pekoe (Bigelow)	1 cup	1	tr
Orange Spice and Tea (Celestial Seasonings)	1 cup	tr	tr
Peppermint Stick (Bigelow)	1 cup	1	tr
Plantation Mint (Bigelow)	1 cup	1	tr
Raspberries and Tea (Celestial Seasonings)	1 cup	2	tr
Raspberry Royale (Bigelow)	1 cup	1	tr
Swiss Mint (Celestial Seasonings)	1 cup	tr	tr
instant, sugar sweetened, lemon flavor, powder; as prep w/ water	9 oz	87	tr
instant, unsweetened, lemon flavor powder; as prep w/ water	8 oz	4	0

FOOD	PORTION	CALORIES	FAT
instant, unsweetened powder; as prep w/ water	8 oz	2	0
tea	6 oz	2	0

TEMPEH

tempeh	½ cup	165	6

TEXTURED VEGETABLE PROTEIN
   (*see* MEAT SUBSTITUTE, SOY)

simulated meat products	1 oz	88	1

TILEFISH

cooked	½ fillet (5.3 oz)	220	7
cooked	3 oz	125	4
raw	3 oz	81	2
raw	½ fillet (6.8 oz)	184	4

TOFU
   (*see also* ICE CREAM, NON-DAIRY)

fried	1 piece (½ oz)	35	3
fuyu, salted & fermented	1 block (⅓ oz)	13	1
koyadofu, dried; frzn	1 piece (½ oz)	82	5
firm, raw	¼ block (3 oz)	118	7
regular, raw	¼ block (4 oz)	88	6

TOFUTTI
   (*see* ICE CREAM, NON-DAIRY)

TOMATO
   (*see also* PIZZA, SPAGHETTI SAUCE)

CANNED Aspic Supreme (S&W)	½ cup	60	0

FOOD	PORTION	CALORIES	FAT
California Sliced (Contadina)	½ cup	40	tr
Crushed Tomatoes in Tomato Puree (Contadina)	½ cup	30	tr
Diced Tomatoes in Rich Puree (S&W)	½ cup	35	0
Italian Paste (Contadina)	2 oz	65	1
Italian Stewed (S&W)	½ cup	35	0
Italian Style (Contadina)	½ cup	25	tr
Italian Style, Stewed (Contadina)	½ cup	35	tr
Italian Style w/ Basil (S&W)	½ cup	25	0
Kosher Tomatoes (Claussen)	1	9	tr
Paste (Contadina)	2 oz	50	tr
Paste (S&W)	6 oz	150	0
Peeled Ready Cut (S&W)	½ cup	25	0
Puree (Contadina)	½ cup	40	0
Puree (S&W)	½ cup	60	0
Sauce (Fresh Chef)	4 oz	160	11
Sauce (S&W)	½ cup	40	0
Sauce, Thick & Zesty (Contadina)	½ cup	40	0
Stewed (Contadina)	½ cup	35	tr

FOOD	PORTION	CALORIES	FAT
Stewed Tomatoes (S&W)	½ cup	35	0
Stewed Tomatoes, 50% Salt Reduced (S&W)	½ cup	35	0
Tomato Sauce (Health Valley)	4 oz	30	0
Tomato Sauce, No Salt Added (Health Valley)	4 oz	30	0
Whole Peeled (Contadina)	½ cup	25	tr
Whole Peeled (S&W)	½ cup	25	0
red, whole	1 cup	47	tr
sauce, spanish style	½ cup	40	tr
stewed	1 cup	68	tr
tomato paste	½ cup	110	1
tomato puree	1 cup	102	tr
tomato sauce	1 cup	74	tr
tomato sauce w/ mushrooms	1 cup	85	tr
tomato sauce w/ onion	½ cup	50	tr
tomato sauce w/ tomato tidbits	½ cup	39	tr
wedges, in tomato juice	1 cup	67	tr
FRESH			
green	1	30	tr
red	1	24	tr
HOME RECIPE			
scalloped	½ cup	88	3
stewed tomatoes	1 cup	59	2
JUICE			
California (S&W)	5½ oz	35	0

FOOD	PORTION	CALORIES	FAT
California (S&W)	6 oz	35	0
Snap-E-Tom Cocktail (Ortega)	6 oz	40	0
Tomato (Campbell)	6 oz	35	0
juice	6 fl oz	32	tr

TOPPINGS
(*see* ICE CREAM TOPPING)

TONGUE

FOOD	PORTION	CALORIES	FAT
beef, raw	4 oz	252	18
beef; simmered	3 oz	241	18
pork, raw	4 oz	254	19
pork; braised	3 oz	230	16

TORTILLA CHIPS
(*see* chips)

TROUT

FOOD	PORTION	CALORIES	FAT
rainbow, raw	3 oz	100	3
rainbow, raw	1 fillet (2.8 oz)	93	3
rainbow; cooked	1 fillet (2.1 oz)	94	3
rainbow; cooked	3 oz	129	4
seatrout, raw	1 fillet (8.4 oz)	248	9
seatrout, raw	3 oz	88	3

TUNA
(*see also* TUNA DISHES)

FOOD	PORTION	CALORIES	FAT
CANNED Chunk Light in Oil (Bumble Bee)	3 oz	200	15

FOOD	PORTION	CALORIES	FAT
Chunk Light in Water (Bumble Bee)	3 oz	90	2
Chunk White in Oil (Bumble Bee)	3 oz	200	15
Chunk White in Water (Bumble Bee)	3 oz	90	2
Solid White in Oil (Bumble Bee)	3 oz	190	10
Solid White in Water (Bumble Bee)	3 oz	90	2
Tuna (Health Valley)	6.5 oz	180	3
Tuna, Diet, No Salt (Health Valley)	6.5 oz	200	3
Tuna Salad (The Spreadables)	¼ can	90	6
light in oil	3 oz	169	7
light in oil	1 can (6 oz)	399	14
light in water	1 can (5.8 oz)	216	1
light in water	3 oz	111	tr
white in oil	3 oz	158	7
white in oil	1 can (6.2 oz)	331	14
white in water	1 can (6 oz)	234	4
white in water	3 oz	116	2
FRESH bluefin, raw	3 oz	122	4
bluefin; cooked	3 oz	157	5
skipjack, raw	3 oz	88	1
skipjack, raw	½ fillet (6.9 oz)	204	2
yellowfin, raw	3 oz	92	1
FROZEN Tuna Pasta Casserole (Mrs. Paul's)	11 oz	290	7

FOOD	PORTION	CALORIES	FAT
READY-TO-USE			
Salad (Wampler Longacre)	1 oz	61	13
tuna salad	3 oz	159	8
tuna salad	1 cup	383	19

TUNA DISHES

FOOD	PORTION	CALORIES	FAT
Tuna Melt (Chefwich)	5 oz	360	14
stuffed green pepper (home recipe)	1 (9.9 oz)	261	13
pattie (home recipe)	1 (3 oz)	228	8

TURBOT

FOOD	PORTION	CALORIES	FAT
european, raw	½ fillet (7.2 oz)	194	6
european, raw	3 oz	81	3

TURKEY

(*see also* DINNER, HOT DOGS, TURKEY DISHES, TURKEY SUBSTITUTE)

FOOD	PORTION	CALORIES	FAT
CANNED			
Turkey Salad (The Spreadables)	¼ can	100	6
turkey w/ broth	½ can (2.5 oz)	116	5
turkey w/ broth	1 can (5 oz)	231	10
FRESH			
Breast (Land O'Lakes)	3 oz	100	1
Breast; cooked (Louis Rich)	1 oz	50	2
Breast Hen w/ wing; cooked (Louis Rich)	1 oz	53	2
Breast Hen w/o back; cooked (Louis Rich)	1 oz	47	2

FOOD	PORTION	CALORIES	FAT
Breast Hen w/o wing; cooked (Louis Rich)	1 oz	53	2
Breast Prime, Young (Shady Brook)	3 oz	140	7
Breast Roast; cooked (Louis Rich)	1 oz	41	tr
Breast Slices; cooked (Louis Rich)	1 oz	44	1
Breast Steaks; cooked (Louis Rich)	1 oz	40	tr
Breast Tenderloins; cooked (Louis Rich)	1 oz	41	tr
Drumsticks (Land O'Lakes)	3 oz	120	5
Drumsticks; cooked (Louis Rich)	1 oz	55	3
Ground; cooked (Louis Rich)	1 oz	61	4
Ground; cooked (Louis Rich)	3.5 oz	217	13
Ground Fresh Lean; cooked (Perdue)	1 oz	40	2
Ground Lean 90% Fat Free; cooked (Louis Rich)	3.5 oz	183	9
Ground Lean 90% Fat Free; cooked (Louis Rich)	1 oz	51	8
Ground Turkey (Bil Mar Foods)	3 oz	163	12
Hindquarters (Land O'Lakes)	3 oz	140	8
Thighs (Land O'Lakes)	3 oz	150	10
Thighs; cooked (Louis Rich)	1 oz	65	4
Whole; cooked (Louis Rich)	3.5 oz	200	10

FOOD	PORTION	CALORIES	FAT
Whole; cooked (Louis Rich)	1 oz	56	3
Wing Drumettes; cooked (Louis Rich)	1 oz	52	2
Wings (Land O'Lakes)	3 oz	120	5
Wings (Shady Brook)	3 oz	130	6
Wings; cooked (Louis Rich)	1 oz	54	3
Young Whole (Land O'Lakes)	3 oz	130	7
Young, Whole, Butter Basted (Land O'Lakes)	3 oz	140	8
Young, Whole, Self-Basting (Land O'Lakes)	3 oz	120	5
back, meat & skin, raw	½ back (1.1 lbs)	940	58
back, meat & skin, raw	1.6 oz	81	5
back, meat & skin; roasted	½ back (13.3 oz)	903	52
breast, meat & skin, raw	½ breast (3.9 lbs)	2700	113
breast, meat & skin, raw	5.4 oz	234	10
breast, meat & skin; roasted	4 oz	217	9
breast, meat & skin; roasted	½ breast (2.9 lbs)	2510	98
dark meat w/ skin, raw	5.3 oz	232	12
dark meat w/ skin, raw	½ turkey (3.9 lbs)	2681	139
dark meat w/ skin; roasted	½ turkey (2.6 lbs)	2553	128
dark meat w/ skin; roasted	3.6 oz	222	11
dark meat w/o skin, raw	4.7 oz	163	5

FOOD	PORTION	CALORIES	FAT
dark meat w/o skin, raw	½ turkey (3.4 lbs)	1879	63
dark meat w/o skin; roasted	1 cup	260	10
dark meat w/o skin; roasted	3.2 oz	167	6
meat & skin, raw	½ turkey (8.5 lbs)	6013	289
meat & skin, raw	11.9 oz	522	25
meat & skin; roasted	½ turkey (6 lbs)	5545	249
meat & skin; roasted	8.4 oz	482	22
meat, raw	½ turkey (7.2 lbs)	3867	89
meat, raw	10 oz	335	8
meat; roasted	7.2 oz	345	10
meat; roasted	1 cup	235	7
leg, meat & skin, raw	2.7 lbs	1736	78
leg, meat & skin, raw	3.8 oz	150	7
leg, meat & skin; roasted	2.5 oz	144	7
leg, meat & skin; roasted	1.8 lbs	1660	78
light meat w/ skin, raw	6.5 oz	288	13
light meat w/ skin, raw	½ turkey (4.7 lbs)	3331	150
light meat w/ skin; roasted	½ turkey (3.4 lbs)	2992	121
light meat w/ skin; roasted	4.8 oz	260	10
light meat w/o skin, raw	5.4 oz	176	2
light meat w/o skin, raw	½ turkey (3.9 lbs)	2023	28
light meat w/o skin; roasted	1 cup	2153	4
light meat w/o skin; roasted	4.1 oz	180	3
neck, meat, raw	1 neck (6.3 oz)	243	10
neck, meat; simmered	1 neck (5.3 oz)	274	11

FOOD	PORTION	CALORIES	FAT
skin, raw	½ turkey (1.3 lbs)	2180	205
skin, raw	1.8 oz	188	18
skin; roasted	½ turkey (1.1 lbs)	1578	139
skin; roasted	1 oz	135	12
whole, meat, skin, giblets & neck, raw	18.4 lbs	12,799	605
whole, meat, skin, giblets & neck; roasted	13.1 lbs	11,873	525
whole, meat, skin, giblets & neck; roasted	10 oz	514	23
wing, meat & skin, raw	1 oz	57	3
wing, meat & skin, raw	12.2 oz	656	39
wing, meat & skin; roasted	8.3 oz	524	27
FROZEN roast, boneless, seasoned, light & dark meat, raw	10 oz	340	6
roast, boneless, seasoned, light & dark meat, raw	2.5 lbs	1358	25
roast, boneless, seasoned, light & dark meat; roasted	1.7 lbs	1213	45
roast, boneless, seasoned, light & dark meat; roasted	6.9 oz	304	11
FROZEN/PREPARED Kibun Turkey Pasta Salad w/ dressing	½ pkg	250	12
Kibun Turkey Pasta Salad w/o dressing	½ pkg	140	2
gravy & turkey	1 cup	160	6
gravy & turkey	1 pkg (5 oz)	95	4
READY-TO-USE Baked Ham (Wampler Longacre)	1 oz	38	tr

FOOD	PORTION	CALORIES	FAT
Baked Ham w/ 12% water (Wampler Longacre)	1 oz	33	tr
Baked Ham w/ 20% water (Wampler Longacre)	1 oz	39	tr
Bologna (Louis Rich)	1 slice (28 g)	59	5
Bologna (Wampler Longacre)	1 oz	56	16
Bologna Mild (Louis Rich)	1 slice (28 g)	61	5
Bologna Red Rind (Mr. Turkey)	1 oz	63	5
Bologna Sliced (Wampler Longacre)	1 oz	57	1
Breast, Barbecued (Louis Rich)	1 oz	36	1
Breast & White Turkey, Deli Chef (Wampler Longacre)	1 oz	35	tr
Breast & White Turkey, No Skin Covering (Wampler Longacre)	1 oz	39	tr
Breast BBQ Quarter (Mr. Turkey)	1 oz	34	1
Breast Fillets w/ Cheese (Land O'Lakes)	5 oz	300	16
Breast Gourmet (Wampler Longacre)	1 oz	31	tr
Breast Gourmet, Browned & Glazed (Wampler Longacre)	1 oz	28	tr
Breast Gourmet, Browned & Roasted (Wampler Longacre)	1 oz	35	tr
Breast Gourmet, Skinless (Wampler Longacre)	1 oz	28	tr
Breast Gourmet, Skinless, Browned & Roasted (Wampler Longacre)	1 oz	31	tr

FOOD	PORTION	CALORIES	FAT
Breast, Hickory Smoked (Louis Rich)	1 oz	31	tr
Breast, Honey Roasted (Louis Rich)	1 slice (28 g)	29	tr
Breast, Mini Gourmet (Wampler Longacre)	1 oz	35	4
Breast, Oven Roasted (Louis Rich)	1 slice (28 g)	31	tr
Breast, Oven Roasted (Louis Rich)	1 oz	30	tr
Breast, Oven Roasted (Oscar Mayer)	1 slice (21 g)	22	tr
Breast, Oven Roasted, Oven Lite (Wampler Longacre)	1 oz	35	tr
Breast, Oven Roasted Quarter (Mr. Turkey)	1 oz	34	1
Breast, Premium (Wampler Longacre)	1 oz	29	tr
Breast, Premium, Browned & Glazed (Wampler Longacre)	1 oz	29	tr
Breast, Premium, Skinless (Wampler Longacre)	1 oz	26	tr
Breast, Premium, Skinless, Browned & Roasted (Wampler Longacre)	1 oz	26	tr
Breast Roll, Sliced (Wampler Longacre)	1 oz	37	tr
Breast Salt Watchers (Wampler Longacre)	1 oz	35	tr
Breast, Skinless Gourmet High Yield (Wampler Longacre)	1 oz	28	tr
Breast, Smoked (Bil Mar Foods)	1 oz	31	tr
Breast, Smoked (Oscar Mayer)	1 slice (21 g)	20	tr

FOOD	PORTION	CALORIES	FAT
Breast, Smoked Chunk (Louis Rich)	1 oz	34	1
Breast, Smoked Gourmet (Wampler Longacre)	1 oz	37	tr
Breast, Smoked Lean-Lite (Wampler Longacre)	1 oz	38	tr
Breast, Smoked, Mini Gourmet (Wampler Longacre)	1 oz	37	tr
Breast, Smoked Quarter (Mr. Turkey)	1 oz	35	1
Breast, Smoked, Sliced (Louis Rich)	1 slice (21 g)	21	tr
Breast, Smoked, Sliced (Wampler Longacre)	1 oz	27	tr
Breasts, Bronze Label (Land O'Lakes)	3 oz	100	4
Breasts, Gold Label, Browned (Land O'Lakes)	3 oz	120	5
Breasts, Gold Label, Skin On (Land O'Lakes)	3 oz	120	4
Breasts, Gold Label, Skinless (Land O'Lakes)	3 oz	90	1
Breasts, Silver Label (Land O'Lakes)	3 oz	100	2
Cheese Patties (Bil Mar Foods)	3 oz	213	13
Chunk Ham w/ 12% water (Wampler Longacre)	1 oz	36	tr
Chunk Ham w/ 20% water (Wampler Longacre)	1 oz	39	tr
Chunk Pastrami (Wampler Longacre)	1 oz	35	tr
Cotto Salami (Louis Rich)	1 slice (28 g)	52	4
Cotto Salami (Mr. Turkey)	1 oz	45	3

FOOD	PORTION	CALORIES	FAT
Dark Smoked Cured (Wampler Longacre)	1 oz	45	tr
Diced Combination Roll (Wampler Longacre)	1 oz	43	tr
Diced Ham w/ 20% water (Wampler Longacre)	1 oz	39	tr
Diced White Roll (Wampler Longacre)	1 oz	43	tr
Diced, White/Dark Mixed (Land O'Lakes)	3 oz	120	6
Ham (Land O'Lakes)	3 oz	100	2
Ham Chopped (Louis Rich)	1 slice (28 g)	42	2
Ham Cured Thigh Meat (Louis Rich)	1 slice (28 g)	34	1
Ham Cured Thigh Meat Square (Louis Rich)	1 slice (21 g)	24	tr
Ham Cured Thigh Meat, Water Added (Louis Rich)	1 slice (28 g)	34	1
Ham Honey Cured (Louis Rich)	1 slice (21 g)	25	tr
Ham, Lean-Lite (Wampler Longacre)	1 oz	36	tr
Ham, Sliced (Wampler Longacre)	1 oz	37	tr
Ham, Smoked Breakfast (Mr. Turkey)	1 oz	33	1
Ham, Smoked, Buffet Style (Bil Mar Foods)	1 oz	32	1
Luncheon Loaf (Louis Rich)	1 slice (28 g)	43	3
Luncheon Loaf, Square Spice (Bil Mar Foods)	1 slice (1 oz)	51	4

FOOD	PORTION	CALORIES	FAT
Nuggets (Mr. Turkey)	1 nugget	33	2
Nuggets, White Breaded; as prep (Wampler Longacre)	1 oz	87	2
Nuggets, White Breaded, Fully Cooked (Wampler Longacre)	1 oz	87	2
Pastrami (Bil Mar Foods)	1 slice (1 oz)	28	tr
Pastrami (Louis Rich)	1 slice (28 g)	33	1
Pastrami (Wampler Longacre)	1 oz	35	tr
Pastrami Sliced (Wampler Longacre)	1 oz	34	tr
Pastrami Square (Louis Rich)	1 slice (23 g)	23	tr
Patties (Land O'Lakes)	2.25 oz	170	11
Patties (Mr. Turkey)	3 oz	195	11
Roast White w/ Gravy (Land O'Lakes)	3 oz	110	5
Roast White/Dark w/ Gravy (Land O'Lakes)	3 oz	120	7
Roasted Thighs (Wampler Longacre)	1 oz	38	6
Roll, Blue Label, Mixed (Land O'Lakes)	3 oz	120	6
Roll, Blue Label, Mixed (Land O'Lakes)	3 oz	110	5
Roll, Breast & White Turkey Deli Chef (Wampler Longacre)	1 oz	39	tr
Roll, Combination Turkey (Wampler Longacre)	1 oz	43	tr

FOOD	PORTION	CALORIES	FAT
Roll, Red Label, Mixed (Land O'Lakes)	3 oz	110	5
Roll, Red Label, White (Land O'Lakes)	3 oz	110	5
Roll, White Turkey (Wampler Longacre)	1 oz	43	tr
Salad (Wampler Longacre)	1 oz	71	1
Salami (Louis Rich)	1 slice (28 g)	52	4
Salami (Wampler Longacre)	1 oz	45	tr
Salami Sliced (Wampler Longacre)	1 oz	46	tr
Smoked (Louis Rich)	1 slice (28 g)	33	1
Sticks (Mr. Turkey)	1 stick	65	4
Summer Sausage (Louis Rich)	1 slice (28 g)	52	4
Turkey (Carl Buddig)	1 oz	50	3
Turkey Bologna (Mr. Turkey)	1 oz	63	5
Turkey Breakfast Sausage; cooked (Louis Rich)	1 (1 oz)	59	4
Turkey Breast (Bil Mar Foods)	1 slice (1 oz)	31	tr
Turkey Breast, Smoked, Sliced (Bil Mar Foods)	1 oz	31	tr
Turkey Ham (Carl Buddig)	1 oz	40	2
Turkey Ham, Smoked (Bil Mar Foods)	1 oz	32	1
Turkey Ham Square, Chopped (Bil Mar Foods)	1 slice (1 oz)	37	2

FOOD	PORTION	CALORIES	FAT
Turkey Ham w/ 20% Water (Wampler Longacre)	1 oz	39	6
Turkey Salami (Carl Buddig)	1 oz	40	2
Turkey Smoked Sausage; cooked (Louis Rich)	1 (1 oz)	55	4
Turkey Smoked Sausage w/ Cheese: cooked (Louis Rich)	1 (1 oz)	58	4
Turkey Sticks (Land O'Lakes)	2 (1 oz each)	150	10
White Meat, Diced (Mr. Turkey)	2 oz	84	2
Whole Smoked (Wampler Longacre)	1 oz	40	tr
bologna	1 slice (28 g)	57	4
breast	1 slice (21 g)	23	tr
breast	1 oz	47	tr
diced, light & dark, seasoned	1 oz	39	2
diced, light & dark, seasoned	½ lb	313	14
ham, thigh meat	1 slice (28 g)	73	3
ham, thigh meat	1 pkg (8 oz)	291	12
pastrami	1 slice (28 g)	80	4
pastrami	1 pkg (8 oz)	320	14
patties, breaded, battered; fried	3.3 oz	266	17
patties, breaded, battered; fried	2.3 oz	181	12
poultry salad sandwich spread	1 Tbsp	109	2
poultry salad sandwich spread	1 oz	238	4
prebasted breast, meat & skin; roasted	3.8 lbs	2175	60
prebasted breast, meat & skin; roasted	½ breast (1.9 lbs)	1087	30
prebasted thigh, meat & skin; roasted	11 oz	494	27

FOOD	PORTION	CALORIES	FAT
prebasted thigh, meat & skin; roasted	2 thighs (1.4 lbs)	990	54
roll, light & dark meat	1 slice (28 g)	42	2
roll, light meat	1 slice (28 g)	42	2
salami; cooked	1 pkg (8 oz)	446	31
salami; cooked	1 slice (28 g)	56	4
turkey loaf, breast meat	2 slices (1.5 oz)	47	1
turkey loaf, breast meat	1 pkg (6 oz)	187	3
turkey sticks, breaded, battered; fried	1 stick (2.3 oz)	178	11
turkey sticks, breaded, battered; fried	2 sticks (4.5 oz)	357	22

TURKEY DISHES
(*see also* DINNER, TURKEY SUBSTITUTE)

stew (home recipe)	¾ cup	336	9
turkey loaf (home recipe)	1 slice (4.7 oz)	263	14

TURKEY SUBSTITUTE

Meatless Turkey (Loma Linda)	2 slices (2 oz)	95	3
Smoked Turkey; frzn (Worthington)	3.5 oz	239	15

TURNIP

CANNED			
Turnip Greens w/ Diced Turnips Seasoned w/ Pork (Luck's)	7.5 oz	90	6
greens	½ cup	17	tr
FRESH			
greens, chopped, raw	½ cup	7	tr

FOOD	PORTION	CALORIES	FAT
greens, chopped; cooked	½ cup	15	tr
cubed, raw	½ cup	18	tr
FROZEN Mashed (Southland)	3.6 oz	90	6
frzn; not prep	10 oz pkg	44	tr
greens & turnips; not prep	10 oz pkg	59	tr
greens; cooked	½ cup	24	tr
greens; not prep	10 oz pkg	62	tr

VANILLA EXTRACT

FOOD	PORTION	CALORIES	FAT
Pure Vanilla Extract (Virginia Dare)	1 tsp	10	0

VEAL
(*see also* BEEF, VEAL DISHES)

FOOD	PORTION	CALORIES	FAT
cutlet, w/ bone, lean & fat; cooked	3 oz	184	9
loin chop, w/ bone, lean & fat; cooked	1 sm (2.9 oz)	190	11
loin chop, w/ bone, lean & fat; cooked	1 med (3.9 oz)	257	15
loin chop, w/ bone, lean only; cooked	1 sm (2.4 oz)	143	5
loin chop, w/ bone, lean only; cooked	1 med (3.3 oz)	194	6
loin roast w/ bone, lean & fat; roasted	3 oz	199	11
loin roast w/ bone, lean only; roasted	3 oz	130	3
rib chop w/ bone, lean & fat; cooked	1 med (3.5 oz)	269	17
round, lean & fat, chopped; cooked	½ cup	151	8
round, lean & fat, ground; cooked	½ cup	119	6
round, patty; cooked	3 oz	184	9

FOOD	PORTION	CALORIES	FAT
shoulder arm roast w/o bone, lean & fat; braised	3 oz	200	11
shoulder arm roast w/o bone, lean only; braised	3 oz	170	5
shoulder arm steak w/ bone, lean only; cooked	3.5 oz	196	5

VEAL DISHES

parmigiana (home recipe)	4.2 oz	279	18
veal loaf (home recipe)	1 slice (4.7 oz)	270	17

VEGETABLES, MIXED
(see also INDIVIDUAL VEGETABLES)

CANNED			
Beets, Pickled w/ Onions (Libby)	½ cup	80	0
Beets Pickled w/ Onions (Seneca)	½ cup	80	0
Garden Salad, Marinated (S&W)	½ cup	60	0
Green Beans & Wax Beans (S&W)	½ cup	20	0
Mixed Vegetables (Hanover)	½ cup	110	0
Mixed Vegetables (Libby)	½ cup	40	0
Mixed Vegetables (Seneca)	½ cup	40	0
Mixed Vegetables, Old Fashioned Harvest Time (S&W)	½ cup	35	0
Okra Creole Gumbo (Trappey's)	½ cup	25	0
Okra Cut & Tomatoes (Trappey's)	½ cup	25	0

FOOD	PORTION	CALORIES	FAT
Okra Cut, Tomatoes & Corn (Trappey's)	½ cup	25	0
Peas & Carrots (Libby)	½ cup	50	0
Peas & Carrots (Seneca)	½ cup	50	0
Succotash (Libby)	½ cup	80	1
Succotash (Seneca)	½ cup	80	1
Succotash, Country Style (S&W)	½ cup	80	1
Sweet Peas & Diced Carrots (S&W)	½ cup	50	0
Sweet Peas w/ Tiny Pearl Onions (S&W)	½ cup	60	1
Vegetable Salad (Hanover)	½ cup	90	0
corn w/ red & green peppers	½ cup	86	1
mixed vegetables	½ cup	44	tr
peas and carrots	½ cup	48	tr
peas and onions	½ cup	30	tr
succotash	½ cup	102	1
FROZEN			
Broccoli, Baby Carrots & Water Chestnuts, Farm Fresh Mixtures (Birds Eye)	¾ cup	45	tr
Broccoli, Carrots & Pasta Twists in Lightly Seasoned Sauce (Birds Eye)	⅔ cup	87	11
Broccoli, Cauliflower & Carrots, Farm Fresh Mixtures (Birds Eye)	¾ cup	33	tr
Broccoli, Cauliflower w/ Creamy Italian Cheese Sauce (Birds Eye)	½ cup	89	6

FOOD	PORTION	CALORIES	FAT
Broccoli, Cauliflower, Carrots w/ Cheese Sauce (Birds Eye)	½ cup	99	5
Broccoli, Corn & Red Peppers, Farm Fresh Mixtures (Birds Eye)	⅔ cup	60	tr
Broccoli Cut & Cauliflower Cut (Hanover)	½ cup	20	0
Brussels Sprouts, Cauliflower & Carrots, Farm Fresh Mixtures (Birds Eye)	¾ cup	40	tr
Caribbean Blend (Hanover)	½ cup	20	0
Carrots, Baby Whole Sweet Peas & Onions Deluxe Vegetable (Birds Eye)	½ cup	48	tr
Cauliflower, Baby Whole Carrots & Snow Peas, Farm Fresh Mixtures (Birds Eye)	⅔ cup	38	tr
Chinese Style International Recipe (Birds Eye)	½ cup	68	4
Chinese Style Stir Fry Vegetable (Birds Eye)	½ cup	36	tr
Chow Mein Style International Recipe (Birds Eye)	½ cup	89	4
Corn, Green Beans & Pasta Curls in Light Cream Sauce (Birds Eye)	½ cup	107	5
Garden Medley (Hanover)	½ cup	20	0
Green Peas & Pearl Onions (Birds Eye)	½ cup	71	tr
Italian Style International Recipe (Birds Eye)	½ cup	101	5
Japanese Style International Recipe (Birds Eye)	½ cup	88	4

FOOD	PORTION	CALORIES	FAT
Japanese Style Stir Fry Vegetables (Birds Eye)	½ cup	29	tr
Mandarin Style International Recipe (Birds Eye)	½ cup	86	4
Medley Vegetable Crisp (Ore Ida)	3 oz	160	9
Mixed Chinese Style Vegetables (La Choy)	½ cup	25	tr
Mixed Vegetables (Birds Eye)	½ cup	58	tr
Mixed Vegetables (Hanover)	½ cup	50	0
Mixed Vegetables w/ Onion Sauce (Birds Eye)	⅓ cup	97	5
New England Style International Recipe (Birds Eye)	½ cup	124	6
Oriental Blend (Hanover)	½ cup	25	0
Pasta Primavera Style International Recipe (Birds Eye)	½ cup	121	5
Peas & Cauliflower in Cream Sauce (Budget Gourmet)	5.75 oz	170	7
Peas & Pearl Onions w/ Cream Sauce (Birds Eye)	½ cup	137	5
Peas & Potatoes w/ Cream Sauce (Birds Eye)	½ cup	126	6
Peas & Water Chestnuts Oriental (Budget Gourmet)	5 oz	120	3
Peppers & Onions (Southland)	2 oz	15	0
Rutabaga-Yellow Turnips (Southland)	4 oz	50	0

FOOD	PORTION	CALORIES	FAT
San Francisco Style International Recipe (Birds Eye)	½ cup	90	4
Soup Mix Vegetables (Southland)	3.2 oz	50	0
Spring Vegetables in Cheese Sauce (Budget Gourmet)	5 oz	90	3
Stew Vegetables (Ore Ida)	3 oz	60	tr
Stew Vegetables (Southland)	4 oz	60	0
Succotash (Hanover)	½ cup	80	0
Summer Vegetables (Hanover)	½ cup	35	0
Vegetables For Soup (Hanover)	½ cup	60	0
Vegetables New England Recipe (Budget Gourmet)	5.5 oz	210	10
mixed; cooked	½ cup	54	tr
mixed; not prep	10 oz pkg	201	1
peas & carrots; cooked	½ cup	38	tr
peas & carrots; not prep	½ cup	37	tr
peas & onions; not prep	½ cup	48	tr
peas and onions; cooked	½ cup	40	tr
succotash	10 oz pkg	265	3
succotash; cooked	½ cup	79	1
HOME RECIPE caponata	¼ cup	28	1
succotash	½ cup	111	tr
JUICE V8 (Campbell)	6 oz	35	0

FOOD	PORTION	CALORIES	FAT
V8, Hot Spicy (Campbell)	6 oz	35	0
V8, No-Salt (Campbell)	6 oz	40	0
Beefamato (Mott's)	6 oz	80	0
Clamato (Mott's)	6 oz	96	0
vegetable cocktail	6 fl oz	34	tr

VINEGAR

FOOD	PORTION	CALORIES	FAT
Apple Cider (White House)	2 Tbsp	4	0
White Distilled (White House)	2 Tbsp	4	0
Wine Vinegar, All Flavors (Regina)	1 oz	4	0

WAFFLES

FROZEN READY-TO-USE

FOOD	PORTION	CALORIES	FAT
Apple & Cinnamon (Aunt Jemima)	2	170	4
Apple Cinnamon (Eggo)	1	130	5
Belgian Chef	1	90	2
Blueberry (Aunt Jemima)	2	170	4
Blueberry (Eggo)	1	130	5
Buttermilk (Aunt Jemima)	2	170	4
Buttermilk (Eggo)	1	130	5

FOOD	PORTION	CALORIES	FAT
Homestyle (Eggo)	1	130	5
Original (Aunt Jemima)	2	170	4
Raisin (Aunt Jemima)	2	200	4
Raisins, Bran & Whole Grain Nutri-Grain (Eggo)	1	130	5
Strawberry (Eggo)	1	130	5
Waffles (Roman Meal)	2	280	14
HOME RECIPE waffle	7" diam	282	19
waffle	9" sq	602	40
MIX mix; as prep w/ egg & milk	1 waffle (2.6 oz)	210	6

WALNUTS

FOOD	PORTION	CALORIES	FAT
Black Walnuts (Planters)	1 oz	190	17
English Walnuts, Whole, Halves or Pieces (Planters)	1 oz	190	20
Walnut Topping (Kraft)	1 Tbsp	90	5
black, dried	1 oz	172	16
black, dried; chopped	1 cup	759	71
english, dried	1 oz	182	18
english, dried; chopped	1 cup	770	74

FOOD	PORTION	CALORIES	FAT

WATERCHESTNUTS

| Water Chestnuts (La Choy) | ¼ cup | 16 | tr |
| chinese, sliced, canned | ½ cup | 35 | tr |

WATERCRESS
(*see also* CRESS)

| chopped; raw | ½ cup | 2 | tr |

WATERMELON

| diced | 1 cup | 50 | 1 |
| seeds, dried | 1 oz | 158 | 13 |

WAX BEANS

Cut Wax Beans (Owatonna)	½ cup	20	0
Golden Cut Premium (S&W)	½ cup	20	0
Wax Beans (Libby)	½ cup	20	0
Wax Beans (Seneca)	½ cup	20	0

WHALE

| raw | 3.5 oz | 156 | 8 |

WHELK (SNAIL)

| cooked | 3 oz | 233 | 1 |
| raw | 3 oz | 117 | tr |

WHIPPED TOPPING
(*see also* CREAM)

| Cool Whip (Non Dairy) | 1 Tbsp | 11 | tr |
| Cool Whip Extra Creamy Dairy | 1 Tbsp | 16 | 1 |

FOOD	PORTION	CALORIES	FAT
D-Zerta; as prep	¼ cup	47	4
D-Zerta w/ Nutrasweet; as prep	1 Tbsp	7	tr
Diamond Crystal	1 Tbsp	4	tr
Dream Whip; as prep	1 Tbsp	9	tr
Real Cream Topping (Kraft)	¼ cup	25	2
Whipped Topping (Kraft)	¼ cup	35	3
Whipped Topping; as prep (Estee)	1 Tbsp	4	tr
cream, pressurized	1 Tbsp	8	tr
cream, pressurized	1 cup	154	13
nondairy, frzn	¼ cup	60	5
nondairy, frzn	1 Tbsp	13	1
nondairy, powdered	1 Tbsp	8	tr
nondairy, pressurized	1 Tbsp	11	1
nondairy, pressurized	¼ cup	46	4

WHITE BEANS

FOOD	PORTION	CALORIES	FAT
CANNED			
white	1 cup	306	1
DRIED			
cooked	1 cup	249	1
raw	1 cup	674	2
small white, raw	1 cup	723	3
small white; cooked	1 cup	253	1

WHITEFISH

FOOD	PORTION	CALORIES	FAT
FRESH			
raw	3 oz	114	5
raw	1 fillet (6.9 oz)	266	12

FOOD	PORTION	CALORIES	FAT
SMOKED			
whitefish	1 oz	39	tr
whitefish	3 oz	92	1

WHITING

cooked	1 fillet (2.5 oz)	83	1
cooked	3 oz	98	1
raw	3 oz	77	1
raw	1 fillet (3.2 oz)	83	1

WINE
(*see also* WINE COOLERS)

dessert	2 oz	90	0
red	3.5 oz	74	0
rose	3.5 oz	73	0
sherry	2 oz	84	0
vermouth, dry	3.5 oz	105	0
vermouth, sweet	3.5 oz	167	0
white	3.5 oz	70	0

WINE COOLERS

Bartles & Jaymes	12 oz	192	0

WINGED BEANS

cooked	1 cup	252	10
raw	1 cup	745	30

WOLF FISH

Atlantic, raw	3 oz	82	2
Atlantic, raw	½ fillet (5.4 oz)	147	4

FOOD	PORTION	CALORIES	FAT

YAM
(see also SWEET POTATO)

FOOD	PORTION	CALORIES	FAT
CANNED			
Candied (S&W)	½ cup	180	0
Yams, Golden Cut in Syrup (Sugary Sam)	½ cup	110	0
Yams, Golden Whole in Heavy Syrup (Trappey's)	½ cup	130	0
Yams, Southern Whole in Extra Heavy Syrup (S&W)	½ cup	139	1
FRESH			
mountain yam, Hawaii; cubed, cooked	½ cup	59	tr
mountain yam, Hawaii, raw; cubed	½ cup	46	tr
yam, cubed; cooked	½ cup	79	tr
FROZEN			
Candied Yams (Mrs. Paul's)	4 oz	200	1
Candied Yams & Apples (Mrs. Paul's)	4 oz	160	0

YARDLONG BEANS

FOOD	PORTION	CALORIES	FAT
cooked	1 cup	202	1
raw	1 cup	580	2

YEAST

FOOD	PORTION	CALORIES	FAT
baker's dry, active	1 pkg (7 g)	20	tr
brewer's dry	1 Tbsp	25	tr

YELLOW BEANS

FOOD	PORTION	CALORIES	FAT
cooked	1 cup	254	2
raw	1 cup	676	5

FOOD	PORTION	CALORIES	FAT

YELLOWEYE BEANS

Yellow Eye Baked Beans (B&M)	⅞ cup	290	7

YELLOWTAIL

raw	3 oz	124	4
raw	½ fillet (6.6 oz)	273	10

YOGURT
(*see also* YOGURT DRINKS, YOGURT FROZEN)

Yoplait yogurt made in and/or distributed from California will have a slightly different fat content to comply with California law.

All Flavors (TCBY)	5 oz	160	3–4
Amaretto Almond Yo Creme (Yoplait)	5 oz	240	10
Apple (La Yogurt)	6 oz	190	4
Apple Cinnamon Breakfast Yogurt (Yoplait)	6 oz	220	4
Apple Original (Yoplait)	4 oz	120	2
Apple Original (Yoplait)	6 oz	190	3
Banana Custard Style (Yoplait)	6 oz	190	4
Banana Fruit-on-the Bottom (Dannon)	8 oz	240	3
Banana Strawberry Non Fat Lite (Colombo)	8 oz	190	tr
Bavarian Chocolate Yo Creme (Yoplait)	5 oz	270	11

FOOD	PORTION	CALORIES	FAT
Berries Breakfast Yogurt (Yoplait)	6 oz	230	4
Black Cherry (Breyers)	8 oz	270	5
Black Cherry, Lowfat (Light N'Lively)	6 oz	180	2
Blueberry (Breyers)	8 oz	260	6
Blueberry (Dannon)	8 oz	200	4
Blueberry (La Yogurt 25)	8 oz	200	0
Blueberry (La Yogurt)	6 oz	190	4
Blueberry (Mountain High)	1 cup	220	6
Blueberry (Yoplait 150)	6 oz	150	0
Blueberry, Custard Style (Yoplait)	6 oz	190	4
Blueberry, Fruit-on-the-Bottom (Dannon)	8 oz	240	3
Blueberry, Fruit-on-the-Bottom (Dannon)	4.4 oz	130	2
Blueberry, Lowfat (Light N'Lively)	6 oz	180	2
Blueberry, Non Fat Lite (Colombo)	8 oz	160	tr
Blueberry, Original (Yoplait)	4 oz	120	2
Blueberry, Original (Yoplait)	6 oz	190	3
Boysenberry, Fruit-on-the-Bottom (Dannon)	8 oz	240	3
Boysenberry, Original (Yoplait)	4 oz	120	2

FOOD	PORTION	CALORIES	FAT
Cherries Jubilee (Yoplait)	5 oz	220	8
Cherry (La Yogurt 25)	8 oz	200	0
Cherry (La Yogurt)	6 oz	190	4
Cherry (Yoplait 150)	6 oz	150	0
Cherry, Custard Style (Yoplait)	6 oz	180	4
Cherry, Fruit-on-the-Bottom (Dannon)	8 oz	240	3
Cherry, Fruit-on-the-Bottom (Dannon)	4.4 oz	130	2
Cherry, Original (Yoplait)	4 oz	120	2
Cherry Vanilla (La Yogurt)	6 oz	190	4
Cherry Vanilla (Lite Line)	1 cup	240	2
Cherry w/ Almonds, Breakfast Yogurt (Yoplait)	6 oz	210	3
Coffee (Dannon)	8 oz	200	3
Coffee, Lowfat (Friendship)	8 oz	210	3
Dutch Apple, Fruit-on-the-Bottom (Dannon)	8 oz	240	3
Exotic Fruit, Fruit-on-the-Bottom (Dannon)	8 oz	240	3
Fruit Cocktail, Non Fat Lite (Colombo)	8 oz	160	tr
Key Lime (La Yogurt)	6 oz	190	4

FOOD	PORTION	CALORIES	FAT
Lemon (Dannon)	8 oz	200	3
Lemon, Custard Style (Yoplait)	6 oz	190	4
Lemon, Original (Yoplait)	4 oz	120	2
Mixed Berries, Extra Smooth (Dannon)	4.4 oz	130	2
Mixed Berries, Fruit-on-the-Bottom (Dannon)	8 oz	240	3
Mixed Berries, Fruit-on-the-Bottom (Dannon)	4.4 oz	130	2
Mixed Berries, Hearty Nuts & Raisins (Dannon)	8 oz	260	3
Mixed Berry (Breyers)	8 oz	270	5
Mixed Berry (La Yogurt)	6 oz	190	4
Mixed Berry, Custard Style (Yoplait)	6 oz	180	4
Mixed Berry, Original (Yoplait)	4 oz	120	2
Orange, Original (Yoplait)	4 oz	120	2
Orchard Fruit, Hearty Nuts & Raisins (Dannon)	8 oz	260	3
Peach (Breyers)	8 oz	270	5
Peach (La Yogurt)	6 oz	190	4
Peach (Lite Line)	1 cup	230	2
Peach (Yoplait 150)	6 oz	150	0

FOOD	PORTION	CALORIES	FAT
Peach, Fruit-on-the-Bottom (Dannon)	8 oz	240	3
Peach, Lowfat (Light N'Lively)	6 oz	180	2
Peach, Non Fat Lite (Colombo)	8 oz	190	tr
Peach, Original (Yoplait)	4 oz	120	2
Pina Colada (La Yogurt)	6 oz	190	4
Pina Colada, Fruit-on-the-Bottom (Dannon)	8 oz	240	3
Pina Colada, Original (Yoplait)	4 oz	120	2
Pineapple (Breyers)	8 oz	270	5
Pineapple, Lowfat (Light N'Lively)	6 oz	180	2
Pineapple, Original (Yoplait)	4 oz	120	2
Plain (Breyers)	8 oz	190	8
Plain (Friendship)	8 oz	170	8
Plain (La Yogurt)	6 oz	140	6
Plain (Mountain High)	1 cup	200	9
Plain (Yoplait)	4 oz	80	2
Plain (Yoplait)	6 oz	120	3
Plain, Low-Fat (Dannon)	8 oz	140	4
Plain, Lowfat (Meadow Gold)	1 cup	160	5

FOOD	PORTION	CALORIES	FAT
Plain, Lowfat, Swiss Style (Lite Line)	1 cup	140	2
Plain, Non-Fat (Dannon)	8 oz	110	0
Raspberries & Cream (Yoplait)	5 oz	230	9
Raspberry (Dannon)	8 oz	200	4
Raspberry (La Yogurt 25)	8 oz	200	0
Raspberry (Yoplait 150)	6 oz	150	0
Raspberry, Custard Style (Yoplait)	6 oz	190	4
Raspberry, Extra Smooth (Dannon)	4.4 oz	130	2
Raspberry, Fruit-on-the-Bottom (Dannon)	8 oz	240	3
Raspberry, Fruit-on-the-Bottom (Dannon)	4.4 oz	130	2
Raspberry, Original (Yoplait)	4 oz	120	2
Raspberry, Sundae Style (Meadow Gold)	1 cup	250	4
Red Raspberry (Breyers)	8 oz	260	6
Red Raspberry, Lowfat (Light N'Lively)	6 oz	170	2
Strawberries, Romanoff (Yoplait)	5 oz	220	8
Strawberry (Breyers)	8 oz	270	5
Strawberry (Dannon)	8 oz	200	4

FOOD	PORTION	CALORIES	FAT
Strawberry (La Yogurt 25)	8 oz	200	0
Strawberry (La Yogurt)	6 oz	190	4
Strawberry (Lite Line)	1 cup	240	2
Strawberry (Yoplait 150)	6 oz	150	0
Strawberry, Banana (Breyers)	8 oz	280	6
Strawberry, Banana (Dannon)	8 oz	200	4
Strawberry-Banana (La Yogurt 25)	8 oz	200	0
Strawberry-Banana (La Yogurt)	6 oz	190	4
Strawberry-Banana (Yoplait 150)	6 oz	150	0
Strawberry, Banana Breakfast Yogurt (Yoplait)	6 oz	240	4
Strawberry Banana, Fruit-on-the-Bottom (Dannon)	4.4oz	130	2
Strawberry Banana, Lowfat (Light N'Lively)	6 oz	200	2
Strawberry-Banana, Original (Yoplait)	4 oz	120	2
Strawberry, Custard Style (Yoplait)	6 oz	190	4
Strawberry, Extra Smooth (Dannon)	4.4 oz	130	2
Strawberry Fruit Cup (La Yogurt)	6 oz	190	4
Strawberry, Fruit-on-the-Bottom (Dannon)	8 oz	240	3

FOOD	PORTION	CALORIES	FAT
Strawberry, Fruit-on-the-Bottom (Dannon)	4.4 oz	130	2
Strawberry, Lowfat (Light N'Lively)	6 oz	180	2
Strawberry, Non Fat Lite (Colombo)	8 oz	190	tr
Strawberry Original (Yoplait)	4 oz	120	2
Strawberry-Rhubarb, Original (Yoplait)	4 oz	120	2
Strawberry w/ Almonds Breakfast Yogurt (Yoplait)	6 oz	210	3
Sunrise Peach Breakfast Yogurt (Yoplait)	6 oz	230	3
Tropical Fruits Breakfast Yogurt (Yoplait)	6 oz	230	4
Tropical Orange (La Yogurt)	6 oz	190	4
Vanilla (Dannon)	8 oz	200	3
Vanilla (Dannon)	4.4 oz	110	2
Vanilla (La Yogurt)	6 oz	160	4
Vanilla Bean (Breyers)	8 oz	230	7
Vanilla, Custard Style (Yoplait)	6 oz	180	4
Vanilla, Hearty Nuts & Raisins (Dannon)	8 oz	270	5
Vanilla, Lowfat (Friendship)	8 oz	210	3
With Fruit, Lowfat (Friendship)	8 oz	230	3

FOOD	PORTION	CALORIES	FAT
coffee, lowfat	1 cup	193	3
coffee, lowfat	4 oz	97	1.4
coffee, lowfat	8 oz	194	2.8
fruit, all flavors, lowfat	1 cup	232	3
fruit, lowfat	4 oz	113	1.3
fruit, lowfat	8 oz	225	2.6
plain	4 oz	70	3.7
plain, lowfat	1 cup	143	4
plain, lowfat	4 oz	72	1.8
plain, lowfat	8 oz	144	3.5
plain, skim milk	1 cup	127	tr
plain, skim milk	4 oz	63	tr
plain, skim milk	8 oz	127	tr
plain, whole milk	1 cup	138	7
vanilla, lowfat	8 oz	194	2.8
vanilla, lowfat	4 oz	97	1.4
vanilla, lowfat	1 cup	193	3

YOGURT DRINKS

FOOD	PORTION	CALORIES	FAT
Exotic Fruit, Dan'up (Dannon)	8 oz	190	4
Mixed Berry, Dan'up (Dannon)	8 oz	190	4
Raspberry, Dan'up (Dannon)	8 oz	190	4
Strawberry, Dan'up (Dannon)	8 oz	190	4.
Strawberry Banana Dan'up (Dannon)	8 oz	190	4

YOGURT, FROZEN

FOOD	PORTION	CALORIES	FAT
Black Cherry (Sealtest)	½ cup	100	2

FOOD	PORTION	CALORIES	FAT
Mixed Berries On-a-Stick (Dannon)	1 bar	50	1
Peach (Sealtest)	½ cup	100	2
Pineapple Coconut On-a-Stick (Dannon)	1 bar	50	1
Raspberry On-a-Stick (Dannon)	1 bar	50	1
Red Raspberry (Sealtest)	½ cup	100	2
Strawberry (Sealtest)	½ cup	100	2
Strawberry On-a-Stick (Dannon)	1 bar	50	1
Strawberry Banana On-a-Stick (Dannon)	1 bar	50	1
Vanilla (Colombo)	4 oz	99	2

YORKSHIRE PUDDING

FOOD	PORTION	CALORIES	FAT
yorkshire pudding (home recipe)	3" sq	171	10

ZABAGLIONE
(*see* CUSTARD)

ZUCCHINI

FOOD	PORTION	CALORIES	FAT
CANNED			
Italian Style (S&W)	½ cup	45	1
Italian style	½ cup	33	tr
FRESH			
sliced; cooked	½ cup	14	tr
sliced, raw	½ cup	9	tr

FOOD	PORTION	CALORIES	FAT
FROZEN			
Light Batter Zucchini Sticks (Mrs. Paul's)	3 oz	200	12
Zucchini Vegetable Crisp (Ore Ida)	3 oz	150	9
Zucchini, Sliced (Southland)	3.2 oz	15	0
cooked	½ cup	19	tr
HOME RECIPE			
croquettes	½ cup	118	6
sticks	½ cup	81	7

PART II

Restaurant, Take-Out and Fast Food Chains

FOOD	PORTION	CALORIES	FAT
BASKIN-ROBBINS			
Chocolate Ice Cream	1 scoop	270	14
Jamoca Almond Fudge Ice Cream	1 scoop	270	14
Low, Lite 'N' Luscious Chocolate Chip	4 oz	80–100	1–2
Low, Lite 'N' Luscious Jamoca Swiss Almond	4 oz	80–100	1–2
Low, Lite 'N' Luscious Strawberry	4 oz	80–100	1–2
Pralines 'N' Cream Ice Cream	1 scoop	280	14
Vanilla Frozen Yogurt	4 oz	124	2
Vanilla Ice Cream	1 scoop	240	14
BURGER KING			
BEVERAGES			
7 UP	1 reg	144	0
Coffee, black	6 oz	2	0
Diet Pepsi	1 reg	1	0
Milk, 2%	8 oz	121	5
Milk, Whole	8 oz	157	9
Orange Juice	6 oz	80	0
Pepsi-Cola	1 reg	159	0
Shake, Chocolate	1 reg	320	12
Shake, Chocolate w/ Syrup Added	1 reg	374	11
Shake, Vanilla	1 reg	321	10
Shake, Vanilla w/ Syrup Added	1 reg	334	10
BREAKFAST SELECTIONS			
Breakfast Croissan'wich w/ Bacon	1	355	21
Breakfast Croissn'wich w/ Ham	1	335	20
Breakfast Croissan'wich w/ Sausage	1	538	41
French Toast Sticks	1 serving	499	29

FOOD	PORTION	CALORIES	FAT
Scrambled Egg Platter	1	468	30
Scrambled Egg Platter w/ Bacon	1	536	36
Scrambled Egg Platter w/ Sausage	1	702	52
DRESSINGS AND SALADS			
Bleu Cheese	3 Tbsp	156	16
House	3 Tbsp	130	13
Italian, Reduced Calorie	3 Tbsp	14	0
Salad w/o Dressing	1 reg	28	0
Thousand Island	3 Tbsp	117	12
MAIN MENU SELECTIONS			
Bacon Double Cheeseburger	1	510	31
Cheeseburger	1	317	15
Chicken Specialty Sandwich	1	688	40
Chicken Tenders	6 pieces	204	10
French Fries	1 reg	227	13
Ham & Cheese Specialty Sandwich	1	471	23
Hamburger	1	275	12
Onion Rings	1 reg	274	16
Whaler Fish Sandwich	1	488	27
Whopper Double Beef	1	863	53
Whopper Double Beef w/ Cheese	1	946	60
Whopper Jr. Sandwich	1	322	17
Whopper Jr. Sandwich w/ Cheese	1	364	20
Whopper Sandwich	1	628	36
Whopper Sandwich w/ Cheese	1	711	43
MISCELLANEOUS			
Apple Pie	1	305	12
Great Danish	1	500	36

FOOD	PORTION	CALORIES	FAT

CARL'S JR.

FOOD	PORTION	CALORIES	FAT
BAKERY SELECTIONS			
Chocolate Cake	1 piece	380	20
Chocolate Chip Cookies	2.5 oz	353	16
Danish	1	300	9
Muffin, Blueberry	1	256	7
Muffin, Bran	1	220	6
BEVERAGES			
Iced Tea	1 reg	2	0
Milk, 2%	10 oz	175	6
Orange Juice	1 sm	94	1
Shake	1 reg	353	7
Soda	1 reg	243	0
Soda, Diet	1 reg	2	0
BREAKFAST ITEMS			
Bacon	2 strips	50	4
English Muffin w/ Margarine	1	180	6
French Toast Dips w/o syrup	1 serving	480	25
Hash Brown Nuggets	1 serving	170	9
Hot Cakes w/ Margarine, w/o Syrup	1 serving	360	12
Sausage	1 patty	190	17
Scrambed Eggs	1 serving	120	9
Sunrise Sandwich w/ Bacon	1	370	19
Sunrise Sandwich w/ Sausage	1	500	32
DRESSINGS AND SALADS			
Blue Cheese Dressing	1 oz	110	11
Chef Salad-to-Go	1	180	7
Chicken Salad-to-Go	1	206	8
Garden Salad-to-Go	1	46	2
House Dressing	1 oz	151	15

FOOD	PORTION	CALORIES	FAT
Italian Dressing	1 oz	120	13
Reduced-Calorie French Dressing	1 oz	38	2
Taco Salad-to-Go	1	356	19
Thousand Island Dressing	1 oz	110	11

REGULAR MENU SELECTIONS

FOOD	PORTION	CALORIES	FAT
American Cheese	½ oz	63	5
California Roast Beef 'n Swiss	1	360	8
Cheeseburger, Double Western Bacon	1	890	53
Cheeseburger, Western Bacon	1	630	33
Chicken Club Sandwich Charbroiler	1	510	22
Chicken Sandwich Charbroiler BBQ	1	320	5
Country Fried Steak Sandwich	1	610	33
Filet of Fish Sandwich	1	550	26
French Fries	1 reg	360	17
Hamburger, Famous Star	1	590	36
Hamburger, Happy Star	1	220	8
Hamburger, Old Time Star	1	400	17
Hamburger, Super Star	1	770	50
Onion Rings	1 serving	310	15
Potato Fiesta	1	550	23
Potato Lite	1	250	3
Potato w/ Bacon & Cheese	1	650	34
Potato w/ Broccoli & Cheese	1	470	17
Potato w/ Cheese	1	550	22
Potato w/ Sour Cream & Chives	1	350	13
Swiss Cheese	½ oz	57	4
Zucchini	1 serving	300	16

SOUPS

FOOD	PORTION	CALORIES	FAT
Boston Clam Chowder	7 oz	140	8

FOOD	PORTION	CALORIES	FAT
Cream of Broccoli	7 oz	140	6
Lumber Jack Mix Vegetable	7 oz	70	3
Old Fashioned Chicken Noodle	7 oz	80	1

CHICK-FIL-A

FOOD	PORTION	CALORIES	FAT
BEVERAGES			
Iced Tea, Unsweetened	9 oz	3	tr
Lemonade	10 oz	124	tr
Orange Juice	6 oz	82	tr
MAIN MENU SELECTIONS			
Carrot-Raisin Salad	2.7 oz	116	5
Carrot-Raisin Salad	13 oz	570	24
Chick-fil-A Nuggets	8 pack	287	15
Chick-fil-A Nuggets	12 pack	430	23
Chick-fil-A Sandwich	1	426	9
Chick-fil-A, no bun	3.6 oz	219	7
Chicken Salad Cup	3.4 oz	309	28
Chicken Salad Sandwich (Wheat)	1	449	26
Cole Slaw	4 oz	175	14
Cole Slaw	15 oz	718	68
Hearty Breast of Chicken Soup	8.5 oz	152	3
Potato Salad	4 oz	198	15
Potato Salad	16 oz	850	64
Waffle Potato Fries	1 reg	270	14
MISCELLANEOUS			
Fudge Brownie w/ Nuts	1	369	19
Ice cream	4.5 oz	134	5
Lemon Pie	1 slice	329	5

FOOD	PORTION	CALORIES	FAT

CHURCH'S FRIED CHICKEN

FOOD	PORTION	CALORIES	FAT
Breast	4.3	278	17
Corn w/ Butter Oil	1 ear	237	9
French Fries	1 reg	138	6
Leg	2.9 oz	147	9
Thigh	4.2 oz	306	22
Wing & Breast	4.8 oz	303	20

DAIRY QUEEN/BRAZIER

FOOD SELECTION

FOOD	PORTION	CALORIES	FAT
All White Chicken Nuggets	1 serving	276	18
BBQ Nugget Sauce	1 pkg	41	tr
Chicken Breast Fillet	1	608	34
Chicken Breast Fillet w/ Cheese	1	661	38
DQ Hounder	1	480	36
DQ Hounder w/ Cheese	1	533	40
DQ Hounder w/ Chili	1	575	41
Double Hamburger	1	530	28
Double Hamburger w/ Cheese	1	650	37
Fish Fillet	1	430	18
Fish Fillet w/ Cheese	1	483	22
French Fries	1 reg	200	10
French Fries	1 lg	320	16
Hot Dog	1	280	16
Hot Dog w/ Cheese	1	330	21
Hot Dog w/ Chili	1	320	20
Onion Rings	1	280	16
Single Hamburger	1	360	16
Single Hamburger w/ Cheese	1	410	20

FOOD	PORTION	CALORIES	FAT
Super Hot Dog	1	520	27
Super Hot Dog w/ Cheese	1	580	34
Super Hot Dog w/ Chili	1	570	32
Triple Hamburger	1	710	45
Triple Hamburger w/ Cheese	1	820	50
ICE CREAM			
Banana Split	1	540	11
Buster Bar	1	460	29
Chipper Sandwich	1	318	7
Cone	1 sm	140	4
Cone	1 reg	240	7
Cone	1 lg	340	10
DQ Sandwich	1	140	4
Dilly Bar	1	210	13
Dipped Cone	1 sm	190	9
Dipped Cone	1 reg	340	16
Dipped Cone	1 lg	510	24
Double Delight	1	490	20
Float	1	410	7
Freeze	1	500	12
Fudge Nut Bar	1	406	25
Heath Blizzard	1	800	24
Hot Fudge Brownie Delight	1	600	25
Malt	1 lg	406	25
Malt	1 sm	520	13
Malt	1 reg	760	18
Mr. Misty	1 sm	190	0
Mr. Misty	1 reg	250	0
Mr. Misty	1 lg	340	0
Mr. Misty Float	1	390	7

FOOD	PORTION	CALORIES	FAT
Mr. Misty Freeze	1	500	12
Mr. Misty Kiss	1	70	0
Parfait	1	430	8
Peanut Buster Parfait	1	740	34
Shake	1 sm (10 oz)	327	13
Shake	1 reg (15 oz)	490	19
Shake	1 lg (17 oz)	710	21
Shake	1 xlg (21 oz)	990	26
Strawberry Shortcake	1	540	12
Sundae	1 sm	190	4
Sundae	1 reg	310	8

DOMINO'S PIZZA

FOOD	PORTION	CALORIES	FAT
10″ PIZZA			
Double Cheese	2 slices	284	11
Double Cheese, Pepperoni	2 slices	331	15
Ground Beef	2 slices	250	8
Ground Beef, Pepperoni	2 slices	297	13
Mushroom Sausage	2 slices	248	9
Pepperoni	2 slices	265	10
Pepperoni, Mushroom	2 slices	267	11
Pepperoni, Sausage	2 slices	293	13
Plain Cheese	2 slices	218	6
Sausage	2 slices	246	8
14″ PIZZA			
Double Cheese	2 slices	365	14
Double Cheese, Pepperoni	2 slices	427	19
Ground Beef	2 slices	321	11
Ground Beef, Pepperoni	2 slices	382	13
Mushroom, Sausage	2 slices	322	11

FOOD	PORTION	CALORIES	FAT
Pepperoni	2 slices	343	13
Pepperoni, Mushroom	2 slices	346	13
Pepperoni, Sausage	2 slices	380	17
Plain Cheese	2 slices	281	7
Sausage	2 slices	318	11
LARGE PIZZA			
Double Cheese	2 slices	700	19
Double Cheese, Pepperoni	2 slices	778	26
Ground Beef	2 slices	527	14
Ground Beef, Pepperoni	2 slices	605	22
Mushroom, Sausage	2 slices	532	15
Pepperoni	2 slices	556	18
Pepperoni, Mushroom	2 slices	550	17
Pepperoni, Sausage	2 slices	606	20
Plain Cheese	2 slices	478	10
Sausage	2 slices	528	15
SMALL PIZZA			
Double Cheese	2 slices	480	16
Double Cheese, Pepperoni	2 slices	453	22
Ground Beef	2 slices	361	12
Ground Beef, Pepperoni	2 slices	431	16
Mushroom Sausage	2 slices	365	13
Pepperoni	2 slices	384	15
Pepperoni, Mushroom	2 slices	388	15
Pepperoni, Sausage	2 slices	431	19
Plain Cheese	2 slices	314	9
Sausage	2 slices	360	13

DRUTHER'S INTERNATIONAL

BREAKFAST SELECTIONS			
Bacon and Egg Biscuit	1	258	16

FOOD	PORTION	CALORIES	FAT
Bacon and Egg Plate; fried	1	721	42
Bacon and Egg Plate; scrambled	1	742	43
Ham And Egg Biscuit	1	217	11
Ham And Egg Plate	1	681	35
Ham and Egg Plate; scrambled	1	703	37
Sausage and Egg Biscuit	1	246	15
Sausage and Egg Plate; fried	1	741	43
Sausage and Egg Plate; scrambled	1	762	45
Two Sausages/Two Biscuits	1 meal	358	22
MAIN MENU SELECTIONS Biscuits and Gravy	1 serving	331	15
Cheeseburger	1	380	18
Chicken Snack, Thigh, Drumstick	1 snack	925	50
Chicken Snack, Wing, Breast	1 snack	970	50
Deluxe Quarter Hamburger	1	660	38
Double Cheeseburger	1	500	26
Eight Piece Chicken Dinner	1	3664	114
Fish and Chips	1 dinner	729	30
Fish Dinner	1	770	31
Fish Sandwich	1	349	14
Hamburger	1	327	13
Three Piece Chicken Dinner, Thigh, Breast, Drumstick	1	1309	67
Three Piece Chicken Dinner, Thigh, Breast, Wing	1	1281	70
Twelve Piece Chicken Dinner	1	5496	171
Two Piece Chicken Dinner, Breast, Wing	1	970	50
Two Piece Chicken Dinner, Thigh, Drumstick	1	925	49

FOOD	PORTION	CALORIES	FAT

DUNKIN' DONUTS
(*see also* DOUGHNUT, WINCHELL'S)

FOOD	PORTION	CALORIES	FAT
CROISSANT			
Almond	1	435	30
Chocolate	1	502	37
Plain	1	291	22
DOUGHNUT			
Apple Filled w/ Cinnamon Sugar	1	219	12
Bavarian Creme Filled	1	226	14
Bavarian Filled w/ Chocolate Frosting	1	231	9
Blueberry Filled	1	196	10
Chocolate Cake Ring w/ Glaze	1	324	21
Chocolate Frosted Yeast Ring	1	246	14
Coconut Coated Cake Ring	1	417	28
French Cruller w/ Glaze	1	201	14
Honey Dipped Coffee Roll	1	348	17
Honey Dipped Cruller	1	370	23
Honey Dipped Yeast Ring	1	208	11
Jelly Filled	1	274	22
Lemon Filled	1	221	11
Munchkin Cake w/ Powdered Sugar	1	69	4
Munchkin Chocolate w/ Glaze	1	88	5
Munchkin Yeast w/ Glaze	1	43	2
Plain Cake Ring	1	319	22
Sugared Jelly Stick	1	332	18
MISCELLANEOUS			
Biscuit	1	332	23
Brownie	1	280	13
Chocolate Chip Cookie	1	129	7
Macaroon	1	351	19

FOOD	PORTION	CALORIES	FAT
MUFFIN			
Apple Spice	1	327	11
Banana Nut	1	327	12
Blueberry	1	263	10
Bran	1	353	13
Cherry	1	317	10
Corn	1	347	13

GODFATHER'S

FOOD	PORTION	CALORIES	FAT
SMALL PIZZA			
Original Cheese	2 slices	480	14
Original Cheese Combo	2 slices	720	30
Stuffed Pie, Pizza Cheese	2 slices	620	22
Stuffed Pie, Pizza Cheese Combo	2 slices	860	40
Thin Crust Cheese	2 slices	360	12
Thin Crust Combo	2 slices	540	26

HARDEE'S

FOOD	PORTION	CALORIES	FAT
BREAKFAST SELECTIONS			
Big Country Breakfast Ham Platter	1	665	38
Big Country Breakfast Platter	1	716	50
Big Country Breakfast Sausage Platter	1	940	70
Biscuit w/ Bacon & Egg	1	405	26
Biscuit w/ Cheese	1	304	16
Biscuit w/ Cinnamon 'N' Raisin	1	276	16
Biscuit w/ Country Ham	1	328	18
Biscuit w/ Egg	1	334	19
Biscuit w/ Sausage	1	426	28
Biscuit w/ Sausage & Egg	1	503	35
Biscuit w/ Steak	1	491	28

FOOD	PORTION	CALORIES	FAT
Biscuit w/ Sugar Cured Ham	1	299	14
Canadian Sunrise	1	489	30
Egg	1 oz	77	6
MAIN MENU SELECTIONS			
American Cheese	½ oz	47	3
Bacon Cheeseburger	1	556	33
Big Deluxe	1	503	29
Biscuit	1	257	12
Biscuit Gravy	4 oz	144	10
Cheeseburger	1	309	13
Cheeseburger, ¼ lb.	1	511	28
Chicken Fillet	1	510	26
Fisherman's Fillet	1	469	20
French Fries	1 reg	239	13
French Fries	1 lg	406	22
Hamburger	1	276	15
Hash Rounds	1	200	13
Hot Ham 'N' Cheese	1	376	15
Mushroom 'n' Swiss	1	512	23
Roast Beef Sandwich	1	312	12
Roast Beef Sandwich, Big	1	440	22
Salad, Chef	1	277	16
Salad, Side	1	21	tr
Turkey Club	1	426	22
MISCELLANEOUS			
Apple Turnover	1	282	14
Big Cookie	1	278	15
Jelly	1 Tbsp	49	tr
Milkshake	11 oz	391	10

FOOD	PORTION	CALORIES	FAT

JACK-IN-THE-BOX

FOOD	PORTION	CALORIES	FAT
BEVERAGES			
Coca-Cola Classic	12 oz	144	0
Coffee, black	8 oz	2	0
Diet Coke	12 oz	8	0
Dr Pepper	12 oz	144	0
Hot Chocolate	8 oz	133	4
Iced Tea	12 oz	3	0
Lowfat Milk	8 oz	122	5
Milk Shake, Chocolate	1 reg	330	7
Milk Shake, Vanilla	1 reg	320	7
Orange Juice	6 oz	80	0
Ramblin' Root Beer	12 oz	176	0
Sprite	12 oz	144	0
BREAKFAST SELECTIONS			
Breakfast Jack	1	307	13
Crescent, Canadian	1	452	31
Crescent, Sausage	1	584	43
Crescent, Supreme	1	547	40
Grape Jelly	1 pkg	38	0
Hash Brown	1	116	7
Hot Apple Turnover	1	410	24
Pancake Platter	1	612	22
Pancake Syrup	1 pkg	121	0
Scrambled Egg Platter	1	662	40
DRESSINGS, SALADS AND SAUCES			
A-1 Steak Sauce	1 pkg	35	tr
BBQ Sauce	1 pkg	39	tr
Bleu Cheese Dressing	1 pkg	131	11

FOOD	PORTION	CALORIES	FAT
Buttermilk House Dressing	1 pkg	181	18
Chef Salad	1	295	18
Guacamole	1 oz	55	5
Mayo-Mustard Sauce	1 pkg	124	13
Mayo-Onion Sauce	1 pkg	143	15
Pasta & Seafood Salad	1	394	22
Reduced-Calorie French Dressing	1 pkg	80	4
Salsa	1 oz	8	tr
Seafood Cocktail Sauce	1 pkg	57	tr
Side Salad	1	51	2
Sweet & Sour Sauce	1 pkg	39	tr
Taco Salad	1	377	24
Thousand Island Dressing	1 pkg	156	15

MAIN MENU SELECTIONS

FOOD	PORTION	CALORIES	FAT
Bacon Cheeseburger	1	705	39
Cheeseburger	1	325	17
Cheesecake	1	309	18
Chicken Strips	4 pieces	349	14
Chicken Strips	6 pieces	523	20
Chicken Supreme	1	524	28
Club Pita (no sauce)	1	277	8
Dinner, Chicken Strip (no sauce)	1	689	30
Dinner, Shrimp (no sauce)	1	731	37
Dinner, Sirloin Steak (no sauce)	1	699	27
Egg Rolls	3 pieces	405	19
Egg Rolls	5 pieces	675	32
Fajita Pita	1	278	7
Fish Supreme	1	554	32
French Fries	1 reg	221	12
French Fries	1 lg	353	19

FOOD	PORTION	CALORIES	FAT
French Fries	1 jumbo	442	24
Ham & Swiss Burger	1	754	49
Hamburger	1	288	13
Hot Club Supreme	1	524	28
Jumbo Jack	1	584	34
Jumbo Jack w/ Cheese	1	677	40
Moby Jack	1	444	25
Monterey Burger	1	865	57
Mushroom Burger	1	470	24
Nachos, Cheese	1 serving	571	35
Nachos, Supreme	1 serving	787	45
Onion Rings	1 serving	383	23
Pizza Pocket	1	497	28
Shrimp	10 pieces	270	16
Shrimp	15 pieces	404	24
Swiss and Bacon Burger	1	678	69
Taco	1	191	11
Taco, Super	1	288	17
Ultimate Cheeseburger	1	942	69

MCDONALD'S

BEVERAGES

Coca-Cola Classic	16 oz	190	0
Diet Coke	16 oz	1	0
Grapefruit Juice	6 oz	80	0
Milk, 2%	8 oz	121	5
Milk Shake, Chocolate	10 oz	388	11
Milk Shake, Strawberry	10 oz	384	10
Milk Shake, Vanilla	10 oz	354	10

FOOD	PORTION	CALORIES	FAT
Orange Drink	16 oz	177	0
Orange Juice	6 oz	80	0
Sprite	16 oz	190	0
BREAKFAST SELECTIONS			
Biscuit w/ Biscuit Spread	1	260	13
Biscuit w/ Sausage	1	440	29
Biscuit w/ Sausage & Egg	1	529	35
Biscuit w/ Bacon, Egg & Cheese	1	449	27
Egg McMuffin	1	293	12
English Muffin w/ Butter	1	169	5
Hashbrown Potatoes	1	131	7
Hotcakes w/ Butter & Syrup	1 portion	413	9
Pork Sausage	1.7 oz	180	16
Sausage McMuffin	1	372	22
Sausage McMuffin w/ Egg	1	451	27
Scrambled Eggs	1 portion	157	11
DESSERTS			
Apple Pie	1	262	15
Cone, Soft Serve	1	144	5
Cookies, Chocolate Chip	1 pkg	325	16
Cookies, McDonaldland	1 pkg	288	9
Danish, Apple	1	389	18
Danish, Cinnamon Raisin	1	445	21
Danish, Iced Cheese	1	395	22
Danish, Raspberry	1	414	16
Sundae, Hot Caramel	1	343	9
Sundae, Hot Fudge	1	313	9
Sundae, Strawberry	1	283	7
DRESSINGS AND SALADS			
Bacon Bits	.1 oz	16	1

FOOD	PORTION	CALORIES	FAT
Bleu Cheese Dressing	½ oz	69	7
Chef Salad	1	231	14
Chicken Salad Oriental	1	141	3
Chow Mein Noodles	.3 oz	45	2
Croutons	.4 oz	52	2
French Dressing	½ oz	58	5
Lite Vinaigrette Dressing	½ oz	15	tr
Oriental Dressing	½ oz	24	tr
Ranch Dressing	½ oz	83	9
Shrimp Salad	1	104	3
Side Salad	1	57	3
Thousand Island Dressing	½ oz	78	8
MAIN MENU SELECTIONS			
Big Mac	1	562	32
Cheeseburger	1	308	14
Chicken McNuggets	1 portion	288	16
Filet-O-Fish	1	442	26
French Fries	1 reg	220	12
French Fries	1 lg	312	16
Hamburger	1	257	10
McD.L.T.	1	674	42
McNuggets Sauce, Barbeque	1 oz	53	tr
McNuggets Sauce, Honey	1 oz	46	0
McNuggets Sauce, Hot Mustard	1 oz	66	4
McNuggets Sauce, Sweet & Sour	1 oz	57	tr
Quarter Pounder	1	517	29

PIZZA HUT

10″ PIZZA Thick 'n Chewy Cheese	3 slices	560	14

FOOD	PORTION	CALORIES	FAT
Thick 'n Chewy Supreme	3 slices	640	22
Thin-n-Crispy Cheese	3 slices	450	15
Thin-n-Crispy Supreme	3 slices	510	21

QUINCY'S FAMILY STEAKHOUSE

FOOD	PORTION	CALORIES	FAT
MAIN MENU SELECTIONS			
Catfish Filets	2	309	12
Chicken Strips	4	318	15
Chili Cheeseburger	1	919	54
Chopped Steaks	6 oz	466	34
Country Style Steak w/ Mushroom Sauce	6 oz	288	19
Hamburger, ¼ lb	1	403	19
Hamburger w/ Cheese	1	451	23
Luncheon Chopped Steak	4 oz	350	25
Ribeye Steak	7 oz	665	60
Shrimp	7	248	12
Sirloin Club	5 oz	283	10
Sirloin Petite	4 oz	446	37
Sirloin Regular	6 oz	649	54
Sirloin Tips	4 oz	236	9
Steak Filet, Extra-Thick	6 oz	331	12
Steak Ribeye, Extra-Thick	9 oz	865	78
Steak, Sirloin, Extra-Thick	8 oz	898	73
Steak, T-Bone	8 oz	1045	95
Steak, T-Bone, Extra-Thick	13 oz	1612	159
SIDE DISHES			
Baked Potato w/o Butter	1	181	tr
Barbecue Beans	1 portion	296	13
Cole Slaw	1 portion	60	5

FOOD	PORTION	CALORIES	FAT
Corn Bread	1 piece	178	6
Country Style Roll	1	70	1
Green Beans	1 portion	40	1
Mushroom Sauce	2 oz	27	tr
Peppers & Onions	1 portion	80	5
Steak Fries	1 portion	426	21
Texas Toast w/o Butter	1 portion	73	tr
SOUP			
Chili w/ Beans	9 oz	346	16
Clam Chowder	9 oz	198	14
Vegetable Beef	9 oz	78	2

RAX

	PORTION	CALORIES	FAT
BEVERAGES			
Cherry Coke	10 oz	120	tr
Coca-Cola	10 oz	120	tr
Coffee, decaf, black	6 oz	2	tr
Coffee, regular, black	6 oz	2	tr
Creamer, Non-Dairy	⅜ oz	14	1
Diet Coke	10 oz	tr	tr
Fanta Root Beer	10 oz	120	tr
Hot Cocoa Mix	10 oz	110	11
Hot Tea	6 oz	tr	tr
Iced Tea	6 oz	tr	tr
Milk, 2%	8 oz	110	4
Milk, Whole	8 oz	150	8
Milkshake, Chocolate	1	560	13
Milkshake, Strawberry	1	560	13
Milkshake, Vanilla	1	500	14
Sprite	10 oz	110	tr

FOOD	PORTION	CALORIES	FAT
MEXICAN BAR			
Banana Pepper Rings	1 Tbsp	2	tr
Cheese Sauce, Nacho	3.5 oz	470	22
Cheese Sauce, Regular	3.5 oz	420	17
Green Onions	¼ cup	10	tr
Japapeno Peppers	1 oz	6	tr
Olives	3.5 oz	110	10
Refried Beans	3 oz	120	4
Sour Topping	3.5 oz	130	11
Spanish Rice	3.5 oz	90	tr
Spicy Meat Sauce	3.5 oz	80	4
Taco Sauce	3.5 oz	30	tr
Taco Shell	1	40	2
Tomatoes	1 oz	6	tr
Tortilla Chips	1 oz	140	7
Tortillas	1	110	2
MISCELLANEOUS			
Chocolate Chip Cookie	1	130	6
Drive-Thru Salad, Chef w/o dressing	1	230	14
Drive-Thru Salad, Garden, w/o dressing	1	160	11
Whipped Topping	1 dip	50	4
PASTA BAR			
Alfredo Sauce	3.5 oz	80	3
Chicken Noodle Soup	3.5 oz	40	tr
Creme of Broccoli Soup	3.5 oz	50	2
Parmesan Cheese Substitute	1 oz	80	4
Pasta Shells	3.5 oz	170	4
Pasta/Vegetable Blend	3.5 oz	100	4
Rainbow Rotine	3.5 oz	180	4
Spaghetti	3.5 oz	140	4

FOOD	PORTION	CALORIES	FAT
Spaghetti Sauce	3.5 oz	80	tr
Spaghetti Sauce w/ Meat	3.5 oz	150	8
POTATOES			
BBQ Potoato	1	730	24
Cheese & Bacon Potato	1	780	28
Cheese & Broccoli Potato	1	760	26
Chili & Cheese Potato	1	700	23
French Fries, salted or unsalted	1 reg	260	13
French Fries, salted or unsalted	1 lg	390	20
Plain	1	270	tr
Plain w/ margarine	1	370	11
Sour Topping Potato	1	400	11
SALAD BAR			
Alfalfa Sprouts	1 oz	8	tr
Applesauce	1 cup	100	tr
Bacon Bits	.5 oz	40	2
Banana Chips	1 oz	100	tr
Beets	1 cup	60	tr
Broccoli	½ cup	16	tr
Cabbage	1 cup	16	tr
Cantaloupe	2 pieces	16	tr
Carrots	¼ cup	8	tr
Cauliflower	½ cup	16	tr
Celery	1 Tbsp	14	tr
Cheddar Cheese Tidbits	1 oz	160	11
Cherry Peppers	1 Tbsp	6	tr
Chow Mein Noodles	1 oz	140	6
Coconut	1 oz	160	11
Cole Slaw	3.5 oz	70	4
Cottage Cheese	1 cup	250	10

FOOD	PORTION	CALORIES	FAT
Crackers (Saltines)	2	16	tr
Croutons	.5 oz	50	tr
Cucumbers	4 slices	2	tr
Eggs	1.5 oz	70	5
Garbanzo Beans	½ cup	360	5
Gelatin, Lime	½ cup	90	tr
Gelatin, Strawberry	½ cup	90	tr
Grapefruit Sections	1 cup	80	tr
Grapes	1 cup	100	tr
Green Peppers	¼ cup	8	tr
Honeydew Melons	2 pieces	25	tr
Kale	1 oz	16	tr
Kidney Beans	1 cup	220	1
Lettuce	1 leaf	2	tr
Macaroni Salad	3.5 oz	160	7
Mushrooms	¼ cup	4	tr
Onions	¼ cup	12	tr
Pasta Salad	3.5 oz	80	1
Peaches	2 slices	16	tr
Peas	1 oz	25	tr
Pickle Spear	1	8	tr
Pineapple canned	3.5 oz	100	tr
Pineapple fresh	1 slice	45	tr
Potato Salad	1 cup	260	7
Pudding, Butterscotch	3.5 oz	140	6
Pudding, Chocolate	3.5 oz	140	6
Pudding, Vanilla	3.5 oz	140	6
Radishes	.5 oz	2	tr
Red Cabbage	¼ cup	4	tr
Sesame Sticks	1 oz	150	10

FOOD	PORTION	CALORIES	FAT
Shredded Imitation Cheddar Cheese	1 oz	90	6
Soynuts	1 oz	120	7
Strawberries	2 oz	18	tr
Sunflower Seeds w/ Raisins	1 oz	130	10
Three Bean Salad	½ cup	100	tr
Tomatoes	1 oz	6	tr
Turkey Bits	2 oz	70	3
Watermelon	2 pieces	18	0
SALAD DRESSING			
Blue Cheese Dressing	1 Tbsp	50	5
French Dressing	1 Tbsp	60	4
Italian Dressing	1 Tbsp	50	4
Lite Blue Cheese Dressing	1 Tbsp	35	3
Lite French Dressing	1 Tbsp	40	2
Lite Italian Dressing	1 Tbsp	30	3
Lite Thousand Island Dressing	1 Tbsp	40	3
Oil	1 Tbsp	130	14
Poppy Seed Dressing	1 Tbsp	60	4
Ranch Dressing	1 Tbsp	45	5
Thousand Island Dressing	1 Tbsp	70	6
Vinegar	1 Tbsp	2	0
SANDWICHES AND INGREDIENTS			
American Cheese	1 slice	60	5
BBC	1	720	49
BBC Sauce	.75 oz	140	16
BBQ Meat Topping	3.25 oz	140	4
BBQ Sandwich	1	420	14
Bacon	1 slice	80	7
Banana Pepper Rings	1 Tbsp	2	tr
Bun	1 sm	180	9

FOOD	PORTION	CALORIES	FAT
Double WB	1	440	24
Fish	3.5 oz	230	12
Fish Sandwich	1	460	17
Ham	2.5 oz	70	2
Ham & Swiss Sandwich	1	430	23
Hamburger	1	130	11
Hamburger Seasoning Salt	1 sprinkle	tr	tr
Horseradish Sauce	.75 oz	10	tr
Kaiser Bun	4"	180	2
Kaiser Bun	6"	280	10
Ketchup	1 Tbsp	6	tr
Mayonnaise	.75 oz	150	16
Mustard	1 Tbsp	4	tr
Onions	3 rings	4	tr
Onions, Diced	¼ cup	18	tr
Philly Beef & Cheese Sandwich	1	470	22
Philly Vegetables	2 oz	30	1
Pickle Slices	4 slices	2	tr
Pickle Spears	1	8	tr
Regular BBQ Sauce	1 oz	40	tr
Roast Beef	2.8 oz	140	9
Roast Beef Sandwich (Uncle Al)	1 sm	260	14
Roast Beef Sandwich	1 reg	320	11
Roast Beef Sandwich	1 lg	570	35
Shredded Lettuce	¼ cup	2	tr
Smokey BBQ Sauce	1 oz	40	tr
Sweet Pickle Relish	1 Tbsp	20	tr
Swiss	1 slice	30	2
Tartar Sauce	.5 oz	50	5

FOOD	PORTION	CALORIES	FAT
Tomato	1 slice	2	tr
Turkey	2.5 oz	80	3
Turkey Bacon Club	1	470	43
Works Burger	1	310	13

RED LOBSTER

All of the following are for a cooked portion unless otherwise noted.

FOOD	PORTION	CALORIES	FAT
Atlantic Cod	1 lunch serving	100	1
Atlantic Ocean Perch	1 lunch serving	130	4
Blacktip Shark	1 lunch serving	150	1
Calamari, breaded & fried	1 lunch serving	360	21
Calico Scallops	1 lunch serving	180	2
Catfish	1 lunch serving	170	10
Cherrystone Clams	1 lunch serving	130	2
Chicken Breast	4 oz before cooking	120	3
Deep Sea Scallops	1 lunch serving	130	2
Flounder	1 lunch serving	100	1
Grouper	1 lunch serving	110	1
Haddock	1 lunch serving	110	1
Halibut	1 lunch serving	110	1
Hamburger	5 oz before cooking	320	23
King Crab Legs	1 lb	170	2
Langostino	1 lunch serving	120	1
Lemon Sole	1 lunch serving	120	1
Mackerel	1 lunch serving	190	12
Maine Lobster	1¼ lb	240	8
Mako Shark	1 lunch serving	140	1
Monkfish	1 lunch serving	110	1
Mussels	3 oz	70	2

FOOD	PORTION	CALORIES	FAT
Norwegian Salmon	1 lunch serving	230	12
Oysters	6 raw	110	4
Pollack	1 lunch serving	120	1
Porterhouse Steak	18 oz before cooking	1420	131
Rainbow Trout	1 lunch serving	170	9
Red Rockfish	1 lunch serving	90	1
Red Snapper	1 lunch serving	110	1
Rock Lobster	1 tail	230	3
Shrimp	8 to 12 pieces	120	2
Sirloin Steak	7 oz before cooking	570	48
Snow Crab Legs	1 lb	150	2
Sockeye Salmon	1 lunch serving	160	4
Strip Steak	7 oz before cooking	690	64
Swordfish	1 lunch serving	100	4
Tilefish	1 lunch serving	100	2
Yellowfin Tuna	1 lunch serving	180	6

ROY ROGERS

BEVERAGES			
Coffee, black	1 reg	0	0
Coke	12 oz	145	0
Diet Coke	12 oz	1	0
Hot Chocolate	6 oz	123	2
Iced Tea	1 reg	0	0
Milk, Whole	8 oz	150	8
Milkshake, Chocolate	1	358	10
Milkshake, Strawberry	1	315	10
Milkshake, Vanilla	1	306	11

FOOD	PORTION	CALORIES	FAT
Orange Juice	7 oz	99	tr
Orange Juice	10 oz	136	tr
BREAKFAST SELECTIONS			
Breakfast Crescent Sandwich	1	401	27
Breakfast Crescent Sandwich w/ Bacon	1	431	30
Breakfast Crescent Sandwich w/ Ham	1	442	29
Breakfast Crescent Sandwich w/ Sausage	1	449	29
Breakfast Crescent Sandwich w/ Sausage	1 lg	608	30
Pancake Platter w/ syrup, butter	1	452	15
Pancake Platter w/ syrup, butter, bacon	1	493	18
Pancake Platter w/ syrup, butter, ham	1	506	17
Pancake Platter w/ syrup, butter, sausage	1	608	30
MAIN MENU SELECTIONS			
Bacon Cheeseburger	1	581	39
Biscuit	1	231	12
Brownie	1	264	11
Cheeseburger	1	563	37
Chicken Breast	4.8 oz	412	24
Chicken Breast & Wing	6.5 oz	604	37
Chicken Leg	1.8 oz	140	8
Chicken Nuggets	6 nuggets	267	17
Chicken Thigh	3.2 oz	296	20
Chicken Thigh & Leg	5 oz	436	28
Chicken Wing	1.7 oz	192	13
Cole Slaw	1 reg	110	7

FOOD	PORTION	CALORIES	FAT
French Fries	1 reg	268	14
French Fries	1 lg	357	18
Hamburger	1	456	28
Hot Topped Potato, Plain	1	211	2
Hot Topped Potato w/ Bacon 'n Cheese	1	397	22
Hot Topped Potato w/ Broccoli 'n Cheese	1	376	18
Hot Topped Potato w/ Oleo	1	274	7
Hot Topped Potato w/ Sour Cream 'n Chives	1	408	21
Hot Topped Potato w/ Taco Beef 'n Cheese	1	463	22
Large Roast Beef Sandwich	1	360	12
Large Roast Beef Sandwich w/ Cheese	1	467	21
Macaroni Salad	1 reg	186	11
Potato Salad	1 reg	107	6
RR Bar Burger	1	611	39
Roast Beef Sandwich	1	317	10
Roast Beef Sandwich w/ Cheese	1	424	19
MISCELLANEOUS Apple Danish	1	249	12
Brownie	1	264	11
Caramel Sundae	1	293	9
Cheese Danish	1	254	12
Cherry Danish	1	271	14
Hot Fudge Sundae	1	337	13
Strawberry Shortcake	1	447	19
Strawberry Sundae	1	216	7

FOOD	PORTION	CALORIES	FAT
SALAD BAR			
Bacon Bits	1 Tbsp	33	1
Bacon 'n Tomato Dressing	2 Tbsp	136	12
Beets, Sliced	¼ cup	16	0
Blue Cheese Dressing	2 Tbsp	150	16
Broccoli	½ cup	20	0
Carrots	¼ cup	42	0
Lo-Cal Italian Dressing	2 Tbsp	70	6
Ranch Dressing	2 Tbsp	155	14
Chinese Noodles	¼ cup	55	3
Chopped Egg	2 Tbsp	55	4
Croutons	2 Tbsp	70	0
Cucumbers	5–6 slices	4	0
Green Peas	¼ cup	7	0
Green Peppers	2 Tbsp	4	0
Lettuce	1 cup	10	0
Mushrooms	¼ cup	5	0
Shredded Cheddar Cheese	¼ cup	112	9
Sunflower Seeds	2 Tbsp	157	9
Thousand Island Dressing	2 Tbsp	160	16
Tomatoes	3 slices	20	0

SHAKEY'S
(see also DOMINO'S PIZZA, GODFATHER'S, PIZZA HUT)

FOOD	PORTION	CALORIES	FAT
MAIN MENU SELECTIONS			
3 Piece Fried Chicken & Potatoes	1	947	56
5 Piece Fried Chicken & Potatoes	1	1700	90
Hot Ham & Cheese	1	550	21
Potatoes	15 pieces	950	36
Spaghetti w/ Meat Sauce & Garlic Bread	1 serving	940	33
Super Hot Hero	1	810	44

FOOD	PORTION	CALORIES	FAT
PIZZA			
Homestyle Shakey's Special	1 slice	384	21
Homestyle Cheese	1 slice	303	14
Homestyle w/ Onion, Green Peppers, Olives, Mushrooms	1 slice	320	15
Homestyle w/ Pepperoni	1 slice	343	15
Homestyle w/ Sausage, Mushrooms	1 slice	343	17
Homestyle w/ Sausage, Pepperoni	1 slice	374	20
Thick Crust, Cheese Only	1 slice	170	5
Thick Crust, Shakey's Special	1 slice	208	8
Thick Crust w/ Pepperoni	1 slice	185	6
Thick Crust w/ Sausage, Mushrooms	1 slice	179	6
Thick Crust w/ Sausage, Pepperoni	1 slice	177	8
Thick Crust w/ Green Peppers, Black Olives, Mushrooms	1 slice	162	4
Thin Crust, Cheese Only	1 slice	133	5
Thin Crust, Shakey's Special	1 slice	171	9
Thin Crust w/ Onion, Green Peppers, Black Olives, Mushrooms	1 slice	125	5
Thin Crust w/ Pepperoni	1 slice	148	7
Thin Crust w/ Sausage, Mushroom	1 slice	141	6
Thin Crust w/ Sausage, Pepperoni	1 slice	166	8
TACO BELL			
Bellbeefer	1	312	13
Bellbeefer, Green	1	306	13
Burrito Double Beef, Supreme, Green	1	459	23
Burrito Supreme Platter	1	774	37
Burrito Supreme Platter, Green	1	762	37
Burrito, Bean	1	360	11
Burrito, Bean, Green	1	354	11

FOOD	PORTION	CALORIES	FAT
Burrito, Beef	1	402	17
Burrito, Beef, Green	1	396	17
Burrito, Combo	1	381	14
Burrito, Combo, Green	1	375	14
Burrito, Double Beef Supreme	1	464	23
Burrito, Supreme	1	422	19
Burrito, Supreme, Green	1	416	19
Cinnamon Crispas	1	266	16
Enchirito	1	382	20
Enchirito, Green	1	370	20
Fabulous Steak Fajita	1	235	11
Fabulous Steak Fajita w/ Guacamole	1	269	13
Fabulous Steak Fajita w/ Sour Cream	1	281	15
Mexican Pizza	1	714	48
Nachos	1	356	19
Nachos Bellgrande	1	719	41
Pico De Gallo	1	8	tr
Pintos & Cheese	1	194	9
Pintos & Cheese, Green	1	189	9
Ranch Dressing	2½ oz	236	25
Salsa	3 oz	18	tr
Seafood Salad w/ Ranch Dressing	1	884	66
Seafood Salad w/o Dressing	1	648	41
Seafood Salad w/o Dressing & Shell	1	216	11
Taco	1	184	11
Taco Bellgrande	1	351	22
Taco Bellgrande Platter	1	1002	51
Taco Bellgrande Platter, Green	1	990	51
Taco Light	1	411	29
Taco Light Platter	1	1062	58

FOOD	PORTION	CALORIES	FAT
Taco Light Platter, Green	1	1051	58
Taco Salad w/ Ranch Dressing	1	1167	87
Taco Salad w/ Salsa	1	949	62
Taco Salad w/o Beans	1	822	57
Taco Salad w/o Salsa	1	931	62
Taco Salad w/o Shell	1	524	32
Taco Sauce	1 pkg	2	tr
Taco Sauce, Hot	1 pkg	3	tr
Taco, Soft	1	228	12
Tostada	1	243	11
Tostada, Beefy	1	322	20
Tostada, Beefy, Green	1	316	20
Tostada, Green	1	238	11

TACO JOHN'S

FOOD	PORTION	CALORIES	FAT
Apple Grande	1	257	8
Bean Burrito	1	249	6
Beef Burrito	1	355	18
Chimi	1	487	19
Churro	1	122	7
Combo Burrito	1	302	12
Enchilada	1	379	18
Nachos	1 serving	407	19
Potato Ole	1 lg	414	6
Refried Beans	1 serving	331	6
Smothered Burrito w/ Green Chili	1	405	24
Smothered Burrito w/ Texas Chili	1	518	24
Softshell	1	276	13
Super Burrito	1	434	11
Super Nachos	1 serving	657	34

FOOD	PORTION	CALORIES	FAT
Super Taco Bravo	1	485	20
Super Taco Salad	1	450	18
Taco	1	228	13
Taco Burger	1	332	14
Texas Chili	1 serving	430	22
Tostada	1	228	13

WENDY'S

All Wendy's sandwiches are custom-made. The following list of sandwich toppings allows you to calculate the fat and calories in any sandwich you order.

BEVERAGES			
Coca-Cola	8 oz	100	0
Coffee, black	6 oz	2	tr
Creamer, Non-Dairy	⅜ oz	14	1
Half & Half	⅜ oz	14	1
Diet Coke	8 oz	0	0
Diet Pepsi	8 oz	0	0
Dr Pepper	8 oz	100	0
Hot Chocolate	6 oz	110	1
Lemonade	12 oz	160	tr
Milk, 2%	8 oz	110	4
Milk, Chocolate	8 oz	190	8
Milk, Whole	8 oz	140	8
Mountain Dew	8 oz	110	0
Orange Juice	6 oz	80	tr
Pepsi-Cola	8 oz	110	tr
Slice, Lemon-Lime	8 oz	100	0
Slice, Mandarin Orange	8 oz	110	0
Tea, Hot	6 oz	0	0
Tea, Iced	12 oz	0	0

FOOD	PORTION	CALORIES	FAT
BREAKFAST SELECTIONS			
Bacon	1 strip	30	2
Biscuit, Buttermilk	1	320	17
Breakfast Potatoes	1	360	22
Breakfast Sandwich	1	370	19
Egg, Fried	1 egg	90	6
Eggs, Scrambled	2 eggs	190	12
French Toast	2 slices	400	19
French Toast, Apple Topping	1 pkg	130	tr
French Toast, Blueberry Topping	1 pkg	60	tr
French Toast, w/ Syrup	1 pkg	140	tr
Grape Jelly	1 pkg	40	tr
Omelet #1	1	290	21
Omelet #2	1	250	17
Omelet #3	1	280	19
Omelet #4	1	210	15
Sausage Gravy	6 oz	440	36
Sausage Patty	1	200	18
Toast, Wheat w/ Margarine	2 slices	190	8
Toast, White	2 slices	250	9
GARDEN SPOT SALAD BAR			
Alfalfa Sprouts	1 oz	8	tr
American Cheese	1 oz	90	7
Bacon Bits	1 tsp	10	tr
Blueberries	1 Tbsp	6	tr
Blue Cheese Dressing	1 Tbsp	60	7
Breadsticks	2	35	1
Broccoli	½ cup	12	tr
Cantaloupe	2 pieces (2 oz)	18	tr

FOOD	PORTION	CALORIES	FAT
Carrots	¼ cup	10	tr
Cauliflower	½ cup	12	tr
Celery	1 Tbsp	tr	tr
Celery Seed Dressing	1 Tbsp	70	6
Cheddar Cheese, Imitation	1 oz	80	6
Cherry Tomatoes, Pickled	1 Tbsp	14	tr
Chow Mein Noodles	½ oz	70	4
Cole Slaw	¼ cup	80	5
Cottage Cheese	½ cup	110	4
Croutons	½ oz	60	3
Cucumbers	4 slices	2	tr
Eggs, Hard Cooked, Chopped	1 Tbsp	30	2
French Style Dressing	1 Tbsp	70	5
Golden Italian Dressing	1 Tbsp	50	4
Grapefruit	2 oz	10	tr
Grapes	¼ cup	30	tr
Green Peas	1 oz	25	tr
Green Peppers	¼ cup	8	tr
Honeydew Melon	2 pieces (2 oz)	20	tr
Jalapeno Peppers	1 Tbsp	9	tr
Lettuce	1 cup	8	tr
Mozzarella Cheese, Imitation	1 oz	90	7
Mushrooms	¼ cup	4	tr
Oil	1 Tbsp	120	14
Oranges	2 oz	25	tr
Parmesan, Grated	1 oz	130	9
Pasta Salad	¼ cup	130	6
Peaches	2 pieces	17	tr
Pepper Rings, Pickled	1 Tbsp	2	tr
Pineapple Chunks	½ cup	70	tr

FOOD	PORTION	CALORIES	FAT
Provolone Cheese	1 oz	90	7
Radishes	½ oz	2	tr
Ranch Dressing	1 Tbsp	50	6
Red Cabbage	¼	4	tr
Red Onions	3 rings	2	tr
Reduced-Calorie Bacon/Tomato Dressing	1 Tbsp	45	4
Reduced-Calorie Creamy Cucumber Dressing	1 Tbsp	50	5
Reduced-Calorie Italian Dressing	1 Tbsp	25	2
Reduced-Calorie Thousand Island Dressing	1 Tbsp	54	4
Saltines	1 pkg	25	tr
Strawberries	2 oz	18	tr
Sunflower Seeds and Raisins	1 oz	140	10
Swiss Cheese, Imitation	1 oz	90	7
Thousand Island Dressing	1 Tbsp	70	7
Tomatoes	1 oz	6	tr
Turkey Ham	¼ cup	50	2
Watermelon	2 pieces (2 oz)	18	tr
Wine Vinegar	1 Tbsp	2	tr
MAIN MENU SELECTION ¼-lb Single, Hamburger Patty, no bun	1	210	14
Big Classic	1	470	25
Bun, Kaiser	1	180	2
Bun, Multi-Grain	1	140	3
Bun, White	1	140	2
Chicken Breast Fillet	1	200	10
Chicken Fried Steak	1	580	41
Chili	1 reg	240	8

FOOD	PORTION	CALORIES	FAT
Crispy Chicken Nuggets; cooked in animal/vegetable oil	6 pieces	290	21
Crispy Chicken Nuggets; cooked in vegetable oil	6 pieces	310	21
Fish Fillet	1	210	11
French Fries; cooked in vegetable oil	1 reg	300	15
French Fries; cooked in animal/vegetable oil	1 reg	310	15
Hot Chili Seasoning	1 pkg	7	tr
Kid's Meal, Hamburger	1	200	9
Nuggets Sauce, Barbecue	1 pkg	50	tr
Nuggets Sauce, Honey	1 pkg	45	tr
Nuggets Sauce, Sweet & Sour	1 pkg	45	tr
Nuggets Sauce, Sweet Mustard	1 pkg	50	1
Taco Salad	1	430	19
Taco Sauce	1 pkg	10	tr
Tartar Sauce	1 Tbsp	80	9
MISCELLANEOUS			
Apple Danish	1	360	14
Chocolate Chip Cookie	1	320	17
Cinnamon Raisin Danish	1	410	18
Frosty Dairy Dessert	1 sm	400	15
HOT STUFFED BAKED POTATOES			
Bacon & Cheese	1	570	30
Broccoli & Cheese	1	500	25
Cheese	1	590	34
Chili & Cheese	1	510	20
Plain	1	250	2
Sour Cream & Chives	1	460	24

FOOD	PORTION	CALORIES	FAT
SANDWICH TOPPINGS			
American Cheese	1 slice	60	6
Bacon	1 strip	30	2
Ketchup	1 tsp	6	tr
Lettuce	1 leaf	2	tr
Mayonnaise	1 Tbsp	90	10
Mustard	1 tsp	4	tr
Onion	3 rings	2	tr
Pickles, Dill	4 slices	2	tr
Tomatoes	1 slice	2	tr

WHITE CASTLE

FOOD	PORTION	CALORIES	FAT
Bun Only	1	74	tr
Cheese Only	.3 oz	31	2
Cheeseburger	1	200	11
Chicken Sandwich	1	186	7
Fish Sandwich w/o Tartar Sauce	1	155	5
French Fries	1 reg	301	15
Hamburger	1	161	8
Onion Rings	1 reg	245	13
Sausage & Egg Sandwich	1	322	22
Sausage Sandwich	1	196	12

WINCHELL'S DONUTS

FOOD	PORTION	CALORIES	FAT
Apple Fritter	1	580	37
Cinnamon Crumb	1	240	11
Cinnamon Roll	1	360	21
Glazed Jelly	1	300	13
Glazed Round	1	210	12
Glazed Twist	1	210	11

FOOD	PORTION	CALORIES	FAT
Iced Chocolate Bar	1	220	11
Iced Chocolate Cake	1	230	10
Iced Chocolate Devil's	1	240	12
Iced Chocolate French	1	220	13
Iced Chocolate Raised	1	210	10
Plain	1	200	11
Plain Donut Hole	1	50	3